NURSING RESEARCH

NURSING RESEARCH

Building Evidence for Practice

Dr R. Bincy

Vice Principal, Government College of Nursing
Thiruvananthapuram

Viva Books

New Delhi | Mumbai | Chennai | Kolkata | Bengaluru | Hyderabad | Kochi | Guwahati

First Published 2012
Reprinted 2013, 2014

Viva Books Private Limited

- 4737/23, Ansari Road, Daryaganj, New Delhi 110 002
  Tel. 42242200, 23258325, 23283121, Email: vivadelhi@vivagroupindia.net
- 76, Service Industries, Shirvane, Sector 1, Nerul, Navi Mumbai 400 706
  Tel. 27721273, 27721274, Email: vivamumbai@vivagroupindia.net
- Megh Tower, Old No. 307, New No. 165, Poonamallee High Road, Maduravoyal
  Chennai - 600 095, Tel : 23780991, 23780992, Email: vivachennai@vivagroupindia.net
- B-103, Jindal Towers, 21/1A/3 Darga Road, Kolkata 700 017
  Tel. 22816713, Email: vivakolkata@vivagroupindia.net
- 7, GF, Sovereign Park Aptts., 56-58, K. R. Road, Basavanagudi, Bengaluru 560 004
  Tel. 26607409, Email: vivabangalore@vivagroupindia.net
- 101-102, Moghal Marc Apartments, 3-4-637 to 641, Narayanguda, Hyderabad 500 029
  Tel. 27564481, Email: vivahyderabad@vivagroupindia.net
- First Floor, Beevi Towers, SRM Road, Kaloor, Kochi 682 018
  Tel. 0484-2403055, 2403056, Email: vivakochi@vivagroupindia.net
- 232, GNB Road, Beside UCO Bank, Silpukhuri, Guwahati 781 003
  Tel. 0361-2666386, Email: vivaguwahati@vivagroupindia.net

www.vivagroupindia.com

ISBN: 978-81-309-1775-7

Published by Vinod Vasishtha for Viva Books Private Limited, 4737/23 Ansari Road, Daryaganj, New Delhi 110 002.

Printed and bound by Raj Press, R-3, Inderpuri, New Delhi 110 012.

G0000/D1200

This book is dedicated to my beloved parents
late Mr. P.K. Raveendran and L. Vijayamma (Rtd. teachers)

CONTENTS

FOREWORD

The emphasis today is on knowledge obtained through meticulous work based on well-designed scientific investigation. The knowledge base so obtained is proactive.

Increased importance is being attached to providing sound training, both conceptual and practical, including analytical skills to researchers in nursing. In recent days evidence-based practice has gained abundant significance in the field of Nursing Research. The prerequisite in this context is access to well-written books.

The nursing curriculum prescribed by Indian Nursing Council at undergraduate, postgraduate and post basic Diploma in clinical speciality programme has Nursing Research as a core subject. There are numerous books available on the subject.

I am happy that Dr. R. Bincy, with her vast experience as an academician and a research guide, has done a commendable piece of work to bring out a comprehensive book titled *Nursing Research: Building Evidence for Practice*. The volume is comprehensive in its coverage, provides adequate introduction and grounding both on the conceptual planning, data collection and analysis. The sequencing of the chapters is in logical order and I am sure it will be a pathfinder to students in their journey through research. Overviewing the current scenario in nursing education and nursing practices I have great pleasure to proclaim the emergence of an extremely helpful book with several unique features.

Professionalism and scientific temper in the book should be lauded.

Dr. R. Bincy has my appreciation as well as best wishes.

Prof. Chandrakanthi
Dean, Ananthapuri College of Nursing
Thiruvananthapuram

Former President
Indian Nursing Council
New Delhi

Former Principal
Govt. College of Nursing
Thiruvananthapuram

PREFACE

In nursing, research is synonymous with evidence which is used to support nursing practice. As in any profession here also continuous attempts should be embarked upon to reach out to the horizons of ever-growing knowledge which is to be utilized in catering to the growing requirements in this area. Nursing research is the means through which such a generation and enrichment of knowledge is facilitated. When the evidence acquired through research is put into practice, it eventually encompasses all nurses in terms of their participation.

It is natural that nurses who engage themselves in research activities can achieve academic laurels, but the prime motive must be providing best quality care to patients. As per Polit and Hungler (2010) research allows nurses to question their practice, find answers and then implement into their area.

It is noticed that research is an important professional responsibility. Thus through research, the knowledge base is being widened and improved, state-of-the-art nursing care is extended to the patients thereby nourishing the growth of the profession and establishing the key role of nurses in the health care team.

There are different expectations regarding research skills needed by nursing students at different levels. The aim of this book is to provide nursing students at all levels with a solid understanding of nursing research and its role in contemporary nursing practice. The disseminating use of nursing research findings depend on knowledge of research process, nursing knowledge and positive attitudes towards nursing research. Active involvement in the learning process is amply highlighted in this book.

Through long years of my teaching and guiding researches both at graduate and postgraduate levels, I have become increasingly dismayed at the appearance of voluminous research books. Usually, students are given more to read about research, but little by way of experience in research. In fact, this worked throughout in my mind while I was at work in the making of this book. Empowering students to the best possible extent in acquiring the most updated practical knowledge, thus, is my real concern in publishing this work.

I am of the view that nurse scientists are assuming the responsibility of writing for a practice audience as well as a research audience.

Actually, I started writing this book in order to emphasize certain vital aspects of nursing research in just a few words. But after interacting with my friends and students, it so happened that the diversion of the book went on expanding.

I have immense pleasure and satisfaction in presenting this text on "Nursing Research: Building Evidence for Practice" to our nursing community.

A sincere attempt has been made not only to give enough exposure of nursing research for the better understanding of research concept by the students but also to enable the faculty to handle the subject more effectively in teaching institutions.

Two new chapters have been added and access to websites is also ensured. Throughout the book, I have adopted an innovative approach and practical examples and tips interspersed whenever found necessary.

Errors might be there. Please feel free to bring such instances, if any, to my notice so that they could be avoided in future.

Dr. R. Bincy

ACKNOWLEDGEMENTS

I am grateful to Lord Almighty for having showered his grace and blessings in the accomplishment of this work.

It takes a team of many people and a lot of hard work to create a quality textbook. I am indebted to all who provided the assistance, encouragement and constructive criticism leading to the formidable task of preparation of this book. Experts from widely diversified academic disciplines volunteered valuable suggestions and critique for this work.

I extend from the bottom of my heart sincere words of reverence to my mentor Dr. Y.M. Fazil Marickar, Principal of Azeezia Medical College, Kollam, retired Professor and Head of Department of Surgery, Medical College, Thiruvananthapuram who taught me the basic lessons of research and encouraging relentlessly to keep updated myself, which helped to fortify my carrier.

With gratitude I remember the distinguished authors I have referred to. I acknowledge my deep gratitude to Prof. Y. Prasanna Kumary, Deputy Director of Nursing Education, Kerala for her constant encouragement and motivation. I place on record the new vistas given to me by her in organizing national and international conferences which paved a strong platform in shaping my self-confidence in the sphere of Nursing Research.

I greatly value the favour extended by Prof. Valsa K. Panicker, Principal, College of Nursing, Thiruvananthapuram, for her unremitting support for writing this book.

I am particularly indebted to our three reviewers who have been with me throughout the entire period of manuscript preparation Mr. Shine Lal, Prof. A. Raja, my brother, and Prof. Sampath, my sister. I thank Miss Biji, Diana, Deepa, Mr. Arun Kumar R., Mr. Mourian and Sindu, who devoted their extensive time for the development of this book.

I place on record my deep gratitude to all my teachers and students who gave me timely encouragement and unstinting support for completing this book credibly.

I am also obliged to Mr. Babu M.K. and Mr. Oommen P. Mathew for their help and scholastic suggestions for chapters on statistics.

I am extremely thankful to Mr. Baby Joseph for editing the manuscript.

Cover design of the book was done by Mr. Sananda Raj. I acknowledge him for the beautiful drawing.

I am extremely thankful to Viva Books especially to Mr. Sreetilak, Mr. Pradeep and Mr. John Paul for their total involvement in the publication of this book.

Special thanks are due, to my beloved husband Dr. Ramesh Kumar, for his continuous support and scholastic suggestions, and for editing the manuscript. My son Akhil deserves a warm pat for computer assistance and for his robust encouragement.

In fact this list is not complete. There are many more who lent me their hands in this endeavour. Let me profusely thank each and every one of them for the services rendered to me.

CHAPTER

1

CONCEPT OF NURSING RESEARCH

Key terms

★ Basic research ★ Applied research ★ Qualitative research ★ Quantitative research ★ Nursing research ★ Empirical data ★ Research utilization ★ Outcome research ★ Evidence-based nursing practice

⊙ Outline

- ★ Research and nursing research
- ★ Research and problem-solving
- ★ Characteristics of good research
- ★ Types of research
- ★ Qualities of a researcher
- ★ Purposes of nursing research
- ★ Role of nurses in research
- ★ Problems and issues in nursing research
- ★ Future of nursing research

⊙ Objectives

On completion of this chapter, you will be able to:

- ★ define nursing research
- ★ identify the importance of the outcomes of research
- ★ discuss the history and scope of nursing research
- ★ enumerate the types of research
- ★ interpret problems and issues in nursing research
- ★ appreciate the future of nursing research

Introduction

Research is of paramount importance in opening up new vistas of knowledge. Changes occur in fraction of a second, and thus factual understanding in any topic undergoes rapid change. Today's knowledge becomes redundant by the next day. This holds true in any science or profession and so in nursing. The concept of a nurse playing second fiddle in health care delivery system has become obsolete.

The nurse has grown as an independent and integral entity in the medical crew. This was made possible on account of hard work and commitment put forth by researchers in the field of nursing world over. In nursing, research should always be exercised to facilitate evidence-based practice. Glimpses of this have been evidenced since the time of Florence

Nightingale. Many nurses now work as researchers in Universities and in health care institutions. Research cannot only add to our knowledge base but also can bring about qualitative improvement in the health care delivery system. This also helps in bridging the gap between newer findings and putting them into practice for the benefit of mankind. Research enables health care providers to look at the patient as a human being and gives reverence to his valuable life. After going through a process of caring, he comes out as a new and refined man to which evidence-based nursing has contributed to the core.

Nurses need to have good observation skills, i.e. a purposeful, reflective and questioning mind. Nursing research has tremendous impact on professional nursing practice. The pertinence of professional nursing practice increases with improvement in other spheres of health care delivery system. So it makes mandatory for each nursing professional to practice evidence-based nursing. Research in nursing holds the key to this cause.

Nursing research is an integral component of an undergraduate student's curriculum. The role of research project is a means of inquiry through formulating questions and finding answers to them, thereby enabling the students to add to their knowledge.

Research and Nursing Research

Meaning of research

Research is an organized investigation of a problem. Generally, it is an attempt to get solution to problems. The word 'research' derives from the French word '*re-cerche*', which means to search again. It is a careful 'search' or systematic inquiry towards increasing the sum of knowledge. It helps the progress of life. Research is a matter of raising a question and trying to find answer to it. The goal of all research is progress-based development for comfortable life.

What is research?

The *Advanced Learner's Dictionary of Current English* lays down the meaning of research as a careful investigation or inquiry especially through search for new facts in any branch of knowledge using different sources of knowledge to carry out enquiry.

The word research means to search again or 'to examine carefully'. More specifically, research is a diligent, systematic inquiry or study that develops new knowledge. Diligent, systematic study indicates planning, organization and persistence. The ultimate aim of research is the development of an empirical body of knowledge for a discipline or profession. Research is a scientific process. It is defined as a systematic search for answers to questions about facts and relationships between facts.

1. Some researches discover the need or truth whereas some others establish relationships between two or more facts.
2. It is scientific because the results are verifiable; i.e. if you do it again under the same condition, you will get similar result.
3. Systematic method has an order and it follows an acceptable procedure for doing the research.

Definitions of research

Research is the planned and systematic query through scientific methods for the solution of the problem.

Research is defined as a systematic and objective analysis and recording of controlled observation that may lead to the development of generalization of principles, theories, resulting in prediction and possible ultimate control of events.

—J.W. Best

It is a careful inquiry or examination seeking facts or principles, a diligent investigation to ascertain something.

—Clifford Woody

Research in its broadest sense is an attempt to gain solutions to problems; more precisely it is the collection of data in a rigorously-controlled situation for the purpose of prediction or explanation.

—Treece and Treece

Research and Problem-solving

Research is taken as a more formal, systematic and intensive process of carrying out the scientific method of analysis.

Problem-solving is a systematic approach to the solution or alleviation of problems characterized by sequential execution of the following observation through action processes.

Approaches to problem-solving include:

1. Inductive approach
2. Deductive approach
3. Analytic approach
4. Synthetic approach

Table 1.1 Comparison between research and problem-solving

Research	Problem-solving
1. Selecting a research topic.	1. Identifying the problem.
2. Data are quantitative or qualitative and analyzed using statistical tools.	2. No statistical analysis.
3. Control factors other than the variable under study.	3. No controls are imposed.
4. Research findings are generalizable to a population.	4. Generalization is not possible.
5. Replication and verification of the findings are possible.	5. Entails no such requirements.
6. Researcher will disseminate the research findings.	6. Evaluation, revision and utilization of the findings in specific situations. No dissemination and generalization of the finding.
7. It is a finding process.	7. It is a learning and problem-solving process.

Steps in Problem-solving

According to John Dewey, there are seven steps for a scientific method of problem-solving:

1. Recognizing, selecting and stating the specific problem.
2. Defining the problem: To state exactly what the actual problem is, i.e. identifying the problem in definite terms.
3. Collecting relevant information from all possible sources for a possible solution of the problem.
4. Formulation of hypothesis and possible solutions.
5. Evaluation of hypothesis for possible solutions.
6. Verifying the validity of the derived conclusions by employing them as a solution for various similar problems.
7. Choosing alternative actions if unsuccessful or until successful solutions are derived.

Characteristics of Good Research

Research is a scientific and systematic process. Most of the descriptions and definitions of research as given in various reference books emphasize this characteristic. Sound research possesses the following features:

1. *It focuses on the generation of knowledge*: Good research contributes to advancement of scientific knowledge.
2. *Problem-solving*: Research starts with the problem. The main objective of research is to discover the cause-and-effect relationship between variables. It directs a solution for the problem.
3. *It demands accurate observation and description*: It emphasizes the fact that research result must be free from any subjective bias and prejudices.
4. *Originality*: It is the hallmark of real research. For any research project, some level of originality is most indispensable. Existing material is used with a new interpretation.
5. *Empirical*: Research is related basically to one or more aspects of real situation and deals with concrete data that provides a basis for external validity to research results.
6. *Logical*: This shows that research is guided by the rules of logical reasoning, and logical process of induction and deduction is of great value in research. Deduction is the process of reasoning from some premise to a conclusion which follows from that very premise.

7. *Replicable*: This characteristic allows research results to be verified by replicating the study, thereby building a sound basis for decisions.
8. *Theory development and testing in a discipline*: Theory development and testing is a systematic process of enquiring in a discipline.
9. *Appropriate methodology*: Use of suitable methodology depends on several factors such as variables to be studied.
10. *Conducted on representative sample*: Representative sample and good sample size are required for getting generalization of research evidence.
11. *Good data collection tools*: Good research result will be obtained only if we use valid and reliable tools.
12. *Carefully recorded and reported*: Research finding has precious value. So it should be recorded. The research findings should be published in journals and media.
13. *Written research findings and the report are made available to the sentiency of associates or other scholars*: Other researchers will have information necessary to analyze, evaluate and replicate the study.

Qualities of a Good Researcher

Globally, the number of nurses who pursue research is less. The current era of nursing demands more nurse researchers who will empower the body of knowledge of nursing. Researchers must acquire the qualities listed in table.

A researcher should be:

1. Inquisitive
2. Reasonably intelligent
3. Imaginative and creative
4. A good observer and critic
5. Optimistic
6. Dedicated and committed
7. Hang-up free and healthy
8. Hard-working

9. Patient
10. Innovative and curious
11. Unbiased

Inquisitive: A researcher must have more of an inquiring attitude than having an inquiring nature. A researcher must have an untiring instinct to search for new avenues of knowledge and integrate it into practice.

Reasonably intelligent: A researcher should be intelligent enough to sense the trends and issues happening around.

Imaginative and creative: A researcher should always be open to the environment and perceive changes in the environment, and think and imagine his own perspective creatively to find ways and means to tackle the problem.

A good observer and critic: A researcher should be a keen observer of his surroundings and critically judge the situation to reach his own conclusion.

Optimistic: A researcher must possess the quality of resilience – resuming its original shape after completion. Thomas Alva Edison, the inventor of electric bulb, tried 999 times without a result. But on the very next attempt, he could achieve this great invention. Even then he was optimistic to say, "I learned 999 ways of how to learn from a mistake".

Dedicated and committed: A researcher should be willing enough to give his heart and soul for the sake of research in bringing out a fruitful outcome for the society.

Hang-up free and healthy: A researcher must be self-motivated, enthusiastic and energetic to pursue a research.

Hard-working: A researcher must be diligent and meticulous enough to attain the goal.

Patient: A researcher has to face many obstacles during the tenure of his work. He should wait and work with utmost expectation till he gains the goal.

Innovative and curious: A researcher should always be ready to take up novel challenges and should possess unending curiosity to explore new vistas of knowledge.

Unbiased: The researcher should not be subjected to or get influenced by personal prejudices and assumptions in the research.

Meaning of Nursing Research

Nursing research is one area of research which includes the breadth and depth of the discipline of nursing; the rehabilitative, therapeutic, preventive and promotive aspects of nursing; as well as the preparation of practitioners and personnel involved in total nursing spheres.

The Commission on Nursing Research of the ANA (1981) views nursing research as follows: Nursing research develops knowledge about health and promotion of health over the full span, care of persons with health problems and disabilities and nursing actions to enhance the ability of individuals to respond effectively to actual or potential health problems.

International Nursing Council of Nurses (1986) supports the need for nursing research as a means of improving the health and welfare of the people. Nursing research is a way to identify new knowledge, improve professional education and practice and use of resources effectively. The scientific base for nursing practice is referred to as nursing science.

Nursing science uses systematic inquiry to develop knowledge that will allow nurses to promote, maintain and restore the status of health in human beings. Nursing research refers to the use of systematic, controlled, empirical and critical investigation in attempting to discover or confirm facts that relate to specific problems or questions about the practice of nursing.

Definition of Nursing Research

- Nursing research is the application of systematic inquiry to discover or confirm facts that relate to specific problems in nursing practice.
- Nursing research is a systematic inquiry designed to develop trustworthy evidence about issues of importance to the nursing profession, including nursing practice, education, administration and informatics.
- The Commission on Nursing Research of the ANA (1981) has defined that, nursing research develops knowledge about health and promotion of health over the full life-span, care of persons with

health problems and disabilities and nursing actions to enhance the ability of individuals to respond effectively to actual or potential health problems.

- Nursing research is a process in which the researcher scientifically collects data to be used in the clinical, administrative or instructional area in order to find solutions to nursing problems; evaluate nursing practices, procedures, policies or curriculum; assess the needs of patients, staff or students; and to make decisions to change or continue various nursing processes which in turn advances the scientific knowledge in nursing field.
- *"A scientific process that validates and refines existing knowledge and generates new knowledge that directly and indirectly influences clinical nursing practice."* (Burns and Grove, 2005)
- *"Nursing research is a way to identify new knowledge, improve professional education and practices and use of resources effectively."* (International Council of Nurses, 1986)
- *"A systematic inquiry designed to develop knowledge about issues of importance to the nursing profession, including nursing practice, education and administration and informatics."* (Polit & Beck, 2005)
- *"A systematic, objective process of analyzing phenomena of importance to nursing."* (Rose Marie Niewiadomy, 2008)

History of Nursing Research

Florence Nightingale's Legacy

Florence Nightingale (1850–1910) was the first nurse to be described as a researcher. Her greatest contributions to nursing as a science were her outstanding work as a statistician, her *Notes on Nursing*, her work during the Crimean War, and her establishment of St. Thomas School of Nursing. Nightingale was a statistician who presented her work carefully and clearly, and through such systematic work she became known as an agent of change and a reformer.

Development of nursing research in Western countries

1864 – National Red Cross was established.

1873 – Linda Richards became known as America's first trained nurse.

1900 – The *American Journal of Nursing* was first published in this year.

1902 – The first Nursing Act was passed.

1924 – The first Nursing Doctoral Programme was developed.

1940 – Nurses from the United States served in the World War II.

1950 – A Code of Ethics was adopted by ANA.

1952 – *Nursing Research* the official research journal of ANA is published.

1953 – Institute of Research and Service in Nursing Education, Colombia University.

1954 – Ph.D. programme was introduced in nursing education.

1960 – Reordering of Nursing Research, which aims to improve the quality of patient care, was done.

1973 – ANA started certification programmes for nurses in specific areas.

1994 – The publication of qualitative research journal was started.

1997 – The Foundation of Canadian Health Services was developed.

2001 – Nurse anesthetists gained independent perspective authority.

2004 – The publication of *World Views on Evidence-Based Nursing Journal* was started.

Development of nursing research in India

1964 – Dr. Marie Ferguson, a public health nurse who joined RAK College of Nursing, New Delhi, was able to create greater appreciation and understanding and value of research in nursing for nursing practice, administration and education. She had conducted a valuable study on "Activity Study to Define Nursing and Non-nursing Functions of Nurses in Selected Health Institutes of India."

1966 – A research section was started by Trained Nurses Association of India, under the guidance of Chairwoman Ms. Margareta Craig namely

"Time Utilization Study" with the help of Ms. Anna Gupta, Principal, RAK College of Nursing, ably directed by Dr. Sulochana Krishnan.

1976 – A seminar on Nursing Research for educationists was organized at Delhi, Mussoorie (Uttarakhand) and Yercaud (Tamil Nadu) by Dr. Aparna Bhaduri and Dr. Marce Farrell.

1981 – Dr. Farrell and Dr. Bhaduri's book *Health Research: A Community-based Approach* was published by World Health Organization (WHO).

1982 – The major development during this period was the organization of the national conference "Nursing Research in India: Prospect and Retrospect". It was held at the Bangalore College of Nursing. Here arose some comments like the necessity of forming research cells, the role of research guides to encourage and allot time for student researchers, to include nursing research on state, central government budgets and also on the budgets of other agencies and organization, etc.

1984 – The University Grants Commission conducted a workshop on nursing research. The nursing school teachers all over India participated in this workshop. Another workshop on "Nursing Process" was conducted by Dr. Marie Farrell at Leelabai Thackersey College of Nursing, SNDT Women's University, Bombay, which was sponsored by the WHO.

1986 – During this year NRSI was developed to promote nursing research. Dr. Indrajit Walia was the President and Mrs. Uma Handa was the Secretary. The Committee conducts conferences annually.

1998 – Mr. R. Rajaratnam, Senior Nursing Tutor of National Institute of Mental Health and Neuroscience (NIMHANS), organized a nursing research interest section.

2002 – During this period, the revised versions of Indian Nursing Council for General Nursing and Midwifery course and Post Basic B.Sc. Nursing were included in Nursing Research as a subject.

2004 – Jain & Co., Noida, started publishing *Nightingale Nursing Times*.

2005 – The National Institute of Nursing Education, PGIMER, Chandigarh, published a research-based journal namely *Nursing and Midwifery Research Journal*.

The Indian Nursing Council constituted National Consortium Ph.D. Nursing Programme under the leadership of Shri T. Dileep Kumar, President INC, New Delhi. WHO also supported this programme.

2009 – During this period, the Central Institute of Nursing Research (CIN) came into existence under the supervision of the Trained Nurses Association of India in New Delhi. Ph.D. Nursing was started by IGNOU.

2010 – Baba Farid University of Health Sciences in Faridkot, Punjab started Ph.D. programme in nursing.

History of nursing research in Kerala

Kerala leads in nursing research also as in other areas of education.

2004 – Nursing Research Society of India (NRSI), a state-level conference of nursing research, was convened at the Nursing College, Calicut.

Ph.D. was taken by the following nursing personnel:

1. Dr. Jolly Jose (Jawaharlal Nehru University, New Delhi, 1996)
2. Dr. Mary Lucitta (Kerala University, 1999)
3. Dr. C. Rema Devi (Kerala University, 2003)
4. Dr. R. Bincy (Kerala University, 2004)
5. Dr. Asuma Beevi (Calicut University, 2004)

Several other nursing personnel took Ph.D. from reputed universities in Kerala.

2008 – Govt. College of Nursing, Thiruvananthapuram, was upgraded as a research centre.

2010 – An international conference on "Challenges in Clinical Nursing Research" under the leadership of Prof. Y. Prasanna Kumari and Dr. R. Bincy was held in Government College of Nursing, Thiruvananthapuram.

2011 – A state-level conference on "Paradigms in Experimental Research" was conducted in Government College of Nursing, Thiruvananthapuram.

2011 – A separate Ethical Committee was formulated for Nursing Research in Kerala.

Universities in Kerala conducting research programmes in nursing

1. University of Kerala
2. University of Calicut
3. MG University, Kottayam

4. WHO and INC – Ph.D. Consortium, Ng College, Thiruvananthapuram as Centre
5. Kerala University of Health Sciences (KUHS)

M.Phil. in nursing

1. Clinical Epidemiology, Medical College, Thiruvananthapuram
2. MG University, Kottayam

Purposes of Nursing Research

Nursing research has a tremendous influence on current and future professional nursing practice. Inquiry-search answers the what, where, when, how and why of various phenomena and enlightens us. Nursing research helps to maintain the accuracy of different nursing, educational and administrative techniques. The major purposes of research are:

1. *Description*: In descriptive or explorative studies, a careful and deliberative description is often essential as a basis for the development of theories, e.g. "Assessment of Knowledge and Management of Minor Disorders of Pregnancy". Here, a detailed description of the research topic is explored. Analysis of that situation may reveal relevant factors which were undetected.
2. *Exploration*: This is an extension of descriptive research and is more directly oriented towards the discovery of relationship, e.g. "An Exploratory Study to Identify the Predisposing Factors for the Development of Diabetic Foot Ulcer". Here the investigator observes, describes and explores the phenomenon of interest, i.e. diabetic foot ulcer.
3. *Explanation*: Research offers an understanding of the underlying cause of phenomenon, and explains how or why a phenomenon exists, e.g. "Determining the Incidence and Identifying the Contributing Factors of Nosocomial Infection".
4. *Prediction and control*: Research may either predict causality or find a correlation between specified factors, e.g. "Cigarette Smoking Causes Coronary Artery Diseases".
5. *Discover knowledge of the discipline*: One can gain the knowledge of nursing actions to enhance individual's ability and respond

effectively to actual or potential health problems, as well as develop knowledge about health and promotion of health over the full life span.

6. *Finding answers to questions or finding solutions to a problem.*
7. *Discovering and interpreting new facts that will help improve our knowledge and ability to handle situations and events.*
8. *Establishes generalization and general laws and contributes to theory building in various fields of knowledge.*
9. *It helps in formulating a phenomenon or to achieve new knowledge and enabling to handle situations or events.*
10. *It facilitates the development of clinical interventions, improves health outcomes and contributes to optimal care delivery. It is necessary for continuing improvement that promotes optimal nursing care.*
11. *Identification*: Research helps in formulating phenomenon or to achieve novel insight into it.
12. *Promote evidence-based nursing*: Research is vital to nursing profession and is necessary for continual improvement that promotes optimal nursing care. Research results will be applied in nursing care. This will ensure the credibility of nursing profession, provide accountability in nursing practice, and determine control over the elements of practice.
13. *Document the cost effectiveness of nursing care*: Recognize a nursing care practice that makes a difference in cost and financial benefits of nursing care.
14. *Develop nursing theories and principles.*

Significance of Nursing Research

Nursing research is a key element in providing appropriate nursing care. It allows the multitude of questions that surface in daily nursing practice to be answered. The nurse relying on nursing research to guide practice can be reasonably confident that an essential element in competent nursing practice has been met.

1. Research will help the development and generation of knowledge in each area of specialization.

2. It is helpful in evidence-based practice. Research findings give first-hand experience on which evidence-based nursing practice can be build upon.
3. Improvement in nursing education and nursing management is possible through research studies.
4. Research will help in standardization and refining nursing practice.
5. Strengthen the profession by generating knowledge through scientific studies.
6. Through evidence-based nursing, cost-effective care can be rendered to clients.
7. Research results will help to provide answers to guide practitioner in the decision-making process.
8. It enables the administrator to take prompt decisions on health-related problems.
9. It is essential for molding attitudes, intellectual competencies and technical skills.

Role of Nurses in Research

In 1981, the ANA Commission on Nursing Research outlined the role of various levels of nurses related to nursing research.

(a) Graduate nurses are primarily consumers of nursing research.
   1. Be able to evaluate research in terms of its applicability to nursing practice-research utilization
   2. Conducting small research
   3. Be able to identify problems for future investigations
   4. Offer clinical expertise to improve a proposed research plan
   5. To incorporate research findings to practice
   6. Participate in a journal club
   7. Attend research presentations

(b) Masters-prepared nurses
   1. Conduct investigations
   2. Assist others with their research
   3. Help to apply research to practice

(c) Doctoral-prepared nurses

1. Direct research projects
2. Provide leadership in conducting research and disseminating research findings

In carrying out research work, one gains valuable experience and training in planning and in conducting, analyzing and presenting an independent research project.

Also, on a general level one will learn about conventions and requirements of nursing research which will equip oneself for further research and for communication within the scientific field of nursing.

Scope of Nursing Research

The scope of nursing research is to enhance the various research activities and to strengthen the body of knowledge in nursing practice, education and administration. The areas of nursing research may be classified under the following headings.

1. Research in clinical nursing (service)
2. Research in nursing education
3. Research in nursing administration

Research in clinical nursing (service)

In order to improve the quality of nursing care, research is required. In clinical nursing, some important researchable areas are:

1. Risk reduction interventions for vulnerable and minority groups
2. Problems of the old age

According to the International Council of Nurses (ICN), the priority areas of nursing research include:

1. Health promotion and prevention of illness
2. Control of symptoms
3. Patients living with chronic conditions
4. Enhancing quality of life
5. Assessing client's problems

6. Providing and testing nursing care interventions
7. Measuring the outcomes of care

Priority areas in Oncology Nursing as proposed by Oncology Nursing Society (2005–2009) include:

1. Cancer symptoms and side effects
2. Individual and family-focused psycho-social and behavioural research
3. Health promotion; primary and secondary prevention
4. Late effects of cancer treatment and long-term survivorship issues for patients and their families
5. Nursing-sensitive patient outcome
6. Factors affecting the clinical application of already created evidence-based guidelines for cancer patients

Priority areas in medical surgical nursing

1. Prevention of risk factors of coronary artery disease
2. Effect of diet and exercise on control of cholesterol
3. Effect of pre-operative exercises on post-operative complications
4. Problems of patient on ventilator
5. Effect of yoga on asthma
6. First-aid management of patients with head injury
7. Role of care-givers in degenerative diseases like Parkinson's Disease, Multiple Sclerosis, GBS, etc.
8. Effect of constrained, induced movement therapy for motor performance of patient with stroke
9. QOL of patients with nephrotic syndrome, renal failure and kidney transplantation
10. Predisposing factors of osteoporosis
11. Relaxation therapy and life-style modifications in gastro-esophageal reflux disease/alcoholic liver diseases
12. Risk factors of diabetic foot ulcer
13. ICU-psychosis: Predisposing factors and prevention

Research in nursing education

Research is also applicable to nursing education. A nurse researcher has the role of a mentor and an educator. This will help improve teaching and learning methods in nursing discipline.

Priority areas in nursing education

1. Compiling the effects of different teaching methods
2. Curriculum of graduate and post-graduate courses
3. Stress of nursing students during training
4. Effect of innovative teaching aids
5. Strict discipline
6. Handling problematic students in nursing
7. Generating evaluation methods to judge the teaching-learning process

Research in nursing administration

Research can influence nursing administration also. Practical problems and issues can be solved with the help of research.

1. Employee satisfaction
2. Measures to reduce the workload of staff nurses
3. Decision-making technique
4. Assertive behaviour of nursing personnel
5. Compare the effect of different communication patterns
6. Comparison of patient assignments
7. Workload of staff nurses
8. Health problems of nursing personnel
9. Infection rates in ICU and general wards
10. ICU psychosis
11. Stress of nurses working in ICUs
12. Measures to prevent frequent turnout of staff
13. Analysis of the roles and responsibilities of nurse practitioners in various specialties

14. Comparison of different communication models in clinical setting

Problems of care-givers

(a) Stress and fatigue
(b) Burn-out syndrome
(c) Orthopedic problems
(d) Back pain for staff working in neuro-ICU
(e) Psychological problems

Problems and Issues in Nursing Research

Many challenges, problems and issues are encountered when conducting research in nursing. Some major problems are as listed below:

1. *Inadequate knowledge of research methodology is one of the main problems for many researchers.*
2. *Lack of qualified research guide or supervisor*: The number of investigators is high, but qualified guides are very less. It is a real problem today.
3. *Difficulty in controlling external variables*: It is very difficult to control the external variables while measuring the effect of an independent variable on a dependent variable.
4. *Lack of time*: Because of the heavy workload, nurses experience lack of time for conducting research studies.
5. *Lack of standardized tools*: Even though self-prepared research tools are the best instruments for assessment of research variables, standardized tools are required for research studies. These tools are not adequately present. The validity and reliability of the tools are also a concern.
6. *Reliability of disciplined research*: In nursing, research questions can be solved by different approaches. Sometimes, it may be difficult to decide the best approach to solve a problem. Repeated attempts to solve a similar question with identical answers may increase the value of generated evidence.

7. *Studying many variables*: The measurement of many variables in a single attempt will be required in some studies. Studying multiple data in a single instance causes difficulty in data collection, analysis and interpretation of data. In addition, the study will be a hectic process for the researcher and needs lot of time, energy and money to handle these data.
8. *Ethical problems*: Studies in nursing deals with human beings where safeguarding their rights is of prime concern. Often it may very difficult to approve the ethical aspects of a study and thus several problems remain to be studied.
9. *Lack of support from the administrative set-up*: Lack of encouragement and being unable to avail leave from duty for conducting research are real hurdles for the researchers.
10. *Financial constraints*: Proper funding is not available for nurses to carry out research studies.

Research for Professional Uplift

Nursing in India has to accomplish more to occupy the position of a full-fledged profession. Research is the only answer to fulfill the lacunae. The under-mentioned areas are priorities warranting research to address the issues.

1. Assertiveness
2. Evidenced-based nursing
3. Authority
4. Credibility and acceptance
5. Moving with the tide of change
6. Constant refreshment of knowledge sector
7. Social accountability and obligation

Future of Nursing Research

The future of nursing research is exciting and promising. A major challenge in attempting to answer the myriad of questions faced by nurses is to continue to develop a philosophy of nursing science that is consistent with the values of the discipline (Philips 1988; Riegil et al, 1992). In research methods, new disciplinary collaboration and dissemination of findings are significant. The future trend of nursing research should be geared to solving the pressing clinical nursing problems. The present priority areas for supporting nursing research are:

1. To encourage multi-disciplinary collaboration for doing research
2. To create a post of nurse researcher in various departments of hospitals

SUMMARY

The ultimate goal of any profession is to provide service of a high quality to its clients. Research represents a critically important tool for adding more knowledge to a profession. Research is a higher level of learning. Nursing research helps for increased professionalism, accountability, social relevance and decision-making in nursing practice.

Essentially, nursing research is about patients and providing best quality care for them (Watson, 1998). The quality of nursing care is greatly influenced by research findings. When nursing practice is evidence-based, patients are more likely to receive proper care that is safe and effective; it promotes comfort and facilitates the best outcomes. Incorporating research into practice ensures a solid basis for nursing practice. As Polit and Hungler (1997) suggested, research allows nurses to question their practice, find answers and thus to implement them in their area.

MULTIPLE CHOICE QUESTIONS

1. The ultimate purpose for conducting nursing research is to ___________.
   (a) broaden one's knowledge base
   (b) promote evidence based care for patients
   (c) find out explanations to theories
   (d) enhance the growth of nursing profession

2. Most objective and reliable source of nursing knowledge is __________.
   (a) tradition
   (b) authority/experts
   (c) trial and error
   (d) scientific research
3. Which of the following is conducted to develop test and refine theories and generate new knowledge?
   (a) basic research/Pure research
   (b) applied research
   (c) qualitative research
   (d) quantitative research
4. The nurses make clinical decisions based on the best research evidence, their clinical expertise and the health care preferences of their patients/clients – this is termed as __________.
   (a) empirical data
   (b) evidence-based nursing practice
   (c) basic research
   (d) qualitative research
5. The research concerned with objectivity, tight controls over the research situations, and the ability to generalize findings is __________.
   (a) qualitative research
   (b) quantitative research
   (c) outcome research
   (d) applied research
6. Research utilization means __________.
   (a) increasing knowledge
   (b) problem solving
   (c) stimulate more research
   (d) implementation of findings from specific research studies

7. The process where the knowledge based on objective evidence (information/data) observed through our senses is called __________.
   (a) investigation
   (b) empiricism
   (c) assumption
   (d) evaluation
8. Which of the following reasons contribute to the importance for research in nursing?
   (a) build a body of nursing knowledge
   (b) validate improvements in nursing practice
   (c) make health care efficient as well as cost effective
   (d) all the above

ANSWER KEY

1. (b) 2. (d) 3. (a) 4. (b) 5. (b) 6. (d) 7. (b) 8. (d)

REVIEW QUESTIONS

1. Define nursing research.
2. Discuss the significance of nursing research.
3. Describe the scope of nursing research.
4. Write short notes on:
   (a) Purposes of nursing research
   (b) Trends in nursing research
   (c) Problems and issues in nursing research

REFERENCES

Abdullah, F.G., & Levine, E. (1965). Better patient care through nursing research. New York: Macmillan.

________. (1994). Preparing nursing research for the 21st century. New York: Springer.

Arford, P.H. (2004). Working with human research protections. *Journal of Nursing Scholarship*, 35, 265–271.

Bayley, E.W., Machean, S.L., Desy, P., & McMahon, M. (2004). ENA's Delphi study on national research priorities for emergency nurses in the United States. *Journal of Emergency Nursing*, 30, 12–21.

Berger, A.M., Berry, S.L., Christopher, K.A., Greene, A.L., Maliski, S., & Swenson, K.K., et al. (2005). Oncology Nursing Society year 2004 research priorities survey. *Oncology Nursing Forum*, 32, 281–290.

Bonifazi, W.L. (2004). Cruelty and courage: Nurses in the Nasi era. *Nurse Week*, 24–26.

Bourdeaux, L., Matthews, L., Richards, N.L., San Augustine, G., Thomas, P., & Veltigan, S. (2005). Comparative study of case management programme for patients with syncope. *Journal of Nursing Care Quality*, 20, 140–144.

Brooten, D., Kumar, S., Brown, L.P., Butts, P., Finkler, S.A., & Bakewell-Sachs, S. et al. (1986). A randomized clinical trial of early hospital discharge and home follow-up of very-low-birth-weight infants. *New England Journal of Medicine*, 315, 934–939.

Brown, J., Tanner, C., & Padrick, K. (1984). Nursing's search for scientific knowledge. *Nursing Research*, 33, 26–32.

Burns, N., & Grove, S.K. (2005). The practice of nursing research: Conduct, critique and utilisation (5th ed.). St. Louis, MO: Elsevier Saunders.

Centres for Disease Control and Prevention. (2006). The Tuskgee Timeline. Retrieved May 18, 2006 from http://www.cdc.gov/nchstp/od/tuskegee/time.ht.

Colling, J. (2004). Procedures, ethics and funding sources. *Urologic Nursing*, 24, 130–133.

Crane, P.B., Letvak, S., Lewallen, L., Hu, J., & Jones, E. (2004). Inclusion of women in nursing research. *Nursing Research*, 53, 227–232.

Downs, F.S. (1994). Hitching the research wagon to theory [editorial]. *Nursing Research*, 45, 195.

Duffery, L., Hepburn, K., Christenson, R., & Brugge-Wiger, P. (1989). A research agenda in care for patients with Alzheimer's disease. *Journal of Nursing Scholarship*, 21, 254–257.

Erlen, J.A. (2000). "Conflict of Interest". An ethical dilemma for the nurse researcher. *Orthopaedic Nursing*, 19, 74–77.

Ferguson, L.A. (1996). Enhancing health care to underserved populations. *AAOHN Journal*, 44, 332–335.

Fitzpatrick, J.J. (1999). Lateness is not greatness. *Nursing and Health Care Perspectives*, 20, 231.

_________. (2004). Making a commitment to go public [editorial]. *Applied Nursing Research*, 17, 223.

Grady, P. (2005). Statement before Congress by Dr. Patricia A. Grady on the FY 2005 budget. Retrieved August 24, 2005 from http://ninr.gov/ninr/about/legislation.html.

_________. (2005). Minutes of the National Advisory Council for Nursing Research, May 17–18, 2005. Retrieved August 28, 2005 from http://ninr.nih.gov/ninr/about/adv-council.html.

Greenberg, M.E. (2000). Telephone nursing: Evidence of client and organizational benefits. *Nursing Economics*, 18, 117–123.

Grier, M. (1982). Editorial. *Research in Nursing and Health*, 5, 111.

Habel, M. (2005). Can you answer patients' questions about clinical trials? *Nurse Week-South Central Edition*, 23–25.

Harden, J.T., & McFarland, G. (2000). Avoiding gender and minority barriers to NIH funding. *Journal of Nursing Scholarship*, 32, 83–86.

Hayter, J. (1979). Issues related to human subjects. In F. Downs & J. Fleming (Eds.). Issues in nursing research (107–147). New York: Appleton-Century-Crofts.

Henderson, V. (1956). Research in nursing practice- when? *Nursing Research*, 4, 99.

Hilpala, S.I., Meyer, K.A., Wallace, T.O., & Zaremba, J.A. (2005). Profile of an admission nurse. *Nursing Management*, 36, 44–47.

Jacobson, S.F., Chu, N.L., Pascucci, M.A., & Gaskins, S.W. (2004). Characteristics of nursing research on race, ethnicity and culture. *Journal of Multicultural Nursing and Health*, 10(3), 6–12.

Katz, K. (1972). Experimentation with human beings. New York: Russell Sage.

Kennedy, M.S. (2004). Not your grandma's nursing research [editorial]. *American Journal of Nursing*, 104, 11.

Kerlinger, F. (1986). Foundations of behavioural research (3rd ed.). New York: Holt, Rinehart & Winston.

Krugman, S., Giles, J., & Hammond, J. (1971). Viral hepatitis, type B (MS-2 strain): Studies on active immunization. *Journal of the American Medical Association*, 217, 41–45.

Lake, E.T. (2006). Multilevel models in health outcomes research: Part 1: Theory, design and measurement. *Applied Nursing Research*, 19, 51–55.

Leninger, M.M. (1985). Ethnography and ethnonursing: Models and modes of qualitative data analysis. In M.M. Leninger (Ed.). Qualitative research methods in nursing (33–72). Orlando, F.L.: Grune & Stratton.

Marvin, M. (1927). Research in nursing. *American Journal of Nursing*, 27, 331–335.

Milgram, S. (1963). Behavioural study of obedience. *Journal of Abnormal and Social Psychology*, 67, 371–378.

Myers, G., & Kosinski, M. (2005). Research in the perianesthesia setting: The basics of getting started. *Journal of Peri Anesthesia Nursing*, 20, 35–41.

National Institute of Nursing Research. (2005). Mission statement. Retrieved August 30, 2005, from http://ninr.nih.gov/ninr/research/diversity/mission.html.

Nuremberg Military Tribunals. (1949). Trials of war criminals before the Nuremberg Military tribunals under Control Council Law No. 10. (Publication No. 1949-841584, Vol. 2). Washington, D.C.: US Government Printing Office.

Office of Research Integrity Annual Report. (2004). Retrieved August 24, 2005 from http://ori.dhhs.gov.

Olsen, D.P., & Mahrenholz, D. (2000). IRB-identified ethical issues in nursing research. *Journal of Professional Nursing*, 16, 140–148.

Oman, K.S., Krugman, M.E., & Fink, R.M. (2003). Nursing research secrets. Philadelphia: Hanley & Belfus.

Paul, J.M., Phillips, T.A., Widime, M.D., & Hollenbeak, C.S. (2004). Cost-effectiveness of postnatal home nursing visits for prevention of hospital care for jaundice and dehydration. *Pediatrics*, 114, 1015–1022.

Polit, D.F., & Beck, C.T. (2004). Nursing research: Principles and methods. (7th ed.). Philadelphia: Lippincott Williams & Wilkins.

Pullen, L., Tuck, I., & Wallace, D.C. (1999). Research priorities in mental health nursing. *Issues in Mental Health Nursing*, 20, 217–227.

Rankin, M., & Esteves, M.D. (1996). How to access a research study? *American Journal of Nursing*, 96, 33–36.

Rittenmeyer, P. (1982). The evaluation of nursing research. *Western Journal of Nursing Research*, 4, 223–225.

Salmond, S.W. (1994). Orthopaedic nursing research priorities. A Delphi study. *Orthopaedic Nursing*, 13, 31–45.

Sedlack, C., Ross, D., Arslanian, C., & Taggart, H. (1998). Orthopaedic nursing research priorities: A replication and extension. *Orthopaedic Nursing*, 17(2), 51–58.

Sigma Theta Tan International Honor Society for Nursing. (2005). The Society's Vision and Mission. Retrieved August 28, 2005 from http://www.nursingsociety.org/about/overview.html.

Silva, M.C. (1995). Ethical guidelines in the conduct, dissemination, and implementation of nursing research. Washington, D.C.: American Nurses Association.

Simmons, L.W., & Henderson, V. (1964). Nursing research: A survey and assessment. New York: Appleton-Century-Crofts.

Simpson, M. (1985). Therapeutic play and cooperation of preschoolers during physical examinations. Unpublished master's thesis. Texas Woman's University, Denton.

Tusker-Allen, S. (2003). Nursing education as a respected area of research [editorial]. *The Association of Black Nursing Faculty Journal*, 14, 115.

Ulrich, B. (2005). Intersecting worlds. Nursing and NASA. *Nurse Week-South Central Edition*, 3.

Williams, S. (2005). The science of care. *Nurse Week-South Central Edition*, 10.

CHAPTER

2

INITIATING RESEARCH AND OVERCOMING OBSTACLES

Key terms

- ★ Barriers of research
- ★ Research diary
- ★ Support for research
- ★ Research supervisor

⊙ Outline

- ★ Significance
- ★ Special nature of research
- ★ Types of barriers for research
- ★ Measures to overcome initial obstacles

⊙ Objectives

On completion of this chapter, you will be able to:

- ★ recognize the significance of initiating research
- ★ identify the types of barriers for research
- ★ understand the measures to overcome obstacles of research

Introduction

Nursing research is mandate for the development of nursing profession. It provides an ideal platform for knowledge base, and satisfies our curiosity to encourage self-reliance and confidence.

Researchers face many obstacles and difficulties during their research work. For eminent researchers like Madame Curie and Albert Einstein, research was not a bed of roses for them. Determination is a key to success in research. Being aware of the possible problems and the ways of overcoming initial obstacles will facilitate the research process.

The man who graduates today and stops learning tomorrow is uneducated the day after.

—Newton D. Baker

Check Points... *Special nature of research*

1. Require patience
2. Stressful
3. Time consuming
4. Needs hard work and commitment from researcher
5. Require the help of experts.
6. Consult statistician before starting study
7. Mindset to face any unexpected failures and obstacles
8. Readiness to accept criticism which is a character and part of researcher
9. Researcher requires new knowledge and application of technology.

Barriers for Research

There are many barriers in conducting research. Students of different disciplines often proceed with the research work with a vague idea. Often they experience initial obstacles, unnecessary confusions and sometimes discontinue the research work. If we do a survey to find reasons for stopping research work, many obstacles come to light.

Types of Barriers

There are three types of barriers to the effective conduct of research work.

Personal barriers

Personal barriers include deficiency of research knowledge, lack of material or financial resources, limited individual motivation, and negative research attitude. Positive attitude is a must for successful completion of research work.

Professional barriers

1. Job requirements that may not acknowledge the use or conduct of research

2. Absence of support from nursing and health care colleagues
3. Poor communication of research findings

Organizational barriers

1. Inadequate administrative support for nursing research
2. Lack of resources for conducting researches
3. Difficulty in getting ethical clearance

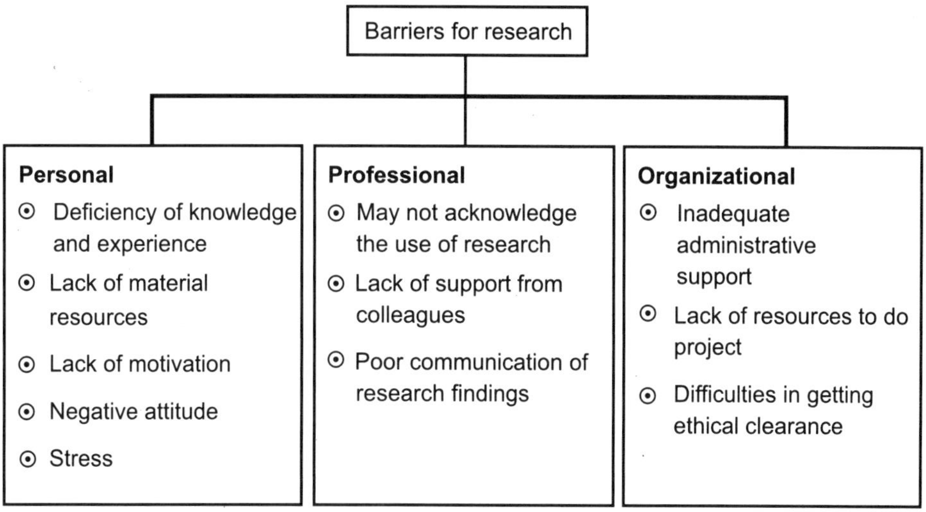

Figure 2.1 Types of barriers for research work

Prerequisites for Research

Develop life skills to initiate research successfully

Researchers need these skills for collection, selection, analysis and presentation of data. It requires the researcher to provide ultimate attention to alternative values, views, meanings and explanations. Research involves the professionalization of these everyday skills.

In educational system, these are commonly understood as core, key, generic or transferable skills, which are used continually by academicians and researchers. These are important skills for research.

Reading: "Reading makes a man." It improves our ideas and thoughts. Books, journals and thesis work are the different sorts of materials for reference.

Listening: It helps the researcher to identify people's voices, their attitudes, emotions, openness and honesty. The researcher would extract useful information from listening to various sources such as friends, family members, colleagues and other modes like television and radio.

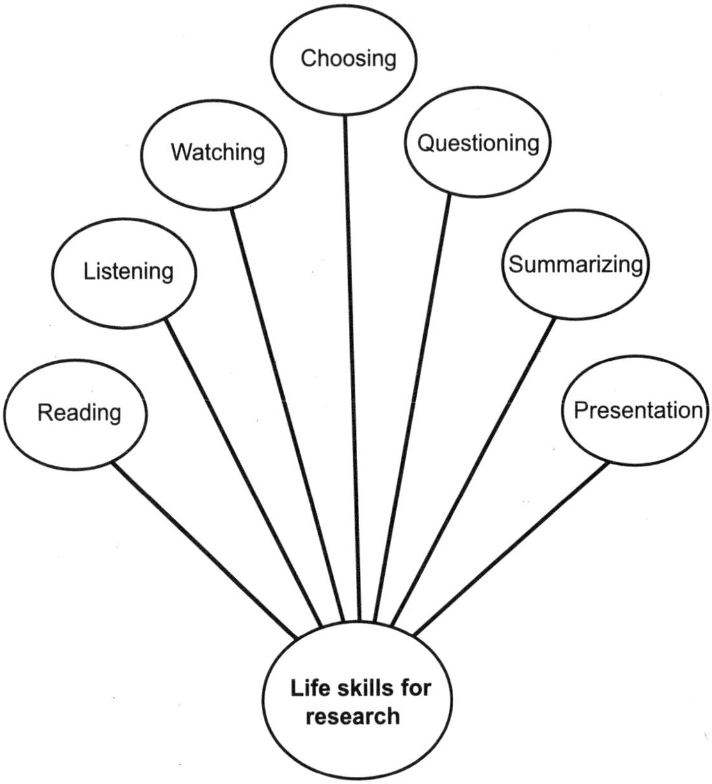

Figure 2.2 Life skills for research

Watching: By watching carefully, one can learn to identify a wide range of usual signals which indicate friendliness, entertainment, unease or danger.

Choosing: A researcher will develop skills of relevance to select topics for research, methods used in research and subjects to be samples.

Questioning: Questioning is an important skill for data collection.

Summarizing: "Keep it short and sweet" (brevity) should be the basic principle of writing in research. In research, the ability to concise is important. A researcher will have a great skill of summarization such as what to leave out, what to stress and what is important. Hence, it is essential that writing skills or aptitude plays a vital role in collecting information as the research progresses.

Presentation: Presentation influences writing. A proper presentation attracts the attention of audience. Reflecting is the most considerable research skill. It gives an idea for thinking carefully what you have done or are doing. In research terms, it is important to reflect upon our own role in the research process.

Need for support

The need for support is an important resource for a researcher. Here arises the applicability of research resources. Resources such as libraries, universities, and availability of technology are vital resources. A researcher utilizes these resources the maximum. Everyone has their own approach regarding a subject. It is hence necessary that the researcher discuss his subject with friends and colleagues. The need for support denotes emotional and personal support rather than academic support. Undertaking research can threaten one's personal, family, work or social life. Be aware of the demands the research project may put on the loved ones of the researcher.

Check Points... *Seeking support*

Answer the following questions.

1. Who can you 'ear bash' about your research?
2. Who will ask you "How is it going"?
3. Who will make you "cups of tea"?
4. Who will give you permission not to do things?

With nobody to take the role of support, a researcher will need to do the above exercise to find them or develop them unless he is unusually confident, organized and self-aware.

Finding the supervisor

The relationship between the researcher and the supervisor is of critical importance during research. A good supervisor and a wonderful supervisory relationship deem to make an efficient research project. A supervisor has personal responsibility for overseeing the progress of student's research projects. Supervisors should have knowledge of specialist areas in which their students are researching as well as a general understanding of the research process and the various strategies possible. The process of supervision differs for each university and subject. The supervisory arrangements have implications of power, attention and dynamics.

Supervisors may come with the job, or they may be chosen by someone, or they may appear to be the only specialist available. Under these circumstances, the research students expect some qualities from their supervisor, and the supervisors also expect some qualities from their students. We have to find out these expectations.

Check Points... *What students expect of their supervisors*

1. To be supervised
2. To read their work well in advance
3. To be available when needed
4. To be friendly, open and supportive
5. To critic constructively
6. To have a good knowledge of their research area.

Check Points... *What supervisors expect of their students*

1. To be independent
2. To produce written work that is not just a first draft
3. To have regular meetings
4. To be honest when reporting upon their progress
5. To follow the advice that they give, when it has been given at their request.
6. To be excited about their work, able to surprise them and fun to be with.

Source: *Phillips and Pugh (2000: Chapter 8 & 11)*

Research diary

Keeping a research diary is important during research work. In this diary, the researcher might record the research progress, feelings, thoughts, insecurities and insights day-by-day as the research continues. Different formats are available for keeping/making a research diary.

The most common is that kept on paper. A researcher might have an option to choose the way whichever is applicable to him. Someone may recommend the researcher to organize the research diary in terms of observational notes, methodological notes, theoretical notes and analytic memos. While keeping a research diary, it reminds of critical incidents and particular aspects of data collection or field work by the researcher. It will serve as a trigger for reflection and physical reminder.

Sections of research diary

There are four sections in a research diary, observes Schalzman and Strauss.

Observational notes: These record events experienced principally through watching and listening. They contain as title interpretation as possible and are reliable as the observer can reconstruct them.

Methodological notes: A statement that reflects an operational act completed or an instruction to oneself, a reminder, or a critique of one's own tactics. It notes the timing, sequencing, stationing, stage-setting or maneuvering. Methodological notes might be thought of as observational notes on the researcher himself and upon the methodological process itself.

Theoretical notes: "Self-conscious, controlled attempts to derive meaning from any one of several observational notes."

Analytic memos: An analytic memo enables the researcher to elaborate upon the inference or to tie up several inferences into a more abstract statement.

Measures to Overcome Initial Obstacles

1. Research is a strenous activity; proper planning of all types of resources is of utmost importance.

2. Always maintain a positive attitude throughout the study.
3. Researchers should be aware of the special nature of research. A comprehensive orientation about the research process is mandatory.
4. The need for support is very important. A researcher needs help and support from team members, family members and colleagues.
5. Keep a research diary.
6. Get help from experts of other disciplines.
7. *Perseverance and hard work*: Investigators should be strong and develop perseverance and tolerance because any trouble or obstacle can happen in any phase of research.
8. Have correct determination, perspective and motivation.
9. Face criticism in each stage of work. It is also a part of the research. Positive and sound mindset is necessary from the beginning to end.

SUMMARY

In this chapter we have had a bird's eye view of the ways of initiating a research project and the measures to overcome the initial obstacles. This step will strengthen a researcher to conduct research confidently.

MULTIPLE CHOICE QUESTION

1. A proper presentation of research report
   (a) attracts the attention of audience
   (b) replicates the research study
   (c) hinders research work
   (d) none of the above
2. The relationship between researcher and supervisor is of critical importance during research
   (a) True
   (b) False

3. In ____________ the researcher might record the research progress, feelings, thoughts, insecurities
   (a) research proposal
   (b) research tool
   (c) research diary
   (d) research design
4. Inadequate administrative support for carrying out research work is an example of
   (a) personal barrier
   (b) professional barrier
   (c) organizational barrier
   (d) none of the above
5. Need for support is an important resource for a researcher during a research project
   (a) no
   (b) yes

ANSWER KEY

1. (a) 2. (a) 3. (c) 4. (c) 5. (b)

REVIEW QUESTIONS

1. (a) Lists the barriers of conducting nursing research.
   (b) Explain the barriers for conducting nursing research.
2. Write short notes on:
   (a) Research diary
   (b) Measures to overcome initial obstacles for conducting research in nursing

REFERENCES

Cobb, A.K. (2000). Acculturation and accommodation in qualitative and quantitative research. *Journal of Professional Nursing*, 16, 188.

Coughlan, M., Cronin, P., & Ryan, F. (2007). Step-by-step guide to critiquing research. Part 1: Quantitative research. *British Journal of Nursing*, 16(11), 658–663.

_________. (2008). Undertaking a literature review. A step-by-step approach. *British Journal of Nursing*, 17(1), 38–43.

Dickinson, F. (2004). Assessing the state of the art: Doing a literature review. *Midwifery Matters*, 101, 6–7.

Dornan, T., Peile, E., & Spencer, J. (2008). On "evidence". *Medical Education*, 42, 232–234.

Duffy, J.R. (2005). Critically appraising quantitative research [Electronic version]. *Nursing and Health Sciences*, 7(4), 281–283.

Dyer, I. (1997). The significance of statistical significance. *Intensive and Critical Care Nursing*, 13, 259–265.

Frame, K. (2003). Reading nursing research. Easy as ABCD. *Journal of School Nursing*, 19(6), 326–329.

Gerrish, K., Ashworth, P., Lacey, A., Bailey, J., & Kendall, S., et al. (2007). Factors influencing the development of evidence-based practice: A research tool. *Journal of Advanced Nursing*, 57(3), 328–338.

Giuffre, M. (1994). Reading research critically: Threats to internal validity. *Journal of Post Anesthesia Nursing*, 995, 303–307.

_________. (1995). Reading research critically: Assessing the validity and reliability of research instrumentation. Part 1: *Journal of Post Anesthesia Nursing*, 10(1), 33–37.

_________. (1995). Reading research critically: Assessing the validity and reliability of research instrumentation. Part 2: *Journal of Post Anesthesia Nursing*, 10(2), 107–112.

Harrell, J.A. (1995). Reading research reports: Should I apply the findings to my practice? *Tar Heel Nurse*, 57(2), 26–27.

Hek, G. (1996). Guidelines on conducting a critical research evaluation. *Nursing Standard*, 11(6), 40–43.

CHAPTER

3

RESEARCH PROCESS

Key terms

★ Research process ★ Assumptions ★ Variables ★ Hypothesis ★ Operational definitions ★ Delimitations and limitations

⊙ Outline

- ★ Introduction
- ★ Definitions
- ★ Stages and steps of research process
- ★ Planning
- ★ Implementation
- ★ Translating research findings into nursing practice
- ★ Summary
- ★ Nursing research on the web
- ★ Review questions

⊙ Objectives

On completion of this chapter, you will be able to:

- ★ define research process
- ★ identify the stages of research process
- ★ recognize the steps of research process

Introduction

Research is a careful inquiry which aimed at searching new facts or verification of established facts under various situations. All research studies have to be designed in a systematic way to yield valid and reliable results. Unless these basic steps are followed, the researcher is bound to get into problems at the time of interpretation of results.

Definition

Research process explains the steps that one needs to follow for conducting research. The basic steps involved in the formulation of a research process can be visualized as follows.

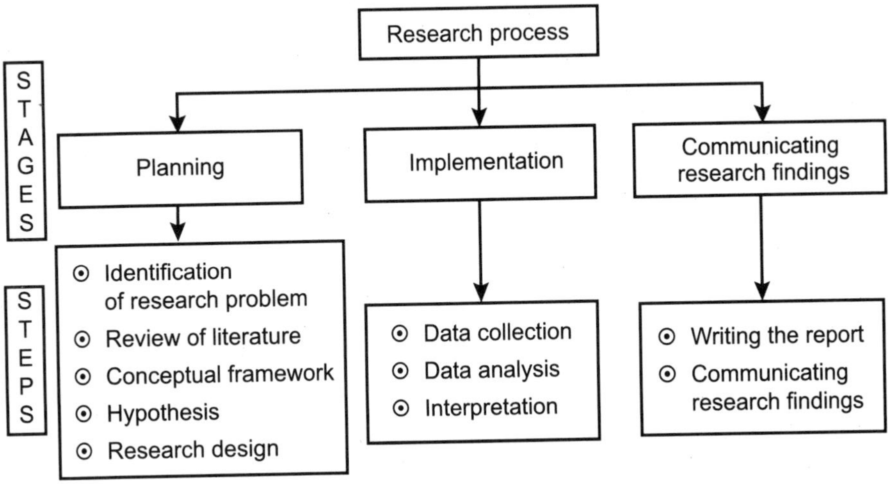

Figure 3.1 Stages and steps of research process

Research Process

A. Planning

1. Identifying Research Problem
2. Searching Literature
3. Developing Theoretical Framework
4. Formulating Hypothesis
5. Design and Planning
6. Research Proposal
7. Identification of Sample and Population
8. Finalizing and Reviewing the Research Plan
9. Pilot Study

B. Implementation stage

10. Collection of Data
11. Preparing Data for Analysis
12. Data Analysis
13. Interpretation or Results

C. Communicating the research findings

14. Evidence-based Nursing

A. Planning

The stages of research process includes a series of independent steps consisting of identification of research problem, review of literature, development of conceptual framework and research designs.

1. *Identification of a Research Problem*

Research starts with identification of a research problem. Initially – select a research area and then a research topic that is of interest to researcher and which contributing nursing. Nursing guides can give guidance for that, but the primary interest must be of the researcher.

- *Operational*: Description of how variables or concepts will be measured or manipulated in a study.
- *Limitation*: They are the theoretical and methodological restrictions in a study that may decrease the generalizability of the findings.
- *Delimitation*: It is the restriction imposed by the researcher himself while conducting the research study.

2. *Searching Literature*

Review of related literature is vital for research studies. Review of research publications should be alone throughout the study, but mostly focused in planning stage. In the initial period it will help to identify a researchable problem and to formulate the research protocol. Review of literature will help to analyze various aspects of the study the strengths and weakness of the study. A thorough review of literature must be followed by a critical review. Through literature review researchers will get an idea regarding concepts, objectives and hypotheses, identify complete theoretical frameworks and research studies that support or reject these, and compare the research designs.

3. *Defining the Theoretical Frameworks*

Theory is the ultimate aim of science when the research is performed in the context of a theoretical framework. Then its findings will have long lasting significance of utility.

4. *Formulating Hypothesis*

It is a cardinal component of research process. It gives direction to carry out the study. Hypothesis is a statement of the researcher's expectations concerning relationship between the variables under investigation. It is the predictions of expected outcome. It states the relationship that the researcher expects to find as a result of the study.

5. *The Design and Planning*

The right decision about the methods to be used to address the research question and test the hypothesis must be arrived at through a careful planning. Research designs can be qualitative as well as quantitative. It may be experimental or descriptive designs such as historical, survey and correlation methods. Research methodology may vary according to the type of research.

Experimental designs describe how the research will be conducted, how the subjects for research are selected and how controls are used.

Descriptive methods like survey design use questionnaires and interview schedules. In nursing studies this method is commonly used. Under historical design the materials are already in existence such as public and private records.

A case study design focuses on an in depth investigation of one unit, a patient, a disease group or an institution. If we are analyzing psychological aspects of clients, this design is the mot suitable one.

6. *Developing Research Protocol for the Interventions*

The research protocol is a written plan of the research to be conducted. It gives clear idea regarding what the investigator intends to do, how he or she plans to do it, details of study sample, study period. Research proposal should be given for the approval of research committee and ethical committee.

7. *Selection of Population and Sample*

Usually, a study is undertaken on a group of human beings who conform to a set of specifications. The decision about the exact nature of the population has to be made on the basis of the problem and objectives under study. The main considerations which are to be kept in mind at the time of taking a decision about the study population is the homogeneity with reference to independent variables.

Data are generally collected from a sample rather than from an entire population. The sample should show all the characteristics of the population. The quality of the sample for quantitative studies depends on how typical or representative the sample is of the population with respect to concerned variables in the study. Sophisticated sampling procedures can produce samples that have a high likelihood of being representative. In a nutshell, the selection of suitable sampling techniques and sampling methods should be proper as it influence the quality of research results.

8. Finalizing and Reviewing the Research Plan

Usually, researchers have their own research plan reviewed by a committee of experts. For the graduate and the post graduate courses in nursing, an institution-based committee will do the appraisal of the research proposal. Research advisors/supervisors give suggestion for finalizing the plan. College level Research Committee should be constituted with research experts, statisticians, medical experts and nursing guides. Then the research plan will be screened by the research committee and ethical committee for final approval.

9. Pilot Study and Making Revisions

A pilot study is a similar version of a proposed study conducted to refine the methodology. It should be as similar to the proposed study as possible using similar subjects, the same setting and the same data collection techniques. In a real situation, the problems or difficulties may arise in the course of research projects. These can be eliminated in the actual study.

B. Implementation Stage

It includes collection of data and analysis of data through descriptive or inferential statistics and interpretation of the results.

10. Data Collection

It is the most time consuming step in the research process, which involves direct or indirect interaction with respondents to gather information related to the topic. It must be carefully planned and implemented to collect data using correct methods, techniques, and tools of data collection.

11. Preparing the Data for Analysis

The data collected are subjected to various types of analyses and interpretation.

12. Analyzing the Data

The data collected are subjected to various types of analyses and interpretations. Data can be analyzed by using descriptive or inferential statistics. The data can be analyzed either by manual calculations or by using statistical software, programs like Statistical Package for Social Sciences (SPSS). Data are presented through tables, graphs and charts to facilitate the interpretation of data.

13. Interpretation of the Results

Interpretation means the process of making sense of the results and of examining the implications of the finding within a broader context.

This is the way of diagnozing the studied result. It produces a valuable meaning to the collected data.

If the findings agree with the formulated research hypothesis the study results are usually clear. If the result is not supported, the investigator should explain it properly. In research studies acceptance and rejection of hypothesis is not a faulty process. Ideally, it is only in the fitness of the things that the researcher finally reviews and criticizes the research work, in preparation for communicating the findings.

C. Communicating the Research Findings

14. Evidence-based Nursing

The final step is the utilization process that is to plan for its utilization in practice setting. Nurse Scientists can contribute to the process through evidence-based nursing. They are translating it into health practices.

SUMMARY

In research process, there are sequential steps that one needs to follow for conducting research. Research process comprises of three stages in planning, implementation, and communication of research findings. Planning includes the steps of conceptualization of research design. Implementation is mainly concerned with data collection, data processing, data analysis and interpretation. The final stage is the communication of research evidence.

MULTIPLE CHOICE QUESTIONS

1. A written or oral summary of a research work is termed as __________.
   (a) abstract (b) research report
   (c) summary (d) none of the above
2. The review of manuscript by professional colleagues who are content or methodological experts is called __________.
   (a) blind review (b) galley proof
   (c) meta analysis (d) peer review
3. The type of review where the reviewers are not aware of the authors identity before the manuscript is evaluated __________.
   (a) peer review (b) presenting research report
   (c) blind review (d) reviewing poster
4. The implementation of research findings into practice is called __________.
   (a) generalization (b) application of research
   (c) triangulation (d) specification
5. The research proposal means __________.
   (a) total plan of research process
   (b) implementing research findings
   (c) recording of research results
   (d) follow up of research studies

6. When both qualitative and quantitative research methods are used simultaneously in the same study, the procedure is called:
   (a) triangulation (b) meta analysis
   (c) multi method (d) methodological plurality

ANSWER KEY

1. (b) 2. (d) 3. (c) 4. (b) 5. (a) 6. (a)

REVIEW QUESTIONS

1. (a) Define research process.
   (b) Explain the elements of research process.
2. Write short notes on:
   (a) Hypothesis
   (b) Pilot study
   (c) Data collection
3. Distinguish between
   (a) Population and sample
   (b) Limitation and delimitation
   (c) Research design and research approach

REFERENCES

Brown, B.E., & Garrison, C.J. (1990). Patterns of symptomatology of adult women incest survivors.

Brown, S.J. (1999). Knowledge for health care practice: A guide to using research evidence. Philadelphia: Saunders.

Browne, A., & Finkelhor, D. (1986). Initial and long-term effects: A review of the research. In D. Finkelhor (Ed.).

Burns, N. (1989). The research process and the nursing process: Distinctly different. Nursing Science Quarterly, 2(4), 157–158. Beverly Hills, CA: Sage.

Burns, N., & Grove, S.K. (2005). The practice of nursing research: Conduct, critique, and utilization (5th ed.).

Follette, N.M., Alexander, P.C., & Follette, W.C. (1991). Individual predictors of outcome in group treatment for incest victims. *Journal of Consulting and Clinical Psychology*, 59, 150–155.

Hulme, P.A., & Grove, S.K. (1994). Symptoms of Female Research in Nursing & Health, 160, 171–178.

I'isbcr, Sir R.A. (1935). The designs of experiments. New York: Hafher.

Ilusiings-Tolsma, M.T., Yucha, C.B., Tompkins, J., Kobson, L., & Szeverenyi, N. (1993). Effect of warm and cold applications on the resolution of IV infiltrations.

Lewis, G.B., & Hecker, J.F. (1991). Radiological examination of failure of intravenous infusions. *British Journal of Surgery*, 78(4), 500–501.

MacCara, M.E. (1983). Extravasation: A hazard of intravenous therapy. Drug Intelligence & Clinical Pharmacy, 17(10), 713–717.

McCarthy, D.O., Lo, C., Nguyen, H., & Ney, D.M. (1997). The effect of protein density of food on food intake and nutritional status of tumor-bearing rats. *Research in Nursing and Health*, 20(2), 131–138.

Melnyk, B.M., & Fineout-Overholt, E. (2005). Evidence-based practice in nursing and healthcare: A guide to best practice. Philadelphia: Lippincott.

Millam, D.A. (1988). Managing complications of IV therapy. *Nursing Research*, 18(3), 34–43.

Miller, D.C. (1991). Handbook of research design in social measurement (5th ed.). Newbury Park, CA: Sage.

Miller, M.A., & Babcock, D.E. (1996). Critical thinking applied to nursing. St. Louis: Mosby.

Moody, L.E., Wilson, M.E., Smyth, K., Schwartz, R.,Tittle, M., & Van Cott, M.L. (1988). Analysis of a decade of nursing practice research: 1977–1986. *Nursing Research*, 37, 374–379.

Myers, S.T. (1982). The search for assumptions. *Western Journal of Nursing Research*, 4(1), 91–98.

Olney, C.M. (2005). The effect of therapeutic back massage in hypertensive persons: A preliminary study. Biological Research for Nursing, 7(2), 98–105.

Prescott, P.A., & Soeken, K.L. (1989). The potential uses of pilot work. *Nursing Research*, 38(1), 60–62.

Rand McNally, & Irosby, L.J. (1990). The abstract: An important first impression. *Journal of Neuroscience Nursing*, 22(3), 192–194.

Raves, E., Hitt, A., Pariza, M.W., Cook, M.E., & McCarthy, D.O. (2005). Conjugated linoleic acid preserves gastrocnemius muscle mass in mice bearing the colon-26 adenocarcinoma. *Research in Nursing & Health*, 28(1), 48–55.

Swanson, E.A., McCloskey, J.C., & Bodensteiner, A. (1991). Publishing opportunities for nurses: A comparison of 92 U.S. journals. Image—*The Journal of Nursing Scholarship*, 23(1), 33–38.

Tornquist, E.M., Funk, S.G., Champagne, M.T., & Wiese, R.A. (1993). Advice on reading research: Overcoming the barriers. *Applied Nursing Research*, 6(4), 177–183.

Van Ort, S. (1981). Research design: Pilot study. In S.D. Krampitz & N. Pavlovich (Eds.). Readings for nursing research (49–53). St. Louis: Mosby.

Whitney, F.W., & Roncoli, M. (1986). Turning clinical problems into research. Heart and Lung: *The Journal of Acute and Critical Care*, 15(1), 57–59.

Whittemore, R. (2005). Combining evidence in nursing research: Methods and implications. *Nursing Research*, 54(1), 56–62. M.A. Williams (1980). Editorial: Assumptions in research.

Wysocki, A.B. (1983). Basic versus applied research: Intrinsic and extrinsic considerations. *Western Journal of Nursing Research*, 5(3), 217–224.

CHAPTER

4

RESEARCH PROBLEM

Key terms

★ Research problem ★ Research purpose ★ Research question
★ Variables ★ Dependent and independent variables

⊙ Outline

- ★ Introduction
- ★ Definition
- ★ Selection of a research problem
- ★ Sources of research problems
- ★ Criteria for the selection of a research problem
- ★ Defining the research problem
- ★ Statement of the research problem
- ★ Summary

⊙ Objectives

On completion of this chapter, you will be able to:

- ★ define a research problem
- ★ identify the sources of nursing research problems
- ★ enumerate the criteria for the selection of a research problem
- ★ understand the format for writing a problem statement

Introduction

One of the important tasks of research is to identify and clearly define the problem you wish to study. If you are unsure what your study was about, others who read your proposal cannot possibly understand anything.

A well-defined problem naturally leads to the statement of research objectives, then to the hypotheses, and then to the methodology for measuring the variables.

What is a Research Problem?

A research is set in motion when a problem is perceived to exist. While problems are the underlying force behind research, not all problems require research. A potential research situation arises when the following conditions exist:

1. A perceived discrepancy between what is and what should be.
2. A question about why the discrepancy exists.
3. At least two possible and plausible answers to the question.

A research problem involves a situation of challenging conditions that can be investigated through systematic studies.

Often a research problem causes the researcher to feel apprehensive, confused and ill at ease. There may be situations the research problem remains unsolved. A research problem is expressed in the context of WHO, WHERE, WHEN and WHY the problem situation arose.

Above all, a research problem addresses a gap in the knowledge base needed for nursing practice.

Definition

A research problem refers to a situation involving difficult conditions that can be investigated through systematic studies.

The identification of a research problem is not an easy exercise. Moreover, it is not possible for one to proceed in an intelligent fashion on a research project unless a clear idea of the problem has been developed.

Often the researchers are in a hurry to identify a problem. It must be remembered that one has to devote many hours in the investigation of the problem that is selected for study. Therefore, research problems have to be carefully identified.

Selection of a Research Problem

The selection of a research problem is the first step to a systematic research. It involves four aspects.

1. Sources of research problems
2. Criteria for the selection of a research problem
3. Defining the research problem
4. Statement of the research problem

Check Points... *Ten things to bear in mind while choosing a research topic*
(1) How much choice you have
(2) Your motivation
(3) Regulation and expectation
(4) Your subject of field of study
(5) Previous examples of research projects
(6) Size of your topic
(7) Time available
(8) Cost of the research
(9) Need for support
(10) Access issues

Sources of Research Problems

Research problems can be derived from different sources. The most common sources are discussed here.

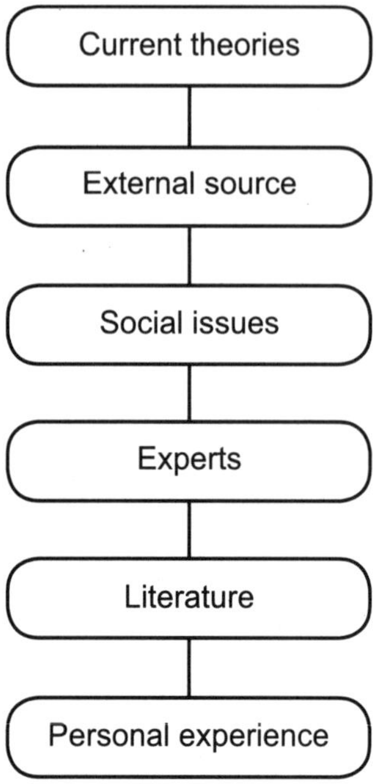

Figure 4.1 Sources of research problems

Personal experience

Direct personal experience is the best source of research problems. We see the problems faced by patients and solutions for those can be identified with research studies. As compared to sources available in literature, direct personal experience accounts a lot for this aspect. From our personal experience and observations, we could identify a topic for study. An example of research problem from personal experience can be:

"Nursing interventions for early healing of diabetic foot ulcer"

For beginners in research, it is advisable to choose a problem that needs a immediate solution or that is interesting and expected to generate more enthusiasm rather than going for abstract and distant problems inferred from theories.

Experiences of senior nurses are also significant. In ward conferences, nurses are encouraged to project important issues/problems that demand scientific investigation.

Literature

Nursing books, journals and other publications are excellent sources of research problems. Research reports and dissertations also contain invaluable suggestions for studies.

Research publications are expected to stimulate reader's imagination and creative work. It provides an idea about setting objectives, hypothesis, research design and strategies for analysis.

Often beginning researchers pay less respect to previous literature fearing blindness. It is sincerely advisable to refer previous research reports available in libraries.

Experts of nursing, medical and subject disciplines

Opinions from experts like doctors, statisticians, administrators, research guides, advisors/mentors, senior researchers and expert teachers are often invaluable for choosing a research problem. A brainstorming session can help generate scores of ideas. You can get your own ideas clarified, sharpened and fully developed into a research question. Experts provide a concrete guidance for starting a meaningful investigation.

Social issues

The existing social and political issues can influence the selection of a research problem. For example, while choosing a research problem dealing with changes in family pattern, domestic violence, stress-related problems, problems of adolescents, child labor, accident prevention, etc., one must consider the status of social and political systems prevalent in the community as a whole. Often an idea for the study may come from the demands of the society; moreover; the study results will contribute to the welfare and development of the public.

External sources

Often a research problem may be generated as a direct suggestion. For example, research guides give students a list of topics to choose a specific one for study. In most cases, such research ideas represent the focus areas of the respective nursing training institutions.

Research scholars can discuss possible research topics with peers, guides and senior research fellows. Research conferences are a very good platform for exchange of ideas.

Current theories

In order to be useful in nursing practice, current theories must be tested through research for their applicability in hospital units, clinics, classrooms and other nursing environments. Nursing research often involves investigating current theories.

A study involving any existing theory may ask such questions as: If the theory is relevant, what kind of behaviour I would expect to find under certain conditions and situations? What kind of evidence would support this theory? An existing theory may be often useful for developing a research problem; usually a part of the theory is tested in a clinical situation.

Criteria for the Selection of a Research Problem

A research problem has to be selected based on the following criteria:

1. Significance and relevance
2. Feasibility
3. Originality
4. Availability of participants
5. Social relevance
6. Applicability of results
7. Ethical considerations

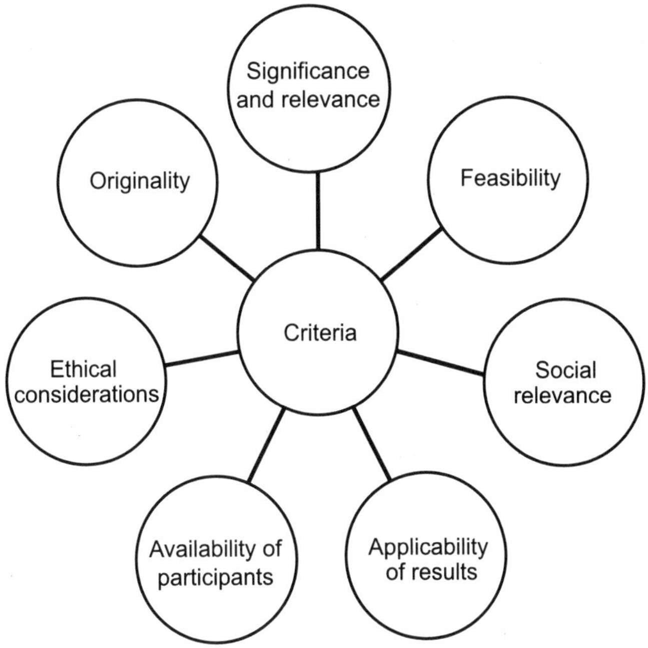

Figure 4.2 Criteria for the selection of a research problem

Significance and relevance

The research problem should be clinically significant; it is meaningless to work on an irrelevant problem. The problem should have the potential to contribute to and extend the scientific body of nursing knowledge.

Feasibility

Availability of subjects, time, facilities, equipment and money, experience of the researcher and ethical considerations are factors a researcher needs to assess in order to decide whether the research problem considered is feasible.

Originality

The problem taken for research should be original because the aim of the research is to bridge the gap in the knowledge base and not add to redundancy. Thus, the researcher must screen the testimonials of previous research available in library in order to avoid replication. In some universities and college libraries, such information can be readily available.

Availability of participants

In a study involving human subjects, the researcher should carefully choose subjects of the desired characteristics. For the research to be fruitful, the identification of subjects is a very important step.

Social relevance

The society expects the outcomes of the research to contribute to its welfare and offer solutions for some practical problems.

Applicability of results

An ideal research problem should produce findings having greater applicability. There should be opportunities available for the implementation of research results.

Ethical considerations

If the investigations would pose unethical demands on the research participants, the research problem may not be feasible. The investigator should, therefore, have a thorough knowledge about the rights of humans or animal subjects.

Defining the Research Problem

Defining the research problem is very important. It involves setting the boundaries within which a researcher shall study the problem with predetermined objectives.

When defining a research problem, the researcher must focus on more specific aspects of the problem.

According to Whitney, defining a problem means to put a fence around it to separate it from other questions related to the situation. A well-defined research problem will enable the researcher to go on the right tracks. It involves three steps:

1. Selecting the research topic
2. Narrowing the topic
3. Evaluating the topic

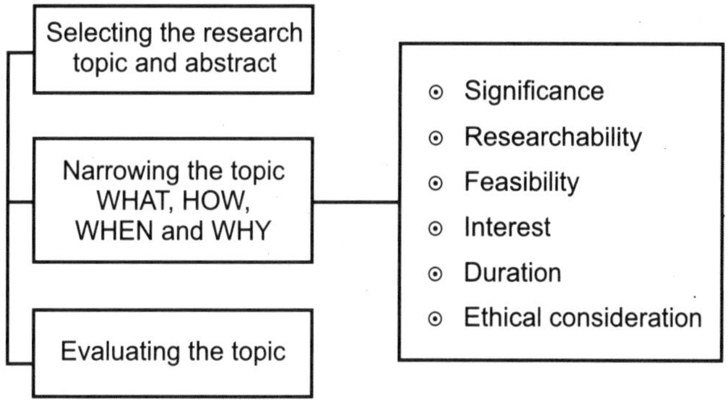

Figure 4.3 Steps for defining the research problem

Statement of the Research Problem

The statement of a research problem is an expression of conditions that need understanding and directions by scientific investigation. The statement of a research problem is necessary to be correct for deriving useful hypothesis. In addition, the statement recognizes the nature of the problem being addressed in the study and typically its context and significance. Thus, a problem statement should be broad to cover the key concerns as well as narrow enough in scope to serve as a guide for study design. The problem statement must address the area of focus, variables (independent and dependent variables), population or participants, setting of the study, and methodology (if implicit or explicit). For example, an experimental study may state the effect of a condition, whereas a descriptive study may be explorative, investigative, correlational, comparative, and so on.

The criteria for the problem statement are:

1. It has to be written in interrogative form.
2. It identifies the population of the study.
3. It includes the variables.
4. It is empirically verifiable.

In expressing the problem statement, the interrogative form is the better way to identify the problem areas of the study. An example of problem statement in interrogative form is:

What are the predisposing factors of metabolic syndrome among inpatients of medical wards of Medical College Hospital, Trivandrum?

Now, compare with the declarative form below:

Assessment of predisposing factors of metabolic syndrome among inpatients of Medical College Hospital, Trivandrum.

The target population group should be clearly identified in the problem statement. For example, "patients with myocardial infarction" has more clarity than simply "patients".

The problem statement can contain variables to be studied. Studies can be classified into the following types based on the variables used:

1. One-variable study
2. Two-variable study
3. Multi-variable study

One-variable study

If the study is exploratory in nature and contains only one variable, it may be called a univariate study. An example of the problem statement of a univariate study might be:

"What are the causes of wound infection?"

The only variable in this question is "causes of wound infection." This type of studies is often the beginning step in a research project.

Two-variable study

When two variables are examined in a study, it can be called a bivariate study.

Multi-variable study

The studies in which more than two variables are examined.

Multivariate Study

Multivariate studies are research studies using more than two variables together. Qualitative studies are usually multivariate studies, which are becoming increasingly common in nursing research studies. For example, 'A study on factors contributing to noncompliance among patients with Chronic kidney disease in selected hospitals of Thirunelveli District, Tamil Nadu'. Here the researcher considers more than two variables which are responsible for noncompliance among chronic kidney disease (CKD) patients.

In most studies there are one or more outcome variables and several explanatory variables together with a variety of variables, which add a characteristic particularly to the situation. Thus for example, in a study of supplementary feeding, growth is the outcome variable and the method of feeding is the explanatory variable. All additional information like mother's age, education, income, type of family and so on, provides the particularity of each mother – infant pair.

In real life, however, several factors act simultaneously. Some may influence the outcome whereas others may be just confounders. In order to obtain a correct assessment of what is happening one has to resort to methods, which would take into account several variables acting together. These are the methods of multivariate analysis. With multivariate analysis the researcher is able to study the effects of several variables acting simultaneously instead of singly.

In most studies the researcher is attempting to describe the relationship between an outcome variable and its several determinants. The purpose may be to measure the sensitivity of a response to its determinants, or to predict the response under varying conditions.

Multivariate methods are based on multiple linear regression, which is a multiple variable approach using the principles of simple linear regression. Multivariate methods have the advantage of bringing more information to bear on a specific outcome. They allow one to take into account the continuing relationship among several variables. This is especially valuable in observational studies where total control is never possible. In case of experimental studies the researcher can exercise some control over intervention and yet total control as in the case of laboratory experiments are never possible.

Advantages

1. They resemble closely to the concepts of the researcher to the data.
2. Easier visualization and interpretation of data is materialized.
3. More data can be analysed simultaneously, adds to providing greater statistical power.
4. The focus is on relationships among variables rather than on isolated individual factors.

Format of the Problem Statement

There are different ways to present the problem statement. A problem statement that examines more than one variable is usually written using correlational or comparative statements.

Objectives

The objective is an important aspect of scientific investigation. It is a statement of what the researcher intends to accomplish through the research. There can be primary and secondary objectives.

Definition

The objective is a statement of what the researcher intends to accomplish. It contains observable and measurable attributes to assess whether the objectives have been achieved.

From practical point of view, it is very important to ensure that the objectives are formulated carefully. It is the stemming force that guides the work.

Objectives should be

1. Properly stated
2. Clearly worded
3. Required objectives

A study can have both primary and secondary objectives depending on their significance. Each objective should be related to the research design and methods.

Usually the study objectives are presented in the first chapter of the dissertation. Another point is that the researcher should check to ensure that research activities are progressing in accordance with the preset objectives. In addition, the researcher should confirm that the research findings represent solutions to the research problem at hand.

SUMMARY

Choosing the right research problem is the determining step to a systematic research. The major sources of research problems include personal experiences, literature, theories and previous research works.

Several criteria should be considered in choosing a problem to study. Ethical issues, significance of the problem, personal motivation, researcher's experience, and feasibility of the study are some criteria.

There are different ways to draw the problem statement – interrogative or declarative form.

The problem statement for quantitative studies often encompasses problem identification, background and scope of the problem, consequences of the problem, and how the proposed study would contribute to the solution of the problem.

MULTIPLE CHOICE QUESTIONS

1. The process that the researcher uses to arrive at the research problem is __________.
   (a) identifying the problem
   (b) formulating the problem
   (c) verifying the problem
   (d) defining the problem
2. Defining the problem means __________.
   (a) identify and state the problem
   (b) define the problems and helps to formulate research objectives
   (c) questions are formed for verifiable, practical and feasible
   (d) specify the problem in detail with precision and directs all research procedures

3. Which of the following are the sources of nursing research problems?
    (a) personal experience
    (b) literature sources
    (c) existing theories
    (d) previous research
    (e) all of the above
4. Feasibility means __________.
    (a) researcher must consider the financial resources available.
    (b) researcher should consider equipment and supplies available.
    (c) availability of subjects, peer support and administrative support should be considered by the researcher.
    (d) researcher needs to be ensure that study can actually be carried out considering time, cost, available instruments and supports.
5. A study of an exploratory nature and contains only one variable is called __________.
    (a) declarative form
    (b) multivariable study
    (c) univariate study
    (d) two-variable study

ANSWER KEY

1. (b) 2. (a) 3. (a) 4. (c) 5. (d)

REVIEW QUESTIONS

1. (a) Define research problem.
   (b) List some sources of research problems.
2. Explain the criteria for the selection of a research problem.
3. Describe the statement of a research problem.
4. What is research objective? Explain the significance of objectives of a research study?

REFERENCES

Anderson, M.A., Clarke, M.M., Halms, L.B., & Foreman, M.D. (2005). Hospital readmission from home health care before and after prospective payment. *Journal of Nursing Scholarship*, 37, 73–79.

Chinn, P.L. (2008). Integrated theory and knowledge development in nursing (7th ed.). St. Louis, MO: Mosby Elsevier.

De Chesnay, M., & Anderson, B.A. (2008). Caring for the vulnerable: Perspectives in nursing theory, practice and research. Sudbury, MA: Jones and Bartlett.

Diers, D. (1971). Finding clinical problems for study. *Journal of Nursing Administration*, 15–18.

Fahs, P.S., Morgan, L.L., & Kalman, M. (2003). A call for replication. *Journal of Nursing Scholarship*, 35, 67–71.

Flaskerus, J.H. (1984). Nursing models as conceptual frameworks for research. *Western Journal of Nursing Research*, 6, 153–155.

Harley, B. (1978). Why a theoretical framework in nursing research? *Western Journal of Nursing Research*, 1(1), 28–41.

Kerlinger, F. (1986). Foundations of behavioural (3rd ed.). New York: Holt, Rinehart & Winston.

Martin, P.A. (1994). The utility of the research problem statement. *Applied Nursing Research*, 7(1), 47–49.

McDonald, D., Monaco, A., Guo, R., Fiano, J., Matney, L., & Turner, G., et al. (2009). The effect of personal relevance on learning stroke symptoms/response. *Western Journal of Nursing Research*, 331(2), 144–152.

McFwan, M., & Mills, E.M. (2007). Theoretical basis for nursing (2nd ed.). Philadelphia: Lippincott, William, S.R. Wilkins.

Meleis, A.I. (1997). Theoretical nursing: Development and progress (3rd ed.). Philadelphia: J.B. Lippincott.

Moody, L.F. (1990). Advancing nursing science through research (vols. 1–2). Newbury Park, CA: Sage.

Musil, C., Warner, C., Zouszniewski, J., Wykle, M.R., & Sanding, T. (2009). Grandmother caregiving, family stress and strain and depressive symptoms. *Western Journal of Nursing Research*, 31(3), 389–408.

Pett, R., Barden, J., & Wheeler, S. (2002). The elaboration likelihood model of persuasion health promotions that yield sustained behavioural change. In R. DiClemente, R. Crosby & M. Kegler (Eds.). Emerging theories in health promotion practice and research. Strategies for improving public health. San Francisco: Jossey-Bass.

Polit, D.F., & Beck, C.T. (2004). Nursing research: Principles and methods (7th ed.). Philadelphia: Lippincott.

Smith, M.C., & Stullenbarger, E. (1991). A prototype for integrative review and meta-analysis of nursing research. *Journal of Advanced Nursing*, 16(11), 1272–1283.

CHAPTER

5

HYPOTHESIS

Key terms

★ Variables ★ Dependent variables ★ Independent variables and complex hypothesis ★ Null and research hypothesis ★ Non-directional and directional hypothesis ★ Hypothesis criteria

⊙ Outline

- Definition
- Significance of hypothesis
- Purposes
- Characteristics
- Sources
- Classification
- Criteria for statement of hypotheses
- Assumption

⊙ Objectives

On completion of this chapter, you will be able to:

- define hypothesis
- recognize the purpose of hypothesis in scientific studies
- identify the sources of rationale for study hypothesis
- list the classification of hypothesis
- mention the criteria to be considered when formulating hypothesis
- recognize the use of assumptions in research

Introduction

Hypothesis is an important and integral component of modern scientific research. It is regarded as an important mental tool and considered as the principal instrument in research. Its main function is to suggest new experiments and observations. Many studies are carried out with deliberate intention of testing hypotheses. In fact the investigator can use the hypothesis to help interpret the significance of an obscure event. Hypotheses can be used as a tool to uncover a new fact.

What is Hypothesis?

Hypothesis is a supposition that appears to explain a group of phenomena and is assumed as a basis of reasoning and experimentation. It is a formal question that intends to be resolved. The expected outcome of a research study will be stated. It depicts the specific relationship to be tested. It translates the research problem and purposes in to clear explanation or prediction of expected results or outcomes of the study.

Definition

Hypothesis may be defined as a statement of prediction of relationship between two or more variables, relates independent variable and dependent variable.

Polit and Beck (2010) define hypothesis as a statement of researcher's expectations about relationships between the variables under investigation.

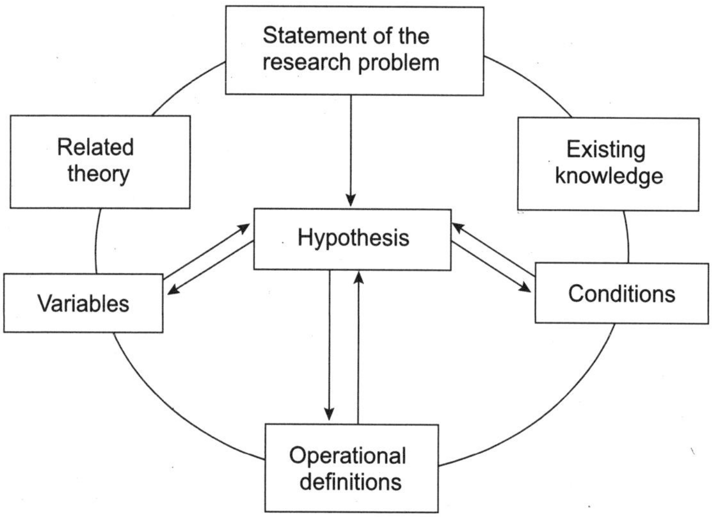

Figure 5.1 Linking hypothesis with other research components

In the literature of research and inference, there are specific meanings for hypotheses. Linking the concept of variables, constraints and operational definitions as shown in Fig. 5.1, we can now state our hypotheses so that it is more specific and gives direction to the research project. Hypothesis is a tentative prediction about the nature of the relationship between two or more variables.

Usually a hypothesis is formulated in experimental research and in some non-experimental correlational studies. There are four elements in a hypothesis.

1. Dependent and independent variables
2. Type of relationship between these variables
3. Direction of change
4. Subjects in the population being studied

Independent and dependent variables

When an experiment is being conducted, some variables are manipulated by the researcher and others are measured from subjects. The former variables are called independent variables and the latter are called dependent variables.

In nursing research, an independent variable may be a particular teaching method like demonstration or computer-assisted instruction, a reward for period of exposure to a new curriculum; whereas a dependent variable may be the test score, the number of scores, or measured speed in performing a task.

Need and Significance of Hypotheses

Hypotheses serve many pertinent functions. A hypothesis gives a definite aspect of the investigation; it guides the direction of the study. It specifies the sources of data; moreover it will help define facts which are relevant. The use of hypothesis thus prevents a blind search and indiscriminate gathering of data. The most appropriate type of research can be adopted using hypothesis. It determines the most appropriate technique of analysis. A hypothesis contributes to the development of theory.

What is a Good Hypothesis?

A good hypothesis should fulfill three conditions. The most elementary requirement is that it should be adequate for its purpose. A descriptive hypothesis clearly states the condition, size or distribution of some variables in terms of values meaningful to the research task. If it is an explanatory hypothesis, it must explain facts that give rise to the need for explanation. Along with hypotheses plus other known and accepted generalizations, one should be able to deduce the original problem condition.

Secondly, the variable, condition or relationship must be testable. A clear implication for testing should be indicated in the stated objectives.

For explanatory hypothesis, there is a third condition. Better hypothesis has a greater range; it explains more facts than do its rivals. When the researcher's aim is to explain, the research hypotheses make predictions about the population and the relationship among variables. Finally the research aim is to predict the hypothesis on the population and cause-and-effect relationship between independent and dependent variables.

Purposes

Hypotheses serve numerous purposes. They are as follows:

1. It provides objectivity to scientific research.
2. Theoretical prepositions can be tested in real world.
3. It guides the researcher to select research design and dictate the type of statistical analysis to be used with data.
4. It serves as a framework for drawing conclusions.

Characteristics of Hypothesis

Hypothesis must possess the following characteristics:

1. Hypothesis should be clear and precise.
2. Hypothesis should be capable of being tested.
3. The relationship between variables should be stated by hypothesis.
4. It should be limited in scope and must be specific. Narrower hypotheses are generally more testable.
5. Simplicity: Hypothesis should be stated in simple terms so that the same is easily understood by all.
6. Hypothesis should be logically consistent.
7. It should be amenable to testing within a realistic time.
8. Hypothesis must explain facts that give rise to the need for explanation.

Sources of Hypotheses

Hypotheses can be derived from various sources like:

1. *Theory*: It gives clues to research by stating what is known. Logical deduction from theory leads to new hypotheses.
2. *Observation*: Direct observation is useful for deriving hypothesis.
3. *Intuition and personal experience*: These may contribute to the formulation of hypothesis. These may in turn direct a person to certain hypotheses more quickly. Nurses can derive many hypotheses from their clinical experience. All knowledge begins with experience, and experience is a source of hypotheses.
4. *Result of previous studies*: The findings of former studies are useful in order to replicate or test the present results.
5. *Continuity of research*: Continuity of research in the same field itself is an important source of hypotheses.

Classification

Hypothesis may be classified as shown in Fig. 5.2.

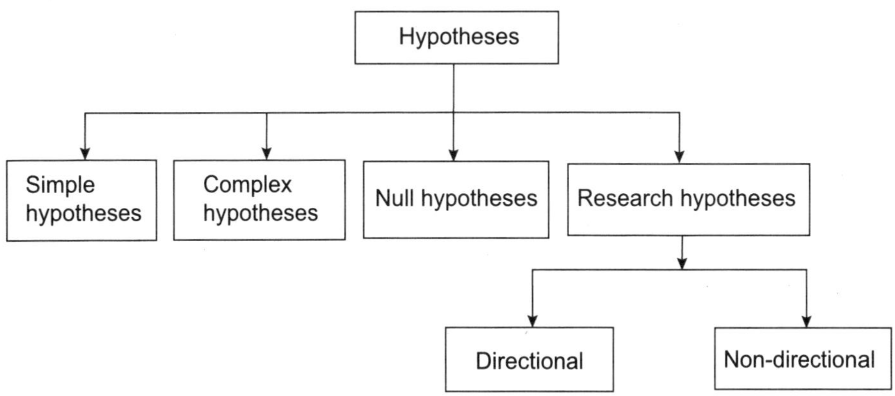

Figure 5.2 Classification of hypotheses

Simple hypothesis

A simple hypothesis concerns the relationship between one independent and one dependent variable. A simple hypothesis is also called bivariate hypothesis.

Complex hypothesis

A complex hypothesis concerns a relationship where two or more independent variables or both are being examined in the same study. A complex hypothesis is also called multivariate hypothesis.

It is possible to divide a complex hypothesis into two or more simple hypotheses. Practically, a hypothesis is either supported totally or it is not supported.

Sometimes complex hypotheses are necessary. Whenever the researcher wants to examine an interaction effect, a complex hypothesis is called for. An interaction effect concerns the action of two variables in conjunction with each other.

Null hypothesis or statistical hypothesis

Null hypothesis (H_0) or statistical hypothesis is used for statistical testing and for interpreting statistical outcomes. Sometimes null hypothesis is not stated as it is the opposite of research hypothesis.

The null hypothesis is also used when the researcher believes there is no relationship between the two variables and when theoretical or empirical information is inadequate to state a research hypothesis. It is non-directional by nature.

Research hypothesis (alternate hypothesis)

Research hypothesis or alternative hypothesis (H_1) states the expected relationship between variables. The research hypothesis is also known as scientific, substantive and theoretical hypothesis. This will be helpful for understanding what the researcher expects to find after analyzing the data. It is directional by nature; it can be descriptive, relational or causal.

Criteria for statement of hypotheses

1. **It should be written in a declarative sentence:** The statement of the problem shows a question about some phenomenon, and the hypothesis depicts an answer or tentative solution to the problem.

   Some modifications in the problem statement can change it into a non-directional research hypothesis.

A problem statement: "Is There a Change in Level of Labour Pain after Listening to Music Therapy?"

The hypothesis: "There is a Change in the Level of Labour Pain after Listening to Music Therapy.

Writing a hypothesis requires more deliberation and consideration of the framework of the hypothesis. An empirical generalization needs to be isolated and then developed into a testable hypothesis that predicts the relationship the researcher expects to find out.

2. **Be written in the present tense:** Hypotheses are tested in the present and should be written in the present tense.

   E.g.: "There is a Positive Relationship between Pelvic Floor Exercise Programme and Stress Incontinence among Antenatal Women"

3. **Contains population:** The population needs to be specifically identified in the hypothesis.

   E.g.: "A Study to Identify Psychosocial Problems of Female Patients in the Age Group of 29–70 Years Who Are Undergoing Mastectomy"

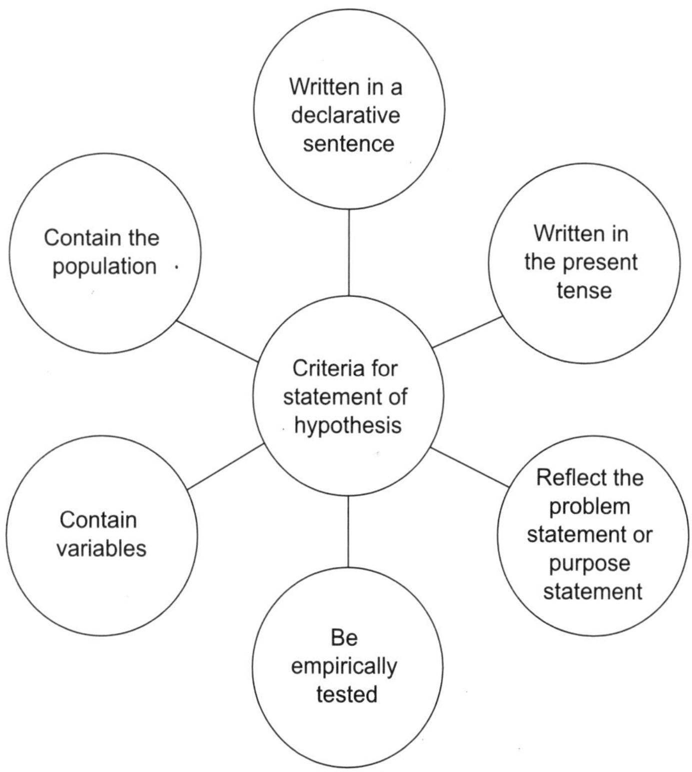

Figure 5.3 Criteria for statement of hypotheses

4. **Contains variables:** A scientific hypothesis, however, contains at least two variables. The hypothesis links two or more variables together. The variables in hypothesis are the same as those in the corresponding problem statement.
5. **Reflect the problem statement or purpose statement:** To reemphasize the point, the hypothesis should contain essentially the same material as the problem statement.
6. **Empirically testable:** A hypothesis that cannot be empirically tested has no scientific relevance. The ability to obtain empirical data should have been determined as you select a research problem.

3A. Directional hypothesis

In directional research hypothesis, the researcher further predicts the type of relationship. It specifies the expected direction of the relationship between independent and dependent variable. This type of research hypothesis has several advantages:

1. It makes clear the researcher's expectation.
2. It allows more precise testing of theoretical proposition and allows the use of one-tailed statistical tests. When one-tailed tests are used, statistical significance is more easily achieved.

3B. Non-directional Hypothesis

In this hypothesis, the researcher merely depicts that a relationship exists. The direction of relationship is not presented. Figure 5.4 illustrates a positive relationship between preoperative teaching and knowledge level of patients regarding post-operative exercise.

E.g.: "A Negative Relationship between Hours of Exercise and Level of Hypercholesterolemia"

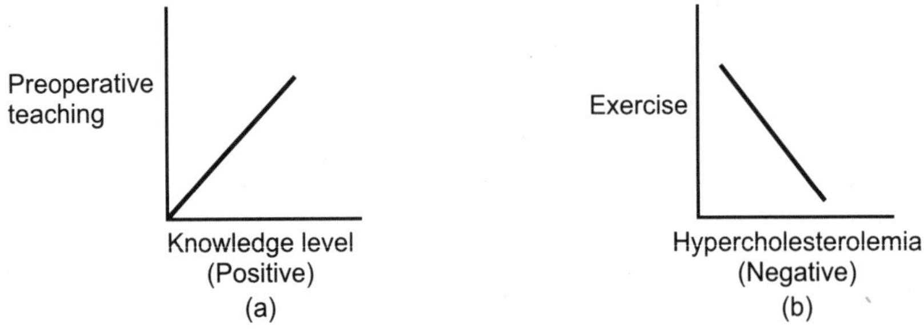

Figure 5.4 Graph showing positive and negative relationships among variables

Guidelines for Evaluating Hypothesis

1. Does the research study contain a hypothesis?
2. Are the hypotheses directly or logically tied to the research problem?
3. Do the hypotheses flow logically from theoretical rationale or review of literature?
4. Does each hypothesis contain at least two variables?
5. Do the hypotheses state a predicted relationship between variables? (between dependent variable and independent variable)
6. Do the hypotheses indicate the nature of population being studied?
7. Is each hypothesis clearly worded and concise?
8. Is it apparent that each hypothesis can be empirically tested?
9. Does each hypothesis contain only one prediction?
10. Is the hypothesis stated as research hypothesis rather than null hypothesis?

Assumptions

Research is built upon assumptions since not everything needed to move forward is known. "One must assume something to learn something." The more the assumptions or the stronger the assumptions that one makes, the more one ensures that his analysis yield clear-cut and interpretable results; at the same time, the researcher more than the empirical observations or records is determining these results.

Definition

An assumption is a realistic expectation of something. It is something that we believe to be true.

An assumption is an act of faith. It will not be tested in your research.

Sharma (2011) defines, assumptions are statements that are taken for granted or are considered true, even though they have not been scientifically tested.

An assumption listed in research paper is often a good source of research topic. An assumption is belief or idea that we hold to be true – often with little or no evidence required. We make assumption everyday in our lives; for example, as I drive on the highway, I assume that other drivers obey traffic signals.

Uses of assumptions in research

1. Assumptions are foundation for research studies.
2. Assumptions are a good source of research topic.
3. They provide the researcher with basic ideas regarding research.
4. They are helpful to develop theories and research instruments for the research project, which will enhance the implementation of research process.

Types of assumptions

Assumptions can be classified into five broad types.

Universal assumptions: Assumptions can be some beliefs of the society, but testing such assumptions is difficult.

E.g.: "Epilepsy is Caused by Evil Spirit and Caused by Divine Power"

Theory-based assumptions: Sometimes the research project can be based on nursing theories. For example, a study based on Pender's Health Promotion model will use theory-based assumptions.

Assumptions needed to conduct a research: Some assumptions may be developed to conduct a particular study.

E.g.: "Childhood Obesity is more Prevalent among Students of Private Schools as Compared to Government Schools"

Warranted assumptions: Research findings or observations are stated along with assumptions.

E.g.: "Regular Physical Activity Reduce Body Mass Index"

Unwarranted assumptions: These are presented without any support of research findings.

E.g.: "Mental Diseases are Cured by Religious Rituals"

Practical examples of assumptions from clinical experience

1. "Counselling Reduce Anxiety of Patients Undergoing Surgery"
2. "Post-operative Exercises Reduce Complications after Surgery"
3. "Cognitive Interventions will Increase the Knowledge Level of Clients"
4. "Balanced Diet will Increase the Resistance for Children"

SUMMARY

Hypothesis is a statement of declaration of the expected outcome of a research study. Often it is called "educated guess" that a researcher proposes for testing. It allows theoretical propositions to be tested in the real world, guides the research design, directs the type of statistical analysis for data, and depicts an understanding of the researcher's expectations about the study before data collection begins. Hypothesis may be categorized as simple or complex. Hypothesis may also be classified as null hypothesis or research hypothesis.

Null hypothesis states that no difference exists between groups or that there is no correlation between variables. But research hypothesis states that a correlation does exist. Research hypothesis can be divided into non-directional and directional hypothesis. Non-directional research hypothesis indicates that a difference exists but does not predict the type.

Research findings of the investigation will either support or fail to support the hypothesis. If hypothesis is accepted, the research hypothesis is supported. Thus, if a theoretical proposition is being tested and support is found for research hypothesis, the theory is also supported. In a descriptive study, hypothesis is not necessary, yet research questions are posed.

MULTIPLE CHOICE QUESTIONS

1. The result of two variables acting in conjunction with each other is __________.
   (a) manipulation (b) interaction effect
   (c) mortality threat (d) history threat
2. Null hypothesis (H_0) is also known as
   (a) statistical Hypothesis (b) research Hypothesis
   (c) alternate Hypothesis (d) directional Hypothesis
3. __________ states the expected relationship between variables
   (a) research hypothesis (b) null hypothesis
   (c) statistical hypothesis (d) directional hypothesis
4. Research hypothesis (H_1) is also called
   (a) null hypothesis (b) statistical Hypothesis
   (c) alternate Hypothesis (d) directional Hypothesis
5. Statement of hypothesis should
   (a) be in past tense (b) contain variables
   (c) be empirically testable (d) b and c

ANSWER KEY

1. (b) 2. (a) 3. (a) 4. (c) 5. (d)

REVIEW QUESTIONS

1. (a) Define hypothesis.
   (b) Explain the significance of hypothesis in nursing research.
2. Differentiate between:
   (a) Hypothesis and assumptions
   (b) Independent and dependent variables
   (c) Simple and complex hypotheses
   (d) Null hypothesis and research hypothesis
   (e) Non-directional and directional hypothesis

3. Explain the elements of a well-stated hypothesis.
4. Write short notes on:
   (a) Null hypothesis
   (b) Assumptions
   (c) Variables
   (d) Sources of hypotheses

REFERENCES

Beveridge, W.B. (1950). The art of scientific investigation. New York: Vintage Books.

Brown, J.S., Tanner, C.A., & Padrick, K.P. (1984). Nursing's search for scientific knowledge. *Nursing Research*, 33(1), 26–32.

Cheng, C., Studdiford, J.S., Chambers, C.V., Diamond, J.J., & Paynter, N. (2002). The reliability of patient self-reported blood pressures. *Journal of Clinical Hypertension*, 4(4), 259–264.

Chinn, P.L., & Kramer, M.K. (1999). Theory and nursing: Integrated knowledge development (5th ed.). St. Louis, MO: Mosby.

Corff, K.E., Seideman, R., Venkataraman, P.S., Lutes, L., & Yates, B. (1995). Facilitated tucking: A nonpharmacological comfort measure for pain in preterm neonates. *Journal of Obstetric, Gynecologic, and Neonatal Nursing*, 24(2), 143–147.

Fagerhaugh, S.Y., & Strauss, A. (1977). Politics of pain management. Menlo Park, CA: Addison-Wesley.

Fawcett, J. (1999). The relationship of theory and research (3rd ed.). Philadelphia: F.A. Davis.

Gerlach, R.W., Gambosi, J.R., & Bowen, R.H. (1990). Cancer survivors' needs reported by survivors and their families. *Journal of Cancer Education*, 5(1), 63–70.

Gillum, R.F. (1996). Epidemiology of hypertension in African American women. *American Heart Journal*, 131(2), 385–395.

Jennings-Dozier, K. (1999). Predicting intentions to obtain a Pap smear among African American and Latina women: Testing the theory of planned behavior. *Nursing Research*, 48(4), 198–205.

Jirovec, M.M., & Kasno, J. (1990). Self-care agency as a function of patient-environmental factors among nursing home residents. *Research in Nursing and Health*, 13(5), 303–309.

Kerlinger, F.N., & Lee, H.B. (2000). Foundations of behavioral research (4th ed.). Fort Worth, TX: Harcourt College Publishers.

McDonald, D.D., Frakes, M., Apostolidis, B., Armstrong, B., Goldblatt, S., & Bernardo, D. (2003). Effect of a psychiatric diagnosis on nursing care for nonpsychiatric problems. *Research in Nursing and Health*, 26(3), 225–232.

Metz, A., Sichel, D., & Goff, D. (1988). Postpartum panic disorder. *Journal of Clinical Psychiatry*, 49(1), 278–279.

Moody, L.E. (1990). Advancing nursing science through research (vol. 1). Newbury Park, CA: Sage.

Moody, L.E., Wilson, M.E., Smyth, K., Schwartz, R., Tittle, M., & Van Cott, M.L. (1988). Analysis of a decade of nursing practice research: 1977–1986. *Nursing Research*, 37(6), 374–379.

Munhall, P.L. (2001). Nursing research: A qualitative perspective (3rd ed.). Sudbury, MA: Jones & Bartlett Publishers and National League for Nursing.

CHAPTER

6

SEARCHING THE LITERATURE

Key terms

★ Abstracts ★ e-journals ★ Primary sources ★ Secondary sources ★ Electronic sources ★ Indices ★ Online journals

⊙ Outline

- ★ Introduction
- ★ Definition
- ★ Purposes
- ★ Characteristics
- ★ Sources
- ★ Performing the literature search
- ★ Preparation of the literature review
- ★ Guidelines for writing the literature review
- ★ Summary
- ★ Nursing research on the web
- ★ Review questions

⊙ Objectives

On completion of the chapter, you will be able to:

- ★ define literature search
- ★ explain the purposes of literature search
- ★ explore the different sources of literature
- ★ understand ways for the preparation of a literature review
- ★ understand the benefits of library services.

Introduction

Searching the literature is a standard activity in a research project. Knowledge drawn from earlier studies is an integral part of research in general.

Before initiating any research, a search of literature for previous studies and experiences related to the proposed investigation should be done.

Definition

Literature search is defined as an account of evidences on a research problem. It involves a systematic and comprehensive review of scholarly publications, audiovisual materials and personal communications. It is the process in which the researchers extend their awareness of scholarly works as well as develop faith in their own investigations.

Purposes of Literature Search

A typical purpose of literature search is to build up research questions. Moreover, it is beneficial to examine the facts already available about the topic you chose to study. Searching the literature has other benefits as follows:

1. To collect definitions of concepts related to the topic;
2. To design research methods, tools and techniques for the studies;
3. To locate ideas useful for the present study or for a new project design;
4. To identify gap or discrepancy in the body of knowledge;
5. To analyze the strengths and weaknesses of research methods and tools used in previous studies;
6. To predict problems that may arise during the research process and to develop ways to overcome them.

In particular, the researcher may be able to locate data useful for comparisons in the present study.

Objectives of Literature Search

For literature search to be effective, the following objectives are important:

1. It should meet the actual purpose of review.
2. It should provide sufficient content for the summary or abstract.
3. The information should be synthesized, analyzed and presented in a logical way.
4. The search should be mainly concerned with primary sources.
5. The review should be supported by an adequate number of sources that form the backbone of the study.
6. Paraphrasing and integration have been ensured to avoid mere quoting of texts.
7. The review should be presented in a logical way together with conclusions of the studies used in review.

Sources of Literature Search

The sources of literature may be of two types:

1. Primary source
2. Secondary source

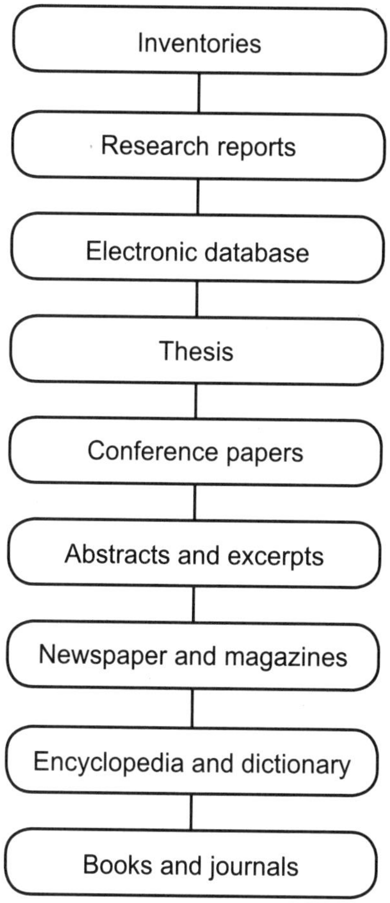

Figure 6.1 Sources of review of literature

Primary source

A primary source is a description available in the original research. Most primary sources are found in published literature. An example of a primary source could be:

An original study on Readers remedy for pressure sores, Cunnel (1986). American Journal of Nursing 86: 923–928.

Secondary source

It is a summary of findings of the research studies conducted by different investigators. Secondary sources often represent a response to or a critical evaluation of a researcher's work. An example of a secondary source could be:

A literature search on gastrointestinal system and bowel management following spinal cord injury, Chen. D. (2000). Physical medicine and rehabilitation clinics of North America, 2:1, 232–233.

Check Points... *Skills essential for the evaluation of literary sources*
(1) Prefer to identify and use primary sources of literature (2) Learn about the critics from senior researchers (3) Prefer to use a secondary source from a revived journal that provides a commentary from the researcher (4) Discuss your assessment of the secondary source with the research guide

Performing the Literature Search

In performing a literature search, the following functions are essential:

1. Using the library
2. Identification of potential sources
3. Selection of relevant sources

Using the library

A library contains a wealth of information. Libraries are a place to look forward to high levels of evidences and reference materials. It is thus important you acquaint yourself with the faculties available in the library you have good access to.

A researcher should spend much of the time in libraries. Librarians can help you to get familiar with cataloging practices, online indices, computers and other reference materials.

In the past, researchers had to travel widely in search of references.

Identification of potential sources

Once a research problem has been identified, the search for literature is the immediate step. However, a strategy has to be developed for selecting the databases to search, identifying the keywords, locating the information and capturing it.

Selecting the keywords is a major task in literature search. Keywords may be phrases or single words. Most databases provide a thesaurus that helps to identify the keywords. Thesaurus can be accessed by logging onto the database. Cropping of words may allow locating more citations related to that keyword. Use of irregular plurals may also be considered. Although the names of authors may be used to perform a search, it may not be necessary to show the names in the list of keywords.

Selection of relevant sources

The ability to search and locate articles on a research topic is an important skill that requires adaptability. With rapid technological changes, many sophisticated methods of searching the literature are being introduced continuously. In the absence of such improved methods, the risk of we presenting outdated information is high. When a search is initiated, each keyword that has been identified is separately searched. Spelling errors can generate unexpected results. Most databases of today quickly indicate the records in which the keyword is present. The most recent records appear first.

Databases usually provide the abstracts of articles in which the keyword is cited. The users should apply intelligence to judge whether the term is useful in relation to the selected topic. References identified may be saved for later use. At this point, one need not attempt to examine all the citations. However, the number of citations found in the search should be noted.

Searching the Electronic Literature

Nowadays most college and university libraries offer students the facility for performing searches in electronic databases. By this way, stacks of bibliographic files can be accessed by using the computer. The development of personal computers together with terminal access systems has made possible for those with little computer exposure to conduct their own literature searches. Access to different databases is made available through several service providers. At present, the most widely used service providers are Aries Knowledge Finder, Ovid, PaperChase, SilverPlatter, and so on. Most bibliographic service providers offer trial access to their databases before subscriptions.

These service providers offer many ways for user-friendly retrieval of bibliographic information. They provide menu-driven, on-screen support systems which work with minimal instructions. Most of the electronic databases of interest to the nursing community are accessible online or via CD-ROMs.

Linking

Linking allows one to connect from one web address to another. For example, a link can be established between a database and an archive of full-text journal articles. In near future, nursing databases will provide links to electronic books. At present, archives of full-text nursing journals are available. However, one drawback here is that most archives are not interlinked.

Index

1. CINAHL (Cumulative Index to Nursing and Allied Health Literature): Accessible at www.cinahl.com, it contains citations of nursing literature published after 1988.
2. MEDLINE (Medical Literature Analysis and Retrieved System Online): It is another electronic source of literature reviews commonly used by nurses.
3. Medline Plus: It is the National Library of Medicines' website for consumer health information.
4. Registry of Nursing Research Sigma: Tau True International Honor Society of Nursing makes this database available through Virginia Henderson International Nursing Library.
5. Cochrane Database of System Reviews: Health care related literature can be searched from this source, available at http://www.cochrane.org.

6. ERIC: The ERIC database is the largest source of educational information, available at http://www.eric.ed.gov.
7. Dissertation Abstracts Online: Abstracts of masters and Ph.D. theses are available here.

Online Journals

Web addresses of some online journals and magazines are as follows:

1. http://www.nursefriendly.com
2. http://www.nsna.org/
3. http://www.healthweb.org
4. http://www.ispub.com/ostia/index.php
5. http://www.nursingworld.org
6. http://www.nursing week.com

Printed Sources

Print versions of literature reviews may be located from nursing research abstracts, dissertation abstracts, etc.

Journals

Journals are a very good source for literature search. Some of the most important nursing research journals are as follows:

1. Clinical Nursing Research
2. Advances in Nursing Science
3. American Journal of Nursing
4. Applied Nursing Research
5. Holistic Nursing Practice
6. International Journal of Nursing Studies
7. Journal of Professional Nursing
8. Journal of Obstetrics, Gynecologic and Neonatal Nursing
9. Nursing Research
10. Research in Nursing and Health
11. Nursing Journal of India

12. Indian Journal of Nursing and Midwifery
13. Nightingale Nursing Times
14. Nursing Sciences Quarterly
15. World Views on Evidence Based Nursing
16. Nursing and Health Care
17. Journal of Qualitative Research
18. Western Journal of Nursing Research

Approaches to Writing a Literature Review

There are different approaches to writing a literature review. In Fig. 6.2, a general outline of steps for writing a thematically organized literature review is shown.

- Identify important publications including earlier works, reports, and other types of literature related to the selected topic. Write a brief summary about each review. Add more similar references from other works.
- Summarize the content of full article.
- Organize the literature under several themes and arrange the themes in a chronological order.
- After a round of cursory reading, researchers now have better understanding about the topic selected, methods and theories. At this point, extensive reading is required to integrate the new readings into the initial drafts of literature review.
- Organize the review into logical segments or sections. Ensure coherence between different segments of the abstract.
- Arrange and integrate the sections using appropriate subheadings.

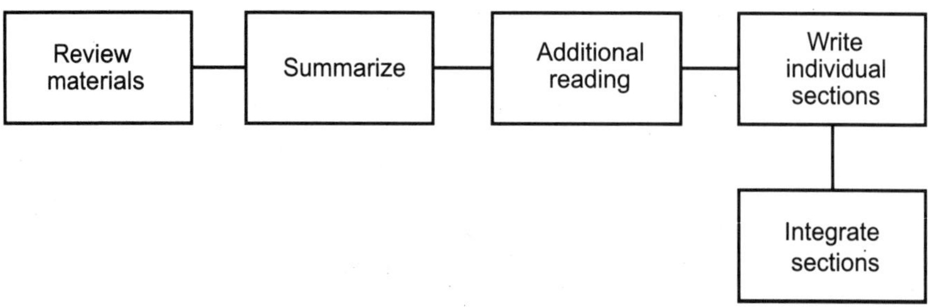

Figure 6.2 Approaches for writing a literature review

Preparation of the Literature Review

In order for a review to be effective, its content, organization and style must be acceptable to its users. An ideal literature review has three essential components:

1. Good beginning
2. Well-structured body
3. Conclusion

Good beginning

A good beginning is possible only if the researcher has well understood the topic and issues connected with it.

Well-structured body

The body of the review gives a description of the purpose and conclusions of individual research articles based on their importance. Research studies can be grouped based on common denominators such as 'qualitative' versus 'quantitative' approaches, conclusions of the authors, and so on.

Conclusion

1. Consider the major contributions of studies under review to the body of knowledge.
2. Evaluate the style and quality of writing.
3. Draw out the methodologies used in the studies.
4. Highlight the relationship between the topic of research study and major areas of study.

Steps in Writing a Literature Review

Preparing a literature review requires a systematic and scientific approach. Not all data collected is presented in the review. Identifying the potential sources, collecting the relevant data, analyzing and organizing the data are important steps for writing an effective review.

Identifying the potential – sources/references

Based on the topic chosen for the study, the researcher should identify potential sources of references.

Locating the relevant references

Once the sources have been identified, the researcher must screen the references to determine the relevance and extent to which it is related to the research question. The researcher should prefer to use only primary sources (descriptions available in original studies).

Abstracting and recording notes

When a review has been selected, it should be read critically. Notes should include the problem statement, methods and procedures, results and conclusions and the full citation.

Organizing the review

Organizing the review could be easy when working with an outline. The outline indicates how the topics have been organized in the review. The outline may be revised many times to make most references fit into it.

Analyzing and integrating the review

The main point of concern in a literature review is to discover the current state of knowledge on the research topic. Hence the review should be made as objective as possible as well as include both supporting and contradicting reports. The review should ultimately represent a critical judgement of the extensiveness and dependability of the information cited.

Writing the review

The review should be reported in the researcher's own words. Paraphrasing can be done and direct quotations should be kept to the minimum. For a significant review, its design, findings and conclusions must be explained in detail.

Guidelines for Writing a Literature Review

The review of literature can be effective if you are careful about the following facts:

1. Prepare an outline of the review.
2. Focus on current topics; preference may be given to the works published in the recent five years. However, former articles are required if your study has historical importance.
3. Collect as many number of articles related to the topic, but you should condense the information into the space available for review.
4. Verify the source of information. You should ensure reliability of the source of evidence.
5. Any reference cited in the review must be included in the bibliography.
6. Any reference mentioned in bibliography must be cited.
7. Use the original source. The reviewer should attempt to cite the original source for each reference.

Check Points... *Phrases to describe study findings*
(1) Author (year) reported that...
(2) Findings of the study showed that...
(3) Results of the study indicated that...
(4) Author (year) analyzed...

8. Be brief and specific. It is suggested not to use lengthy quotes for the purpose of in-depth analysis.
9. Use correct grammar and punctuation. They are hallmarks of a standard thesis.
10. Use past tense for writing the review of literature.

SUMMARY

Searching the literature is important for a research study because it shows what has already been discovered about the topic. Earlier studies are a theoretical or conceptual basic for the study.

Literature sources are classified as primary and secondary. A primary source is a description written by the original investigator; a secondary source is written by someone other than the original investigator. Literature sources can be available in print and electronic versions. Print sources include indices and abstracts. Indices contain references to periodic articles. Abstracts contain brief summaries of articles, and provide the purpose, methods, and major findings of the studies.

MULTIPLE CHOICE QUESTIONS

1. Description of a research study written by the original investigator(s) is ______________.
   (a) primary source
   (b) secondary source
   (c) abstracts
   (d) indexes
2. Which of the following is true?
   (a) a secondary source in the research literature is a summary or description of a research study written by some one other than the study investigator(s).
   (b) indices contain reference materials on periodicals and some books.
   (c) abstracts contain brief summaries of articles.
   (d) all of the above
3. Name the sources which would provide latest information on literature source.
   (a) printed materials (b) CD ROMs
   (c) online data base (d) none of the above

4. The most research articles that appear in medical journals are examples of
   (a) primary source
   (b) secondary source
   (c) external source
   (d) tertiary source
5. By ____________ stacks of bibliographic file can be accessed using computer.
   (a) electronic data base
   (b) textbook
   (c) dissertation
   (d) none of the above
6. Allows an individual to connect from one web address to another.
   (a) video conferencing
   (b) linking
   (c) blog
   (d) flash

ANSWER KEY

1. (a) 2. (d) 3. (c) 4. (a) 5. (a) 6. (b)

REVIEW QUESTIONS

1. (a) Define review of literature.
   (b) Explain the sources of review of literature.
2. Discusses the method of review of literature.
3. What is review of literature? Write the practical application of review of literature.
4. Mention the significance of review of literature.
5. Write the practical application of review of literature.
6. Explain the steps of review of literature in research.

REFERENCES

Amen, K., King, C.R., & Rieger, P.T. (2005). The bane of accurate referencing: How to achieve "Perfection". *Oncology Nursing Forum*, 32, 734–736.

American Psychological Association. (2001). Publication manual of the American Psychological Association (3rd ed.). Washington, D.C.: Author.

Avis, M. (1994). Reading research critically. II. An introduction to appraisal: Assessing the evidence. *Journal of Clinical Nursing*, 3, 271–277.

Beyea, S.C., & Nicott, L.H. (1997). Quantitative and qualitative approaches to nursing research. *AORN Journal*, 66(2), 323–325.

Carr, L.T. (1994). The strengths and weaknesses of qualitative and quantitative research: What method for nursing? *Journal of Advanced Nursing*, 20, 716–721.

Conn, V.S., Isaramalai, S., Rath, S., Jantarakupt, P., Wadhavan, R., & Dash, Y. (2003). Beyond MEDLINE for literature searches. *Journal of Nursing Scholarship*, 35, 177–182.

Cooper, H.M., & Hedger, L.V. (1994). The handbook of research synthesis. London: Sage.

Coopey, M., & Nix, M.P. (2006). Translating research into evidence-based nursing practice and evaluating effectiveness. *Journal of Nursing Care Quality*, 21(3), 195–202.

Coughlan, M., Cronin, P., & Ryan, F. (2007). Step-by-step guide to critiquing research. Part 1: Quantitative research. *British Journal of Nursing*, 16(11), 658–663.

________. (2008). Undertaking a literature review. A step-by-step approach. *British Journal of Nursing*, 17(1), 38–43.

Dickinson, F. (2004). Assessing the state of the art: Doing a literature review. *Midwifery Matters*, 101, 6–7.

Dornan, T., Peile, E., & Spencer, J. (2008). On "evidence". *Medical Education*, 42, 232–234.

Duffy, J.R. (2005). Critically appraising quantitative research [Electronic version]. *Nursing and Health Sciences*, 7(4), 281–283.

Dyer, I. (1997). The significance of statistical significance. *Intensive and Critical Care Nursing*, 13, 259–265.

Frame, K. (2003). Reading nursing research. Easy as ABCD. *Journal of School Nursing*, 19(6), 326–329.

Gerrish, K., Ashworth, P., Lacey, A., Bailey, J., Cooke, J., & Kendall, S., et al. (2007). Factors influencing the development of evidence-based practice: A research tool. *Journal of Advanced Nursing*, 57(3), 328–338.

Giuffre, M. (1994). Reading research critically: Threats to internal validity. *Journal of Post Anesthesia Nursing*, 995, 303–307.

________. (1995). Reading research critically: Assessing the validity and reliability of research instrumentation. Part 1: *Journal of Post Anesthesia Nursing*, 10(1), 33–37.

________. (1995). Reading research critically: Assessing the validity and reliability of research instrumentation. Part 2: *Journal of Post Anesthesia Nursing*, 10(2), 107–112.

Harrell, J.A. (1995). Reading research reports: Should I apply the findings to my practice? *Tar Heel Nurse*, 57(2), 26–27.

Hek, G. (1996). Guidelines on conducting a critical research evaluation. *Nursing Standard*, 11(6), 40–43.

Hinshaw, A.S., & Schepp, K. (1984). Problems in doing nursing research: How to recognize garbage when you see it! *Western Journal of Nursing Research*, 6(1), 126–130.

Houser, J. (2008). Nursing research: Reading, using and creating evidence. Sudbury, MA: Jones and Bartlett.

Jones, S.L., & Cook, C.B. (2000). *Electronic Journals*: Are they a paradigm shift? Online Journal of Issues in Nursing. Available at www.nursingworld.org/ojin/topic11/tpc11_1.htm.

Lemeshow, A.R., Blum, R.E., Berlin, J.A., Stoto, M.A., & Colditz, G.A. (2005). Searching one or two databases was insufficient for meta-analysis of observational studies. *Journal of Clinical Epidemiology*, 58, 867–873.

Lobiondo-Wood, G., & Haber, J. (2010). Nursing research: Methods and critical appraisal for evidence-based practice (7th ed.). St. Louis, MO: Mosby.

Loiselle, C.G., & Profetto-McGrath, J. (2007). Canadian essentials of nursing research (2nd ed.). Philadelphia: Lippincott and Williams.

Luker, K. (2007). Assessing the quality of research: A challenge for nursing. *Nursing Inquiry*, 14(1), 1.

Miracle, V.A. (2004). Making sense of conflicting research findings. *Dimensions of Critical Care Nursing*, 23(5), 230–233.

Mulrow, D. (1994). Systematic reviews: Rationale for systematic reviews. *British Medical Journal*, 309, 597–599.

Norbeck, J. (1978). The research critique: A theoretical approach to skill development and consolidation. *Western Journal of Nursing Research*, 1(4), 296–306.

Oermann, M.H., Mason, N.M., & Wilmes, N.A. (2002). Accuracy of references in general readership nursing journals. *Nurse Educator*, 27, 260–264.

Summers, S. (1991). Defining components of the research process needed to conduct and critique studies. *Journal of Post Anesthesia Nursing*, 6(1), 50–55.

Supino, P.G., & Borer, J. (2007). Teaching clinical research methodology to the academic medical community. A fifteen-year retrospective of a comprehensive curriculum. *Medical Teacher*, 29, 346–352.

Volmink, J., Siegfried, N., Robertson, K., & Gulmezoglu, A.M. (2004). Research synthesis and dissemination as a bridge to knowledge management: The Cochrane Collaboration. *Bulletin of the World Health Organization*, 82(10), 778–783.

Vrabel, M. (2005). Searching for evidence: The value of librarian-clinician collaboration-the librarian's role. *Home Health Care Management and Practice*, 17, 286–292.

Zakon, R.H. (2005). Hobbes' Internet timeline V8.1. Retrieved October 12, 2005 at www.zakon.org/robert/internet/timeline/.

CHAPTER

7

CONCEPTUAL AND THEORETICAL FRAMEWORK

Key terms

★ Concept ★ Conceptual framework ★ Conceptual model ★ Construct ★ Empirical generalization ★ Grand theories ★ Middle-range theories ★ Theoretical framework ★ Theory

⊙ Outline

- ★ Definitions
- ★ Purposes
- ★ Nursing conceptual models
- ★ Theoretical and conceptual frame
- ★ Theory testing in nursing research

⊙ Objectives

On completion of the chapter, you will be able to:

- ★ define theory, concept, construct, proposition, model and conceptual models
- ★ list the purposes of theory in nursing research
- ★ appreciate nursing conceptual models
- ★ distinguish between theoretical and conceptual frameworks
- ★ identify theories in nursing research
- ★ describe theory testing in nursing research

Introduction

In nursing, theory and research provide essential foundation for practice. Conceptual and theoretical framework helps researchers organize findings into a broader conceptual context. Theoretical framework supports a research is much the same way how the skeleton supports the human body. A theoretical framework provides rationale for predictions about the relationships among variables of a research study. This chapter addresses the nature, purpose and process of developing a theoretical framework for a research study.

Important Terminology

Concepts are building blocks of a theory that abstractly describe an object or phenomenon, e.g. health, anxiety.

Constructs are abstractions that are deliberately and systematically invented. Constructs cannot be pragmatic and must be inferred. It is a symbolic representation of an abstract idea that is adapted for a scientific purpose, e.g. health promotion (Pender's model), self-care (Orem's model).

Propositions are statements that elucidate the relationship between concepts.

General propositions are statements that are of high level of abstraction (found in conceptual models).

Specific proposition refers to statements that are at moderate level of abstraction (found in theories).

E.g.: "The Amount of Physical Activity Positively Influences the Level of Muscle Integrity"

Models are representations of the interaction among concepts showing a pattern.

Definition of a Theory

The term theory has a lot of meanings and definitions. Theory is a set of related statements that describes or explains a phenomenon in a systematic way. Theory is defined as an abstract generalization that offers a systematic explanation about how the phenomena are interrelated. Theories are abstract rather than concrete.

Kerlinger's (1986) definition of theory is perhaps the most widely used in research. It takes a basic view of science, i.e. the development of general explanations about natural phenomena through theories.

1. A theory is a set of interrelated constants (concepts) adopted for a scientific purpose; definitions and propositions that present a significant view of explaining and predicting the phenomenon (Kerlinger, 1986).
2. According to Meleis (1985), a theory enables us to explain a "maximum number of observable relationships" by setting limits on what questions to ask and what methods to use to pursue answers to the questions.

3. Theory is a creative and rigorous idea that projects a tentative, purposeful and systematic view of phenomena (Chinn & Kraneer, 1995).

Nursing Theory

Nursing theory is an organized framework of concepts and purposes designed to guide the practice (Jean Watson, 2011).

Definition of Theoretical Framework

Theoretical framework is a frame of reference that is a basis for observations, definitions of concepts, research design, interpretations, and generalizations. It gives guide to systematically identifying logical, precisely defined relationships among and between variables.

Suppose a nurse researcher was interested in studying the effect of educational interventions on lifestyle diseases among *Kudumbasree* women.

Through a review of literature, she could understand the various aspects of lifestyle diseases. Thus, the researcher would be studying the relationship between educational interventions and knowledge of lifestyle diseases.

A research should report clearly the theoretical basis for researcher's prediction about the outcome of the study, study findings and outcome interpretations.

Definition of a Conceptual Model

A model is a representation of interaction among and between concepts showing a pattern. A conceptual model is made up of concepts and propositions. As defined by Fawcett (2000), a conceptual model "gives direction to the search for relevant questions about the phenomena of central interest to a discipline and suggests solutions to practical problems".

Conceptual models are like theories that deal with abstractions that are assembled by virtue of their relevance to a perspective regarding interrelated phenomena but are more loosely structured than theories. They depict the phenomenon of interest and reflect assumptions and philosophic views of model designers, e.g. Pender's health promotion model, Orem's self-care model.

Frameworks in Quantitative Studies

Testing a theory/conceptual model

1. *Theories stimulate new studies:* In testing a theory, researchers deduce implications, develop research hypotheses to test.
2. Using a model/theory as organizing structure
3. Researchers begin with a broad conceptualization of nursing that is consistent with that of other models (stress, health beliefs)
4. Use the models' constructs to provide a broad organizational context

Fitting a problem to a theory

A nurse researcher formulates the problem and attempts to link a theory or model to the problem (conceptualization of a problem on an abstract level).

E.g.: "Weekly Home Visits to Patients with Diabetes Mellitus by Nurses Reduce Development of Complications of Diabetes Mellitus" (theory of reinforcement)

If you begin with a research problem and try to identify a suitable framework, discuss with people who are familiar with a broad range of theoretical perspectives. By open discussion, you will become aware of your own conceptual perspectives to identify an appropriate framework. If you begin with a research question and then subsequently identify a theory or model, be willing to adapt or augment your research problem as you gain greater understanding of the theory.

Developing your own framework

Developing a required framework is not research experience alone, but powers of observation, grasp of a problem, and knowledge of prior research.

An imaginative and sensitive person is able to formulate an original conceptual framework of a study. The basic intellectual process needed is induction, a process of reasoning from particular observations and facts to generalizations.

The inductive process involves integrating one's experience and observations into conclusion. The first step is to formulate a generalized scheme of relevant concepts (concept analysis).

Purposes of Theory in Research

The major purpose of theory is to make research findings meaningful and helpful for generalizability.

Other important purposes are:

1. To help researchers to compile observations and facts into an orderly format.
2. To identify meaningful and relevant areas for research.
3. To guide a researcher about the natural phenomenon and reasons for occurrence of the phenomenon.
4. To provide a foundation for predicting the occurrence of a phenomenon.
5. Acts as an important resource for the development of nursing intervention and to develop clinical practice protocol.
6. Helps to stimulate research and extension of knowledge by providing both direction and motivation.
7. Helps to define concepts and proposed relationships between concepts.
8. To serve as a springboard for advances in knowledge and the accumulation of evidence for practice.
9. To propose credible approaches to health problems.

Use of Theory in Nursing Research

Theory is used in nursing research in three different ways. They are:

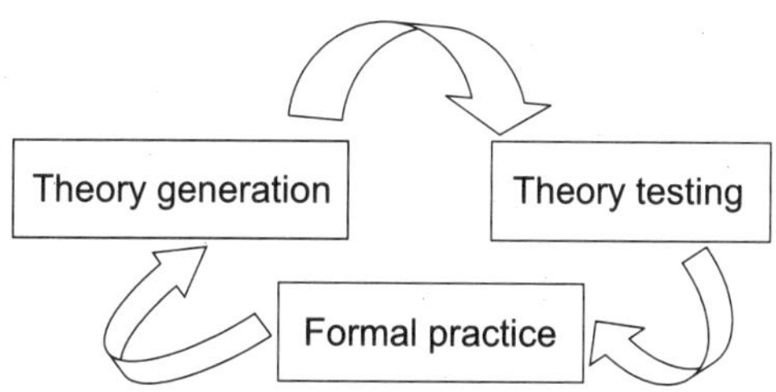

Figure 7.1 Use of theory in research

1. In research studies, there will be minimum use of theory; it is clearly identified as the framework. The researcher neglects the application of theory as a guide to test research variables into practice.
2. Theory is used in moderate amount. Theory is used for descriptive purpose. Theory is incorporated with variables.
3. Theoretical model is adequately used. Hypotheses are derived from assumptions and tested in an appropriate manner. Research results are also analyzed and they offer for or against the theory and possible revision to the theory.

Research is a complex process. Research topics are generated from current, formal nursing practice. Answers to research questions give theory generation via inductive research. The newly generated knowledge will be practiced in nursing service (evidence-based nursing).Then new research questions will arise and this cycle repeats.

Testing and developing theories

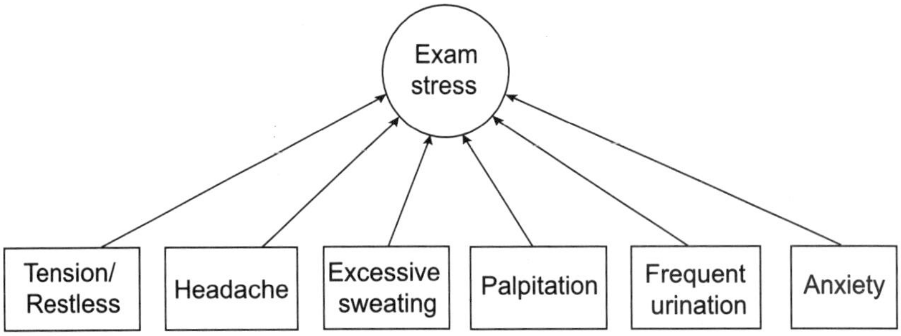

Figure 7.2 Inductive reasoning from observation to theory

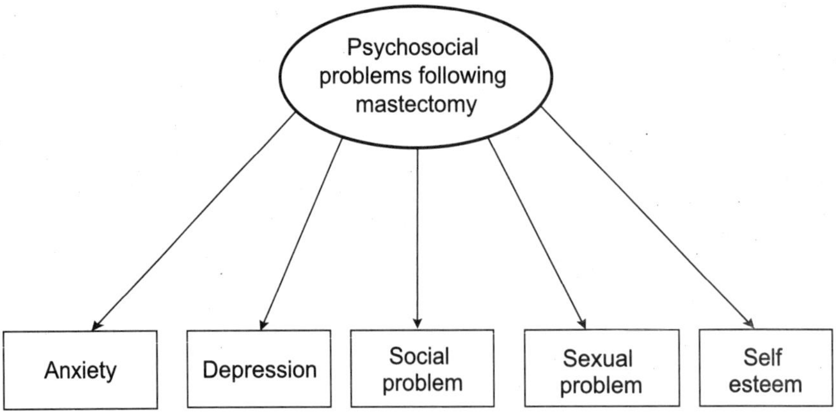

Figure 7.3 Deductive reasoning from theory to observation

Classification of Nursing Theories

Classification based on function

Descriptive theory: It identifies the properties and components of a discipline. It explains specific dimensions or characteristics of individuals, groups, relations or events by summarizing the commonalities found in distinct observation. It identifies meaning and observations and describes what elements exist in that discipline.

Explanatory theory: It identifies how the properties and components relate to each other and accounts for how the discipline functions.

Predictive theory (practice theory): It predicts the relationships between components of a phenomenon and predicts under what conditions it will occur.

Prescriptive theory: It addresses nursing therapeutics and consequences of interventions.

Classification based on generalizability of their principles

Meta theory: It is most abstract and not easy to test. It identifies specific phenomenon through abstract concepts.

Grand theory: It explains large segments of human experience. It is broadest in scope. It is a conceptual framework that defines the broad perspective for nursing practice, e.g. learning theories.

Classification based on principles of discipline

Middle range theory: It is moderately abstract and has a limited number of variables, and can be tested directly. It focuses on a narrow range of experience. Theories with fewer concepts implying to explain a smaller part of the universe are labelled middle range theories, e.g. interpersonal relationship, anxiety.

Practice theory: It traces the outline for practice. Objectives are set, and actions are set to meet the objectives. It explores one particular situation found in nursing. Theories hold the background for observing facts in a sequential manner.

Framework

A framework is the overall conceptual foundation of a study. Every study has got a framework that guides the researcher to proceed. If the framework in a study was developed based on theory, it is referred to as the theoretical framework. A study that has its root in a specified conceptual model is referred to as conceptual framework.

The theoretical framework for a particular research study is made up of concepts and relational statements between the concepts to be examined or tested. When researchers feel to clarify the conceptual foundation of their research variables, it becomes difficult to integrate the research findings. A study should make clear the conceptual definitions of its key variables, thereby providing information about the study's framework.

Conceptual Model/Conceptual Framework

A model, as an abstraction of reality, provides a way to visualize reality to simplify thinking. Conceptual models, like theories, deal with abstractions (concepts) that are assembled by virtue of their relevance to a common theme. It provides a perspective regarding interrelated phenomena that are more loosely structured than theories. It broadly presents an understanding of the phenomena of interest and reflects the assumptions and philosophic views of the model's designer.

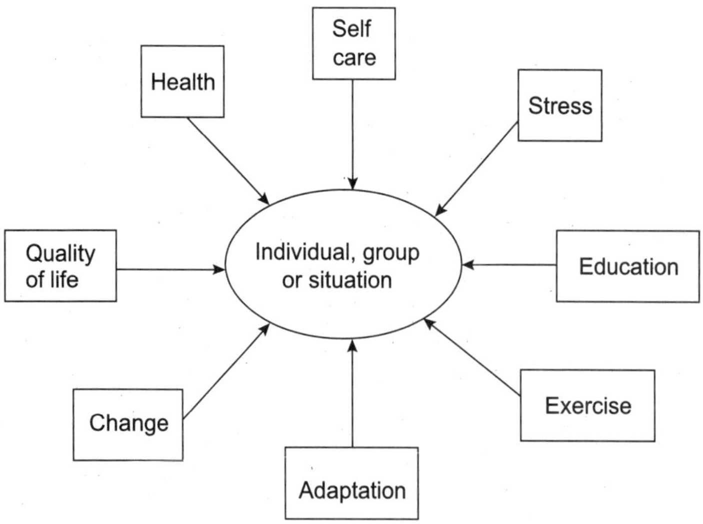

Figure 7.4 Common concepts used in nursing research

According to Fawcett (2000), "A conceptual model gives direction to the research for relevant questions about the phenomenon and suggests solutions to practical problems. These models represent conceptualizations of the nursing process and the nature of nurse-client relationship."

When the models are used in connection with symbolic representation of a conceptualization, it is termed schematic models. Schematic models are visual representation of some aspect of reality. It helps to express abstract ideas in a concise and readily understandable form.

An example of schematic model is 'Pender's Health Promotion Model' that explains and predicts the health promotion component of lifestyle diseases. It is useful in explaining linkages among concepts.

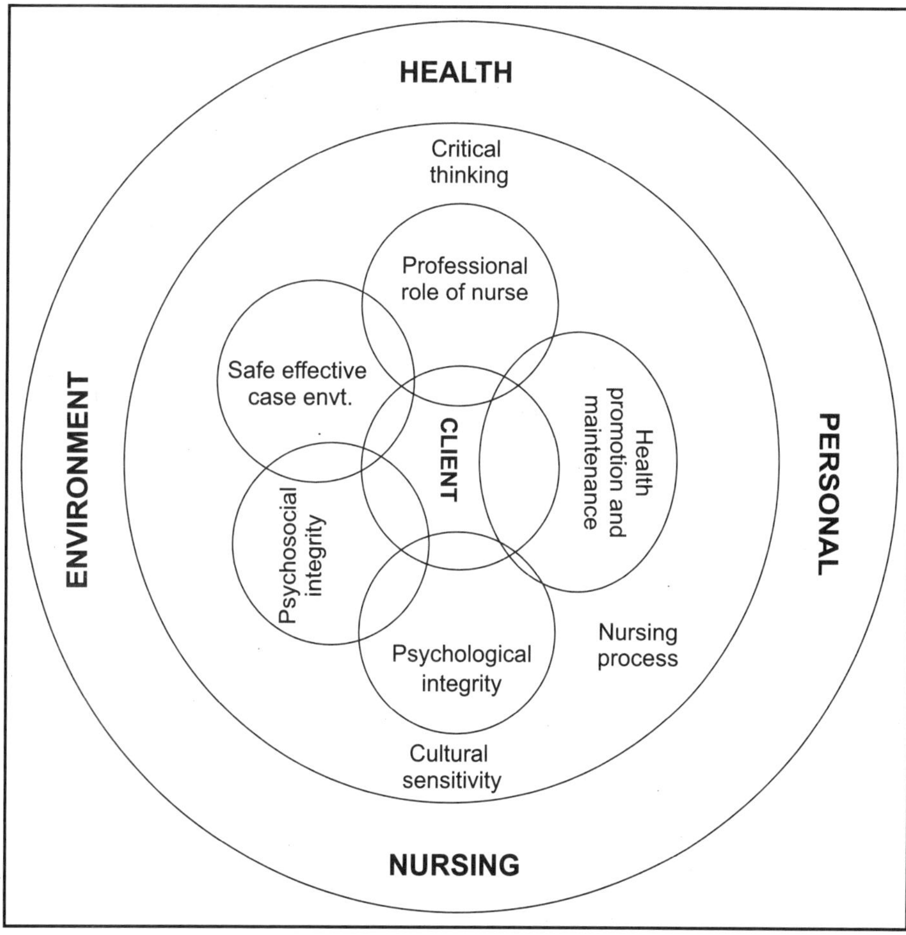

Figure 7.5 Concepts of conceptual model (Fawcett, 2005)

Conceptual Models Used in Nursing Research

Nursing researchers have used both nursing and non-nursing frameworks to provide a conceptual context for their studies. According to Fawcett (2005), four concepts are generally considered central to the discipline of nursing:

1. Person who receives nursing care
2. Environment (society)
3. Nursing (goals, roles and functions)
4. Health

The various conceptual models define these concepts differently and give different emphasis to relationships among them. For example, Sister Callista Roy's Adaptation Model identifies adaptation of patient as a critical phenomenon. Marta Rogers emphasizes the centrality of individual as a unified whole.

A conceptual framework helps nurse researchers in formulating research questions and hypothesis. It is used in research to outline the possible courses of action or to present a preferred approach to an idea or thought.

According to Bordage (2009), the use of conceptual framework in research:

1. allows researchers to build upon one another's work, thereby building a body of knowledge
2. helps accumulate deeper understanding over time and moves a discipline forward

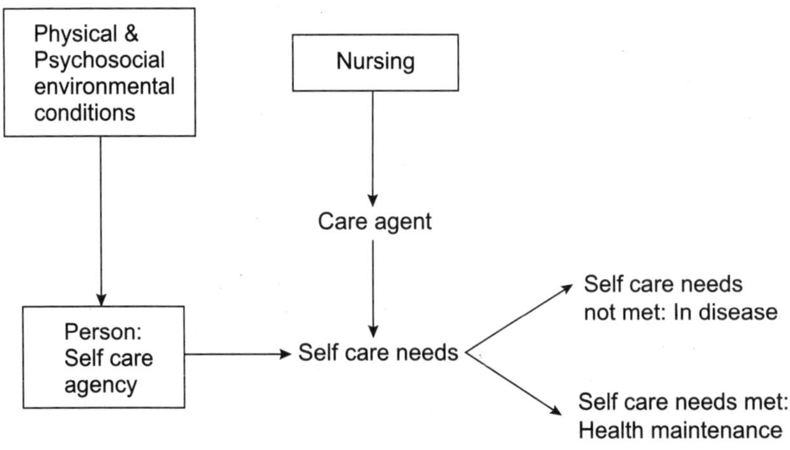

Figure 7.6 Orem's self care model

Figure 7.6 shows how the different nursing models view the four key concepts and their relationship – humans, environment, nursing and health.

Development of Conceptual or Theoretical Framework and Models

A conceptual and theoretical framework acts as an outline to represent a concept or research idea. The basic intellectual process underlying theory development is induction, i.e. reasoning from particular observation and facts to broader generation. The inductive process involves the integrity one has experienced or based into some organized scheme.

For qualitative research, the observations used in the inductive process usually are findings from other studies. The first step in the development of a framework is formulation of a concept.

Steps for Development of Conceptual Framework

Defining the concept

A researcher formulates a generalized scheme of relevant concepts firmly grounded in research literature. These concepts may be based on research problem, variables, previous research findings, existing theories and models. It is also possible to identify concepts from real life situations or clinical experience.

Predict the relationship among variables

General concepts and information help the researcher identify the concepts more empirically in order to establish the relationship between concepts for development of framework. The researcher must read details of the concepts from primary sources, and then a framework based on specific theory can be developed.

Concept mapping

A concept map is a band of diagram that lays out key ideas related to your area and indicates relationships between these areas. Without some kind of 'map' or conceptualization of what might be going on, it would be difficult to design a strong study. Mapping is useful in foreseeing and thinking about information and relationships in differentiation.

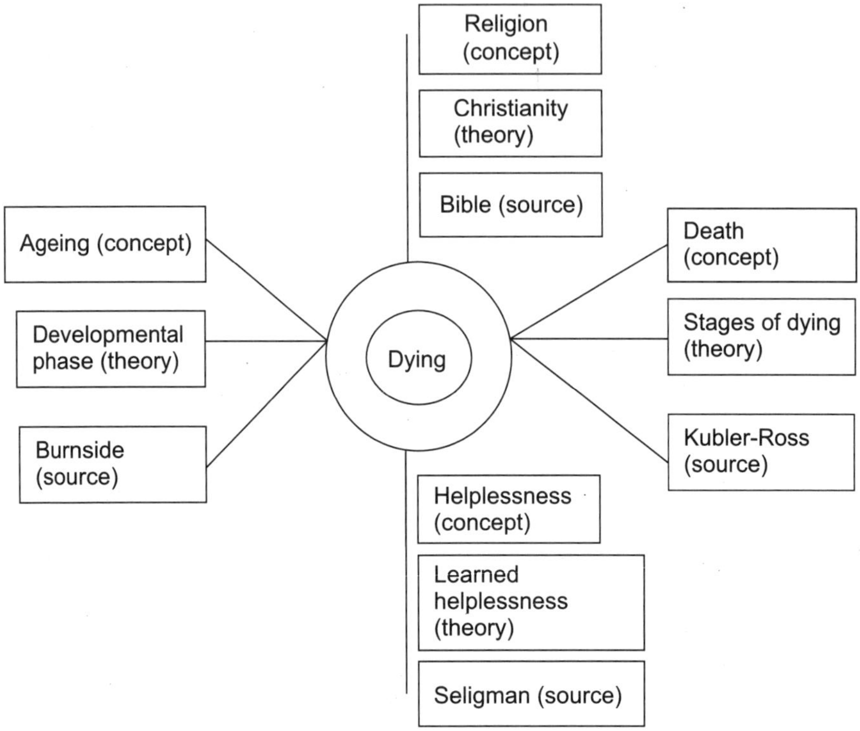

Figure 7.7 A concept map (source)

Testing the relationship between variables

In this step, the relationship between variables is tested.

Evaluating the result

The concepts and constructs act as building blocks for frameworks which are later evaluated for their relevance and relationship to conclude or generalize the facts. A revision may be made before the development of a frame.

Relationships of Theory, Research and Practice

Practice truly relies on theory and research; each one is interrelated. Deckoff et al. claims that, in order for theory to be useful, it must be determined whether it tests reality. In a practice-based discipline such as nursing, clinical practice and reality is consulted through research. In other words, theory provides knowledge about the world of clinical health practice through research.

Maas (2006) describes that when theory, research and practice are in harmony, the discipline is best served, ultimately resulting in better patient outcome.

Rolfe (1998) claims that all practices should be based on research or evidence. There is a hierarchical relationship between theory and practice where research generates knowledge that builds supports or tests theory. The theory must be tested by subjecting deductions from it (hypothesis) to further systematic enquiry. Their research plays a dual and continuing role in theory, building and testing. Those guides generate ideas for research. Research assesses the worth of a theory and provides a foundation for new theories.

Practice should be based on a theory tested through research that is well documented. Parahoo (1997) states, "practice without research is like building castles on slippery ground" and "research without practice is like building castles in air".

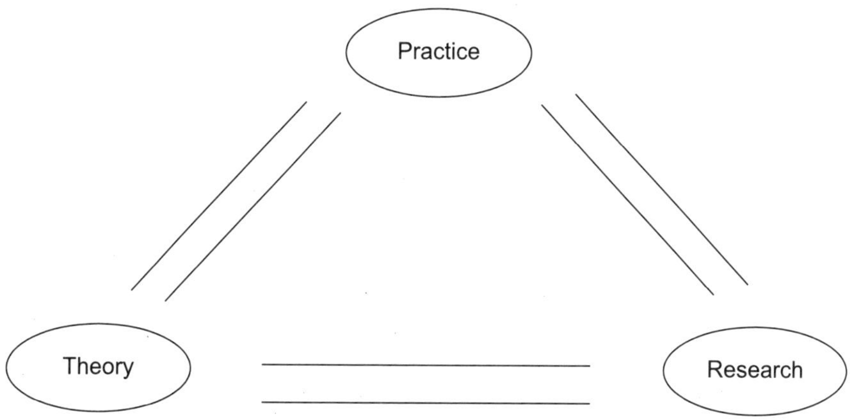

Figure 7.8 Relationship between theory, practice and research

According to Pryjmachuk (1996), research is a link between theory and practice. He believes it to be the key for development of a discipline. He argues that theory is seen as objective evidence derived from research investigations, the results of which are used to guide and regulate practice. Practice based on research evidence helps to render quality care to the patients. Research without theory may result in information or data which does not add to the accumulated knowledge of the discipline. Theory guides the research process, forms research questions and helps in design analysis and interpretation.

Testing theories in research studies

A nurse researcher has the responsibility to develop and test ideas that may be useful to practice (Batcher, 2006). This can be done by deductive and inductive reasoning.

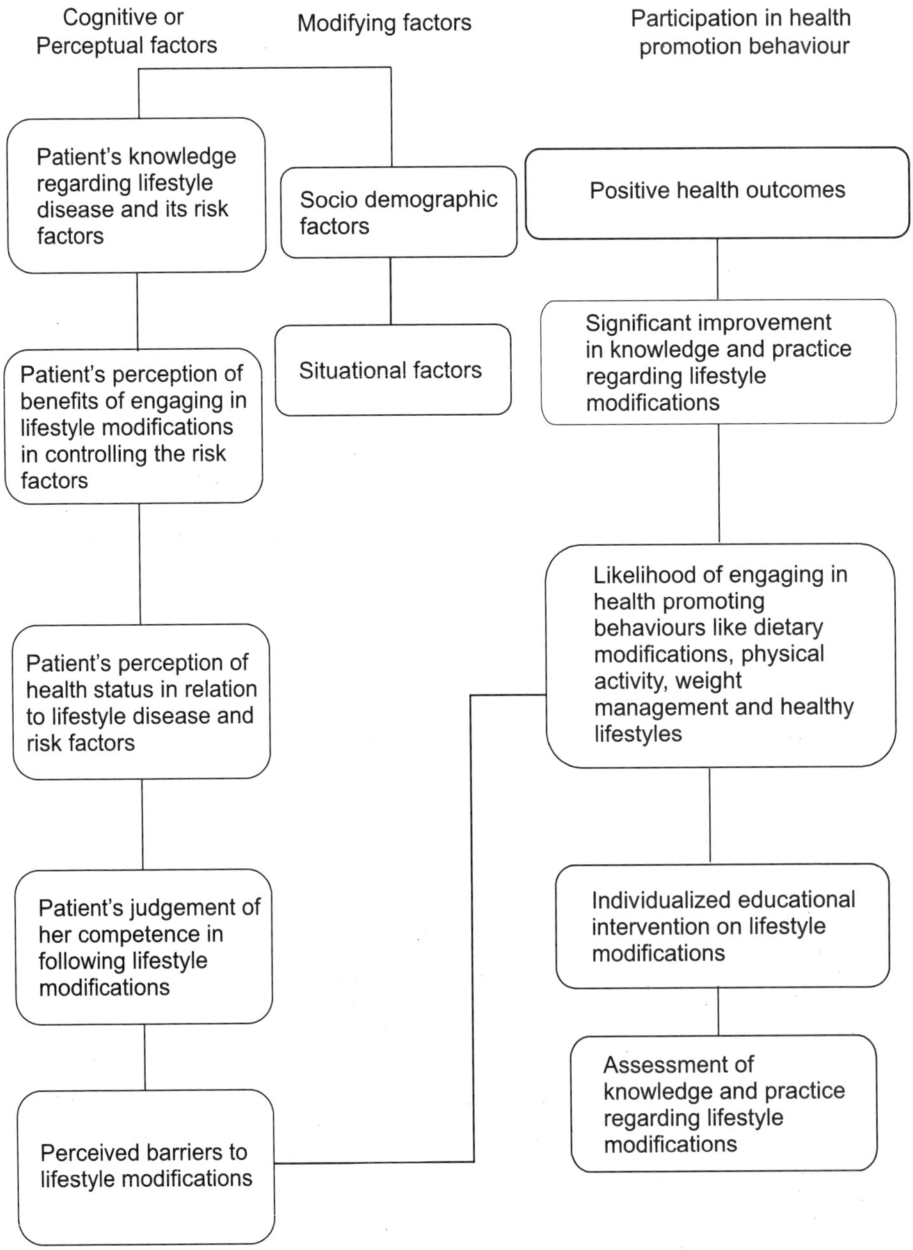

Figure 7.9 Conceptual framework based on Nola J. Pender's health promotion model

Practical considerations for formulating theoretical framework

1. Explain why it is suitable for a particular research problem.
2. Select the framework only after reviewing sufficient literature.
3. Critically analyze and write the framework and describe its application to the present study.
4. Refer how the framework has been used in previous studies.
5. Clearly describe the method of utilization of particular framework in the study.
6. Data collection methods should be outlined and depicted.
7. In the 'discussion' section, describe how the study findings are consistent within the framework.
8. Offer suggestions for practice and further research that are congruent with framework, concepts and proposition.
9. The details may be shown diagrammatically.

SUMMARY

Theoretical and conceptual models guide in understanding the relationship between variables in a scientific way. This rationale provides a clear road map for appraising problems and developing and testing hypothesis. It gives meaning to the research topic and study findings. For developing these frameworks, knowledge may be derived from other disciplines also. As Fawcett (2005) states, framework gives a context for constructing theories that deal with the central phenomena related to nursing, i.e. person, environment, health and nursing.

It is also significant to consider not only clarity and logic of theoretical rationale itself but also whether the operational definitions, tools, methods of data collection, hypothesis and results are consistent with theory.

MULTIPLE CHOICE QUESTIONS

1. A set of related statements that describes or explains phenomena in a systematic way is termed __________.

   (a) propositions (b) concept
   (c) speculation (d) theory

2. The building blocks of theory which is a word picture or mental idea of a phenomenon is __________.

   (a) construct (b) theory
   (c) concept (d) propositions

3. The term used to indicate a phenomenon that cannot be directly observed but must be inferred by certain concrete or less abstract indicators of the phenomena is __________.

   (a) concept (b) theory
   (c) speculation (d) construct

4. A statement or assertion of the relationship between concepts __________.

   (a) proposition (b) hypothesis
   (c) assumption (d) generalization

5. When a similar pattern of events is found in the empirical data of a number of different studies, the pattern is called __________.

   (a) triangulation (b) empirical generalization
   (c) conceptual model (d) speculation

6. In nursing research which of the following reasoning process is used?

   (a) inductive
   (b) deductive
   (c) both inductive and deductive
   (d) neither inductive nor deductive

7. A reasoning process that proceeds from the specific to the general, from empirical data to theory is __________.

   (a) inductive reasoning (b) critical analysis
   (c) conceptualization (d) deductive reasoning

8. Deriving a propositional statement from a theory involves the logical reasoning process called __________.
   (a) conceptualization (b) deduction
   (c) critical analysis (d) induction

ANSWER KEY

1. (d) 2. (c) 3. (d) 4. (a) 5. (b) 6. (c) 7. (a) 8. (b)

REVIEW QUESTIONS

1. (a) Define theory in nursing.
   (b) Explain the role of theory in nursing research.
2. (a) What is conceptual framework?
   (b) Discuss how you develop, use and test conceptual framework.
3. Define conceptualization.
4. (a) What are the characteristics of a theory?
   (b) Explain the significance of theory in nursing research.

REFERENCES

Bergman, R. (1994). Are my outcomes better than yours? *Hospital Health Network*, 68(15).

Bernstein, S.J., & Hill Borne, L. (1993). Clinical indicators: The road to quality care? *Joint Commission Journal on Quality Improvement*, 19(11).

Fink, A. (2009). How to conduct surveys: A step-by-step guide. Beverly Hills, CA: Sage.

Giuffre, M. (1995). Reading research critically: Assessing the validity and reliability of research instrumentation. Part 2: *Journal of Post Anesthesia Nursing*, 10(2), 107–112.

Harrell, J.A. (1995). Reading research reports: Should I apply the findings to my practice? *Tar Heel Nurse*, 57(2), 26–27.

Hek, G. (1996). Guidelines on conducting a critical research evaluation. *Nursing Standard*, 11(6), 40–43.

Hinshaw, A.S., & Schepp, K. (1984). Problems in doing nursing research: How to recognize garbage when you see it! *Western Journal of Nursing Research*, 6(1), 126–130.

Houser, J. (2008). Nursing research: Reading, using and creating evidence. Sudbury, MA: Jones and Bartlett.

Lobiondo-Wood, G., & Haber, J. (2010). Nursing research: Methods and critical appraisal for evidence-based practice. (7th ed.). St. Louis, MO: Mosby.

Loiselle, C.G., & Profetto-McGrath, J. (2007). Canadian essentials of nursing research (2nd ed.). Philadelphia: Lippincott and Williams.

Luker, K. (2007). Assessing the quality of research: A challenge for nursing. *Nursing Inquiry*, 14(1), 1.

May, K. (1991). Interview techniques in qualitative research: Concerns and challenges. In J.M. Morse (Ed). Qualitative nursing research: A contemporary dialogue (Rev. Ed.). Newbury Park, CA: Sage.

Miracle, V.A. (2004). Making sense of conflicting research findings. *Dimensions of Critical Care Nursing*, 23(5), 230–233.

Patton, M.Q. (2002). Qualitative evaluation of research methods (3rd ed.). Newbury Park, CA: Sage.

Payne, S.L. (1951). The art of asking questions. Princeton, NJ: Princeton University Press.

Roberts, B.L., Srour, M.I., & Winkelman, C. (1996). Videotaping: An important research strategy. *Nursing Research*, 45(6).

Woods, D.L., Kovach, C.R., Raff, H., Joosse, L., Basmadjian, A., & Hegadoren, K. (2008). Using saliva to measure endogenous cortisol in nursing home resident with advanced dementia. *Research in Nursing and Health*, 31(3).

CHAPTER

8

ETHICAL CONSIDERATIONS IN NURSING RESEARCH

Key terms

★ Assent ★ Informed consent ★ Anonymity
★ Ethical committee ★ Ethical principles

⊙ Outline

- Definitions
- Historical perspective of ethics in research
- Significance of ethics in nursing research
- Code of ethics in nursing research
- Purposes of ethical principles
- Ethical implications for nursing research
- Guidelines for critiquing the ethical aspects of a study
- Ethical committee
- Responsibilities of the principal investigator
- Role of a clinical nurse in ensuring optimal patient care during the research process

⊙ Objectives

On completion of the chapter, you will be able to:

- enumerate ethical principles
- recognize human ethics committee
- interpret ethical considerations in research
- discuss ethical dilemmas in conducting research

Introduction

Research consists of activities designed to test a hypothesis, permit conclusions to be drawn, and thereby to develop or contribute to the body of knowledge. In each step of research process, the ethical dimension needs to be addressed. Research should cause no harm or distress to any of the subjects involved. It is mandatory that any proposal be reviewed by an unbiased individual or group. 'Deviations' from ethical conduct occur in research as a result of ignorance or failure to reflect critically on problematic traditions, and then a course in research ethics may help reduce the rate of serious deviations by improving the researcher's understanding of ethics and by sensitizing him or her to the issues.

Definitions

Ethics

Ethics are norms for conduct that distinguish between acceptable and unacceptable behaviour. Ethics is defined as a method, procedure or perspective for deciding how to act and for analyzing complex problems and issues. In other words, ethics refers to a system of principles and rules of conduct covering the whole field of moral, political and social science.

Law

Law is a set of rules. It is important to remember that ethics and law are not the same. An action may be legal but unethical.

Code

Set of laws or rules.

Moral

Standards of human behaviour; moral is a custom which can change over time.

Historical Perspective of Ethical Dimensions

German researchers were very much interested in conducting research but their practices were unethical since they used prisoners in military camps as subjects. In the light of brutalities reported during the Second World War, Nuremberg Code was established in 1947. Nuremberg Code lays down the fundamental ethical guidelines for conduct of any type of research. The criteria include:

1. Researcher must inform subjects about the study.
2. Research must be for the good of society.
3. Research must be based on animal experiment, if possible.
4. Researcher must try to avoid injury to research subjects.
5. Researcher must be qualified to conduct research.
6. Subjects or the researcher can stop the study if problems occur.

Codes of Ethics in Nursing Research

1. Nuremberg Code
2. Declaration of Helsinki, 1964
3. ICN Code of Ethics
4. American Nurses Association Code of Ethics
5. Code of Professional Conduct for the Nurse, Midwife, and Health Visitor (UKCC)

Ethical Principles in Nursing Research

Ethical principles are guidelines to decide whether a situation is moral or immoral in nursing practice. Nurses often look toward narrower, more specific ethical principles to guide their judgement and decisions.

Basics Principles Guiding Ethical and Legal Considerations of Research (Belmont Report)

Three principles guide ethical considerations, namely respect of persons, beneficence and justice. These principles guide a researcher in formulating the research question through study design, subject recruitment, protocol initiation, statistical analysis and discussion of findings.

Principle of respect for persons

This principle empowers people with the ability to act independently and gives additional protection to people with diminishing autonomy. Under this principle, a researcher must ensure the following:

1. Subjects have the right to ask for full information about the study.
2. They have the right to quit from the study.
3. Informed consent must be taken from the participants.

Informed consent: Informed consent is one where the participants have a test or procedure performed after they have been fully informed about the test or procedure.

Participants must give the consent voluntarily without coercion or persuasion. Moreover, they must be mentally competent (having mental and psychological capacity to make decisions).

Vulnerable group: Individuals who cannot give consent include children, vulnerable adults, patients who are unconscious or have serious or enduring mental health problems, some older people with memory impairment, and individuals with learning disabilities.

In this situation, a researcher makes an attempt to describe the procedure to the participant in a way understandable by the participant. The description includes potential benefits to the participant as well as possible risks and should not imply any guarantee of results. Nurse researchers frequently seek expressed consent from a participant in a consent form. They are obligated to ensure that the participant is given appropriate information, able to understand the information, and voluntarily agrees to the test or procedure.

Elements of informed consent

1. Researcher's identity and credentials
2. Purpose of the study
3. Investigation process – selection procedure, data collection method
4. Potential benefit and risk to the participants
5. Usability of the study findings
6. Anonymity and confidentiality of the participants
7. Right to withdraw from the study at any time without any penalty
8. Right to clarify doubts
9. Documentation of informed consent

Veracity: Veracity concerns truth-telling and incorporates the concept that individuals should always tell the truth. This principle also compels that truth be completely told.

Fidelity: Fidelity is the researcher's obligation to keep commitments he/she has made. It holds that a researcher faithfully fulfil his/her duties and obligations.

Principle of beneficence

Beneficence means "doing good", while nonmaleficence refers to refraining from doing harm. Nonmaleficence is the principle that obliges us not to inflict harm intentionally or unintentionally.

The principle of beneficence states that the actions one takes should be done in an effort to promote good. The concept of nonmaleficence says that if one cannot do good, then he/she should at least do no harm.

1. The risk of research should never exceed the expected benefits for the subjects from knowledge generated by the research activity.
2. Participants are protected from any harmful effects of the study.
3. They must be protected from physical and psychological consequences caused by the research.
4. Maximum physical, psychological, social and religious comfort should be ensured, and undue disturbance and time utilization of the subjects should be avoided.
5. Researchers should not expose the participants to situations for which they have not been prepared.

Principle of justice

This principle ensures right treatment and maintenance of privacy of the subjects.

1. The selection of participants should be strictly based on research requirement and be fair and non-discriminatory. Any risk and benefits will be equally shared by participants.
2. Non-prejudicial treatment should be offered to individuals who decline to participate or who withdraw from the study after agreeing to participate.
3. Confidentiality should be maintained.
4. The collected data should be used only for the purpose of the study.
5. Vulnerable subjects should be protected.
6. Policy statements should contain ethical consideration for human subjects on whom experiments are to be carried out.

The guidelines of this principle are as follows:

1. The rights of human subjects on whom experiments are to be carried out are sufficiently protected.

2. Potential benefits to the subjects or society are stressed rather than the risks of individuals.
3. Clinical investigations on human subjects should be carried out by a competent researcher only.
4. The competent research follows a procedure for obtaining advice, support and assistance before embarking on a particular clinical research programme.

Ethical implications for nursing research

1. Nurse researchers have to get informed consent from study subjects.
2. *Confidentiality*: Data and information collected from subjects must be kept confidentiality.
3. The collected information should not be used outside the terms of agreement.
4. *Protection of the participants*: Ethics will help for protection of participants from all types of harms.
5. *Research settings*: The researcher must get approval of research settings.
6. A researcher should have a clear idea regarding other members involved in the study.

Guidelines for critiquing ethical aspects of the study

1. The study must be approved by the review board.
2. Informed consent should be obtained from the subjects.
3. There is provision for anonymity or confidentiality.
4. Selection of subjects must not be biased.
5. Participants must not be forced into acting as subjects.
6. The benefits of participation in the study must outweigh the risks involved.
7. Subjects must have the opportunity to ask questions about the study and to contact the researcher when questions arose.
8. Subjects must be told how the results of the study will be used.

Institutional Human Ethics Committee

Every research centre should have a Human Ethics Committee to scrutinize the research proposal and tools, thus ensuring the rights and safety of the subjects. Often a human ethics committee follows the guidelines of 'Standard Operating Procedure' (SOP) laid down by ICMR.

Members of the human ethics committee

The committee constitutes 11 to13 eminent personnel consisting of

1. Medical expert (2 or 3)
2. Nursing expert (2 or 3)
3. Pharmacologist
4. Advocate
5. Educationist
6. Medical social worker
7. Representative from public

Organizational pattern of human ethics committee

The **chairperson** must be a medical expert from outside the research centre and must possess quality research experience.

The **member secretary** must be from nursing department of the research centre. The member secretary plans, organizes and executes ethical decision-making. It is the responsibility of the member secretary to issue ethical clearance as per the decision of the committee.

Before submitting the research proposal and tool to the human ethics committee, it must be submitted to and clearance got from a research committee.

All other experts are members of the committee.

Role of ethics committee

1. Risks to the subjects are minimized.
2. Risks to the subjects are reasonable in relation to the anticipated benefits.

3. Selection of subjects is equitable.
4. Informed consent is sought from each prospective subject or the subject's legally authorized representative.
5. Informed consent is appropriately documented.
6. The data collection process is monitored to ensure the safety of subjects.
7. Adequate provisions are included to protect the privacy of subjects and to maintain the confidentiality of data.
8. Appropriate additional safeguards are included for subjects with diminished autonomy.

Responsibilities of the Principal Investigator

Before starting a research project, the principal investigator is responsible for being familiar with ethical principles, designing the study with consideration of human subjects' rights, obtaining peer review, and establishing a mechanism for securing informed consent. While the study is being conducted, the investigator is responsible for establishing and maintaining communication with all persons involved in the study and for clearing doubts during data collection.

The researcher should share information regarding the purpose, methodology, risks and benefits of the study to the participants. The researcher must provide sufficient information to help nurses functioning in the caregiver's role make appropriate decisions to notify the researcher if the patient's condition changes and continuing in the study appears to place the subject at additional risk. The investigator is responsible for reporting all untoward reactions or protocol changes to the peer review board and caregivers.

When a research study is completed, it is the responsibility of the investigator to submit a final report to the peer review board and, if requested, to the caregivers. The investigator should acknowledge health professionals who assist with research as data collectors or research subjects.

Role of Clinical Nurses in Ensuring Optimal Patient Care during Research Process

A nurse's primary ethical obligation is towards patients, as opposed to any other professional relationship, when there is a conflict of interest.

Medical college hospitals have a plethora of ongoing research studies. The nurses must serve as an advocate in order to prevent patients and their families from being overwhelmed by requests to participate in numerous studies. A professional nurse should advocate the highest quality of health care for patients and their families. In the role of patient advocate, the nurse must judge between the requirements of the study and the changing needs of the patient.

Nurses at bedside are responsible for continually assessing and evaluating patient response to the treatment being provided. On the basis of this assessment and evaluation, the nurse must decide whether it is in the patient's best interest to continue in the study or to suggest to the principal investigator that change may be indicated. Sometimes, changes in patient condition may demand temporary or permanent withdrawal from the study. In making this decision and acting on it, the nurse may experience conflict between obligations to the patient and expectations of the research team.

It is important to remember that the primary responsibility for appropriate conduct of research rests with the principal investigator. Nurses in the patient-advocate role are not responsible for policing the researchers but are responsible for assuring that patients' rights are respected.

SUMMARY

The rights of research subjects in all disciplines must be protected. A research should have deep concern for human welfare and sensitivity for the rights of research subjects.

Human rights, self-determination, privacy, anonymity and confidentiality, fair treatment and protection from discomfort and harm are major concerns in research involving human subjects. The major ethical principles are principle of respect of human dignity, principle of beneficence and principle of justice. An institutional Human Ethics Committee examines studies for ethical concerns with complete level of review.

Nurse scientists act as patient advocates and the advisory involves protecting patients' privacy and dignity. Peculiar attention should be given to the rights of vulnerable groups such as children, elders, and unconscious or sedated patients.

MULTIPLE CHOICE QUESTIONS

1. Which of the following terms refers to a system of principles and rules of conduct?
   (a) justice (b) ethics
   (c) assent (d) anonymity
2. The meeting with research participants that ensures their understanding of the reasons and justification for the procedures used in the study is termed as __________.
   (a) debriefing (b) anonymity
   (c) confidentiality (d) clinical trials
3. The name of the process to obtain agreement of a child to participate in a study is __________.
   (a) assent (b) consent of a minor
   (c) minor agreement (d) none of the above
4. Which of the following criteria for research is not true?
   (a) research must inform subjects about the study.
   (b) researcher must try to avoid injury to research subjects.
   (c) subjects or researcher cannot stop the study if problems occur.
   (d) researcher must be qualified to conduct research.
5. Which of the following is one of the basic principles of research – that means research subjects should be protected from harm?
   (a) anonymity (b) confidentiality
   (c) justice (d) beneficence

6. Which of the following is the principal means for protecting the rights of research subjects?

   (a) anonymity (b) beneficence

   (c) informed consent (d) confidentiality

7. The research studies conducted to evaluate new treatments, new drugs, and new or improved medical equipment is termed __________.

   (a) basic research (b) applied research

   (c) clinical trials (d) qualitative research

ANSWER KEY

1. (b) 2. (a) 3. (a) 4. (c) 5. (d) 6. (c) 7. (c)

REVIEW QUESTIONS

1. List the principles which guide ethical and legal considerations of research.
2. Describe the ethical considerations in research.
3. Explain the ethical issues in health research.
4. Explain the ethical dilemmas in conducting research and discusses the fundamental ethical principles in research.
5. Write short notes on:
   (a) Ethical issues in nursing research
   (b) Role of principal investigator in nursing research
   (c) Human ethics committee

REFERENCES

Amdur, R., & Bankert, E. (Eds). (2002). Institutional Review Board management and function. Boston: Jones & Bartlett.

American Nurses Association. (2001). Code of ethics for nurses with interpretive statements. Washington, D.C.

Arford, P.H. (2004). Working with human research protections. *Journal of Nursing Scholarship*, 35, 265–271.

Beecher, H.K. (1966). Ethics and clinical research. *The New England Journal of Medicine*, 274 (24), 1354–1360.

Bonifazi, W.L. (2004). Cruelty and Courage: Nurses in the Nasi era. *Nurse Week*, 24–26.

Burns, N., & Groves, S.K. (2005). The practice of nursing research: Conduct, critique and utilization. (5th ed.). Philadelphia: Saunders.

Centres for Disease Control and Prevention. (2006). The Tuskgee Timeline. Retrieved May 18, 2006 from http://www.cdc.gov/nchstp/od/tuskegee/time.ht.

Crane, P.B., Letvak, S., Lewallen, L., Hu, J., & Jones, E. (2004). Inclusion of women in nursing research. *Nursing Research*, 53, 237–232.

Emanuel, E.J. (2004). Ending concerns about undue inducement. *A Journal of American Society of Law, Medicine and Ethics*, 32(1), 100–105.

Erlen, J.A. (2000). "Conflict of Interest". An ethical dilemma for the nurse researcher. *Orthopedic Nursing*, 19, 74–77.

Ford, J.S., & Reuter, L.I. (1990). Ethical dilemmas associated with small samples. *Journal of Advanced Nursing*, 15(2).

Friedman, P.J. (1990). Correcting the literature following fraudulent publication. *Journal of the American Medical Association*, 263(10), 1416–1419.

Grady, P. (2005). Statement before Congress by Dr. Patricia A. Grady on the FY 2005 budget. Retrieved August 24, 2005 from http://ninr.gov/ninr/about/legislation.html.

Harden, J.T., & McFarland, G. (2000). Avoiding gender and minority barriers to NIH funding. *Journal of Nursing Scholarship*, 32, 83–86.

Havens, G.A. (2004). Ethical implications for the professional nurse of research involving human subjects. *Journal of Vascular Nursing*, 22(1), 19–23.

Hayter, J. (1979). Issues related to human subjects. In F. Downs & J. Fleming (Eds.). Issues in nursing research (107–147). New York: Appleton-Century-Crofts.

Jacobson, S.F., Chu, N.L., Pascucci, M.A., & Gaskins, S.W. (2004). Characteristics of nursing research on race, ethnicity and culture. *Journal of Multicultural Nursing and Health*, 10(3), 6–12.

Katz, K., (1972). Experimentation with human beings. New York: Russell Sage.

Kelman, H.C. (1967). Human use of human subjects: The problem of deception in social psychological experiments. Psychological experiments. *Psychological Bulletin*, 67(1), 1–11.

Krugman, S., Giles, J., & Hammond, J. (1971). Viral hepatitis, type B (MS-2 strain): Studies on active immunization. *Journal of the American Medical Association*, 217, 41–45.

Milgram, S. (1963). Behavioural study of obedience. *Journal of Abnormal and Social Psychology*, 67, 371–378.

Olsen, D.P., & Mahrenholz, D. (2000). IRB-identified ethical issues in nursing research. *Journal of Professional Nursing*, 16, 140–148.

Silva, M.C. (1995). Ethical guidelines in the conduct, dissemination, and implementation of nursing research. Washington, D.C.: American Nurses Association.

CHAPTER

9

RESEARCH DESIGN

Key terms

★ Research design ★ Descriptive studies ★ Double blind experiment ★ Ex-post-factor studies ★ Validity ★ Hawthorne effect ★ Methodological studies ★ Quasi experimental design ★ Retrospective studies ★ Solomon 4-group design ★ Non-equivalent control group design ★ One-group pre-test–post-test design ★ Post-test only control group design ★ Pre-experimental design ★ Pre-test–post-test control group design ★ Prospective studies ★ Randomization random assignment

⊙ Outline

- ★ Definition
- ★ Purposes
- ★ Elements of research design
- ★ Approach
- ★ Criteria for selecting a research design
- ★ Types of research design
- ★ Characteristics of research design
- ★ Steps of experimental research

⊙ Objectives

On completion of the chapter, you will be able to:

- ★ define research design
- ★ identify the purposes of research design
- ★ enumerate the elements of research design
- ★ recognize the criteria for the selection of research design
- ★ discuss the types of research design

Introduction

An appropriate study design is critical to the investigator's ability to answer the research question. Research design is the overall plan selected by the researcher to carry out the study and find answers to the research questions. Research design is the plan or strategy of investigations in generating and analyzing data for the study. Specific designs will be described and exemplified, and considerations for strengthening the validity and feasibility of the design will be addressed. The best design for the study depends upon the research question. Methodology refers to the study of a method and can include research on any of the related components, including design, sample or instruments.

Definitions of Research Design

Research design is the plan, structure and strategy of a study. The method of a study is the totality of how the study is carried out. Design is a part of the method and includes the sample, setting instruments, and procedure and data analysis. Research is the blueprint, whereas method is a miniature model of the study.

A research design is the determination and statement of the general research approach or strategy adopted for the particular project. It is the heart of planning.

—David J. Luck and Ronald S. Rubin

Research design is the plan, structure and strategy of investigation conceived so as to obtain answers to research questions and to control variance.

—Kerlinger

A research design is the specification of methods and procedure for acquiring the information needed. It is the overall operational pattern or framework of the project that stipulates what information is to be collected from which source and by what procedures.

—Green and Tull

Purposes of Research Design

The important purposes of research design are to:

1. provide information about the study variables measured by the investigator;
2. describe the settings where the findings of a study are likely to be similar when put into practice;
3. be helpful in finding answers to research questions;
4. eliminate bias and to reduce the margin of error in the study.

Elements of Research Design

A good research design includes a proper blend of various elements.

Research approach: It is the plan for research of the study. The study may be qualitative or quantitative. This shows the presence or absence of manipulation and control. A comparison of groups also can be seen from the approach.

Participants: They are individuals involved in research studies who are being observed or recipients of the experiment.

Variables: They are the points of focus of the study that are measured to predict the outcome of the study. There are different types of variables.

Time: The time element specifies when and how often an observation is made in the study, including the duration of the study, the specified days, place and sources of data collection.

Setting: Setting is the place where a study is being carried out, e.g. surgical wards of Medical College Hospital, Thiruvananthapuram.

Tools and methods of data analysis: The knowledge of tools used and methods of data analysis enables the researcher to collect relevant data. If the researcher does not have a formal plan of data analysis, it will result in confusion and hence faulty inferences.

Often students make mistakes in using different methods of analysis. Therefore, a definite plan of analysis is compulsory before proceeding to the study. The role of the investigator is specified in a research design, and depending upon the study topic to decide whether or not to impose control on the variables studied.

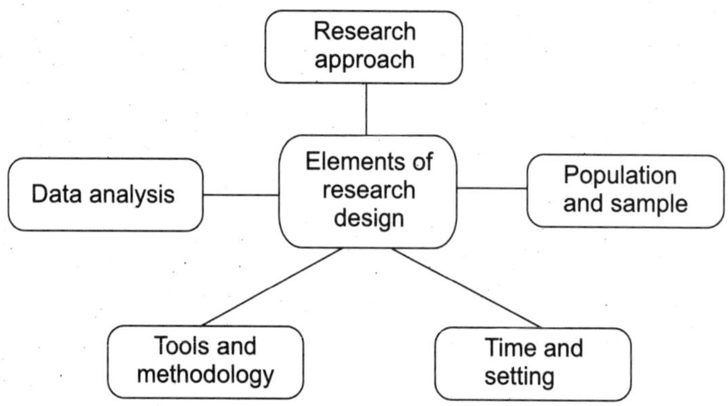

Figure 9.1 Elements of research design

Criteria for Selecting the Research Design

Selecting a suitable research design sets the framework for a superior study. The purpose of the study, theoretical framework, ethical issues, feasibility, validity, accessibility of data, accuracy, level of knowledge, nature of the topic under study, and cost are among many criteria for selecting a research design.

The essential criteria for selecting research design are:

Level of knowledge

The research design is selected based upon the extent of knowledge available on a particular research topic. When little is explored about a topic of interest, a detailed study is possible to be done.

Nature of the topic under study

The research design is selected based on the nature of research problem. Then the researcher can take a decision regarding the research design; e.g., the survey method may be experimental, quasi-experimental and non-experimental, etc.

Purpose of the study

The purpose for which the study is framed forms a part of research design.

Ethical implications and feasibility

The research design selected must be feasible and should not put unethical demands on subjects.

Availability of subjects and facilities

The availability of sufficient sample is a concern in making the research design. The characteristics of subjects, their willingness to participate in the study, and ease in locating the required sample determine the research design. The availability of facility and requirements, necessary tools, equipment and setting of the study are also crucial for research design.

Validity of data

The selected research design must yield valid data.

Accuracy

The research design helps to acquire the most accurate assessment of study variables. A design that permits the researcher to manage the factors that influence the variables maximizes the exactness of the data collected.

Experience of the researcher

Selecting a research question as per the researcher's interest and experience in other similar studies plays a role in opting for the research design.

Cost

The researcher needs to have an estimate of the anticipated cost of the study. The cost should be within the decided budget of the researcher.

Control

The control that the researcher can exercise to minimize the effect of extraneous variables maximizes the precision of results, decreases errors and determines the effectiveness of the study. The selected research design must include a homogenous sample, consistent data collection techniques and randomization for effective control over the study.

The following are guidelines for designing a study:

1. Number and type of participants
2. Selection and assignment of participants to one or more groups
3. Number of observations needed
4. Frequency of data collection

Types of Research Design

Research design can be generally classified as following:

I. Quantitative design

(A) Experimental designs

(a) True experimental designs

Post-test only design (after only design)

Pre-test–Post-test design (before-after design)

Solomon four group

Factorial design
Randomized block design
Cross-over design (repeated measure design)

(b) Quasi-experimental designs
Non-equivalent control group design
Time series design
Multiple time series design

(c) Pre-experimental designs
One shot case study
One group pre-test–post-test

(B) Non-experimental designs
(a) Descriptive design
(b) Survey design
(c) Correlational design (Ex-post-facto design)
(d) Developmental design
(e) Epidemiological design

(C) Other additional research designs
(a) Outcome research
(b) Meta analysis
(c) Methodological studies
(d) Secondary data analysis studies
(e) Evaluation studies
(f) Operational research

II. Qualitative design

(A) Phenomenological design
(B) Ethnographic design
(C) Grounded theory
(D) Historical method
(E) Case study design
(F) Action research

Table 9.1 Comparisons of research designs

Broad categories	Types of research design	Main features
Quantitative Research		
Experimental research designs	(a) True/classical experimental	Independent variable is manipulated in the presence of control group, randomization
	(b) Quasi-experimental	Independent variable is manipulated but absence of either randomization or control group
	(c) Pre-experimental	Independent variable is manipulated but limited control over extraneous variable, no control group and randomization
Non-experimental research designs	Descriptive design	Without imposing any control or manipulation, accurate description of characteristics of individual, situations or group and frequency with which a certain phenomenon occurs in natural setting
	QUALITATIVE RESEARCH	
	Phenomenological studies	This research design examines human experiences through the descriptions provided by the involved people
	Ethnographic	This research design deals with the study of people within their cultural context
	Grounded theory	This research design is developed inductively from a corpus of data acquired by a participant observer
	Historical	This research design deals with the identification, evaluation and synthesis of data from the past
	Case study	This research design studies phenomena, in depth, as a single case example
	Action research	This research design seeks action to improve practices and studies the effect of the action that was taken

Qualitative research design is the systematic, interactive and subjective approach to solve research questions. Qualitative research is concerned with qualitative phenomena. Qualitative research in nursing deals with questions related to human experiences and realities. As it studies problems in natural setting, it gives more insight into the problem studied.

Quantitative research design is the formal, objective, systematic process of testing relationships, and cause and effect between variables. It is based on the measurement of quantity and is applicable to phenomena that can be expressed in terms of quantity.

Both quantitative and qualitative research approaches help to understand the phenomena under study. Though a majority of nursing studies apply quantitative design, qualitative designs are currently in much use supported by new and valuable insights regarding the effectiveness of qualitative studies.

Experimental Research Design

Experimental research deals with cause and effect relationships. The researcher is an active member in experimental research. Experimental research is the most scientifically bound research method. Experimental research is defined as observation under controlled conditions.

Characteristics of True Experimental Design

All true experimental studies include manipulation or control of independent variables (cause) and measurement of dependent variables (effect).

The characteristics of true experiments are the following:

1. Manipulation
2. Control
3. Randomization

Manipulation

In an experimental research, the researcher manipulates the independent variables and studies its effect on the dependent variables. The dependent variables are conditions that get changed with changes in independent variables. In nursing research, the researcher manipulates a nursing intervention and applies it to some subjects while withholding the same from others.

In nursing the commonly used (manipulations) interventions are exercises, teaching, counselling, nutritional interventions, stress reduction techniques and implementation of protocols of nursing.

Control

To ascertain the validity of the design, the researcher must control the extraneous variables. Extraneous variables are those that the researcher is not able to control or that may influence the result of a study. Extraneous variables are also called confounding, intervening variables or study limitations. These variables pose a threat to both external and internal validity of the study variables.

External validity refers to the extent to which the study results can be generalized to other people and settings. Internal validity of an experimental design signifies the degree to which changes in the dependent variable (effect) can be attributed to the independent variable (cause). Internal and external validity are inversely related in an experimental design. So the researcher needs to balance both internal and external validity.

Threats to internal validity

Internal validity of an experimental study is established by Campbell and Stanley (1963) and Cook and Campbell (1979). The major threats to internal validity are:

Selection bias: Selection bias occurs when the researchers, by identifying the differences in the subjects, suitably selects the subjects for the study and manipulates the independent variables accordingly. This bias occurs mainly when the subjects are not randomly assigned to experimental and control groups. For example, in a study to assess the effect of educational programmes to quit smoking among adults, select a group of motivated adults as the experimental group and group with poor motivation to quit smoking as the control group. The results obtained will be in favour of the experimental group who are already motivated to quit smoking.

History: The threat of history occurs when some event other than the experimental intervention occurs during the course of the study. For example, the study is to identify compliance to drug therapy among adult patients with hypertension after a teaching programme. During the course of study, an article comes in a health magazine regarding hypotensive therapy. The researcher noticed that the group had more compliance to drug therapy. The researcher cannot prove that the increase in compliance is only due to the effect of his/her educational programme and not because of the influence of the article in the health magazine.

The threat can be controlled by including at least one simultaneous control or comparison group in a study and by a random selection of subjects.

Maturation: Maturation is a threat that occurs when changes within the subjects during the course of study influence the results. A change in age, height, weight, etc. of the subjects can influence the study results. This can be controlled by adding a comparison group in the study.

Testing: The threat of testing occurs when the subjects are provided with a pre-test or the subjects have baseline knowledge. The subjects may remember the answers and put the right answer in the post-test. For example, in a glycemic control programme, the subjects who were told as having elevated blood sugar level will try to reduce the blood sugar level irrespective of the intervention planned by the researcher.

Instrumentation change: The threat of instrumentation change occurs due to the difference between the pre-test and post-test measurement caused by the change in the accuracy of the instrument or the researcher's ratings rather than the result of experimental intervention. By checking throughout the study, the accuracy of instruments used and by frequently assessing fatigue factors and arranging training sessions for judges, threat factor can be controlled.

Mortality: Mortality is the term used to the situation in which there is wide difference in the dropout rate between the experimental and the control groups. If a group who scored worst in the pre-test dropped out, the final result which concluded that the experimental intervention was very effective may not be generalized. Mortality is difficult to manage, as the participants have the right to abstain from the study whenever they want to. Reducing the duration of the study as well as helping the participants recognizes the importance of their continued participation in the study helps to reduce the threat.

Interactions with selection: This means that a number of previously described threats to validity can interact with selection causing spurious treatment effects, e.g. selection-maturation, selection-history, and selection-instrumentation.

Diffusion or imitation of treatments: It refers to the introduction of a treatment that involves information that the experimental and control group participants may be able to interact with one another, directly or indirectly, and learn about information intended for others.

Compensatory equalization of treatments: This refers to the use of an experimental treatment that has actual potential value to participate in cases in which authorities or participants may be unwilling to tolerate an imposed inequity in the distribution of treatment.

Compensatory rivalry by respondents receiving less desirable treatment: This deals with the fact that the control group participants are disadvantaged by the absence of the treatment in contrast to experimental participants and thus are motivated to compete for equity. Compensatory equalization is mainly a response by administrators, and compensatory rivalry is a response by participants.

Threats to external validity

The major threats to external validity are the experimenter effect, Hawthorne effect and the reactive effect of pre-test.

Hawthorne effect: When the participants know that they are being observed, they behave in a innocent manner. This effect is known as Hawthorne effect. The term was coined as a result of studies on worker productivity at the Hawthorne plant of the Western Electric Company. Hawthorne effect may also pose threat to internal validity. The threat can be controlled by conducting a double-blind study where neither the researcher nor the participants are aware of the particular group in which they are being involved (i.e. either experimental or control group).

Experimenter effect: The threat that occurs when the researcher's characteristics influence the subject's behaviour is termed as experimenter effect. The physical appearance, age, gender, body-build and even facial expressions can influence the subjects. The Rosenthal effect is a term with similar meaning used in non-experimental studies. It refers to the influence of the interviewer on respondent's answers.

Reactive effects of the pre-test: The threat is also termed measurement effect. This occurs when the subjects are already exposed to a pre-test or when they have the knowledge regarding baseline data. Unlike the threat of testing where it acts as the cause for the post-test result, reactive effects act as a catalyst in producing the post-test measurement results.

Interaction of selection and treatment: It refers to the effects obtained that are applicable only to the specific individual who participated in the study.

Interaction of setting and treatment: The threat refers to the effects obtained that are applicable only to the specific setting in which the experiment is conducted.

Interactions of history and treatment: It refers to the effects obtained that are applied only to the specific timeframe within which the study is conducted. Unusual occurrences that coincide with a study period can make an extrapolation of results to other periods of time questionable. Replication of study at different times is the logical approach to counteracting the interaction effect of history.

Randomization

Randomization is a process that ensures that each unit in a target population has an equal chance of being chosen for the study and also that each sample has the equal chance of being selected to either the experimental or control group. Experimental studies are done in carefully controlled conditions, possibly eliminating all the threats that can affect the outcome of the study. Randomization is considered as an important process that reduces bias in the study.

Methods of randomization

1. Flip of a coin for each participant can be used for randomization. The participants can be categorized to control or experimental group depending on the side of the coin.
2. Lot method also can be used. Write the names of the subjects on slips of paper and put the slips into a bowl and then draw lots. The first designated numbers are put into one group and the rest are given to another group.
3. Random table (see Appendix) may be used to facilitate the randomization process. Here blind-folded subjects choose a number from a table of numbers horizontally (rows or columns) till the required number is reached for both experimental and control groups. Computer-assisted random sequences also may be used for the assignment of participants.

Major Steps in Experimental Design

Experimental design involves a series of steps. The important steps are:

1. The population for the study should be identified and defined.
2. Select the required sample by random sampling.
3. Subdivide the sample into experimental and control groups by random sampling.
4. The characteristics of both groups are to be observed and recorded.
5. Implement the independent variable (intervention) into the experimental group, withholding it from the control group.
6. Assess the dependent variable in both the groups after implementation for any changes.
7. Compare the changes and record the differences.
8. Compare the values statistically and identify the significance of the differences.

Symbolic representation of research design

Research designs are expressed in terms of symbols. The symbols used in research design are:

R	=	Random assignment of subjects to groups
O	=	Observation or measurement of dependent variable
X	=	Experimental treatment or intervention
X_1	=	First intervention
X_2	=	Second intervention
O_1	=	First observation
O_2	=	Second observation

In the example,

R	O_1	X	O_2	(Experimental group)
R	O_1		O_2	(Control group)

An observation was made in both randomly selected experimental and control groups after which intervention was given only to the experimental group. Thereafter, a second observation or post-test was conducted in both groups.

Types of Experimental Design

A. True or Classical Experimental Design

The researcher has greater control over true experimental design. Threats to internal validity are greatly reduced in this experimental design. It follows three criteria for an experimental design in order to reduce bias.

1. The researcher manipulates the experimental variables.
2. One experimental and one control group are at least present.
3. Random selection of subjects.

Seven types of true experimental designs are follows:

(a) Post-test only control group

The design is also known as after-only control group design. This design also comprises two groups (experimental and control group) which are randomly assigned. But neither of these groups are previously measured or pre-tested. The design can be represented as:

R	X	O_1	(Experimental)
R		O_1	(Control)

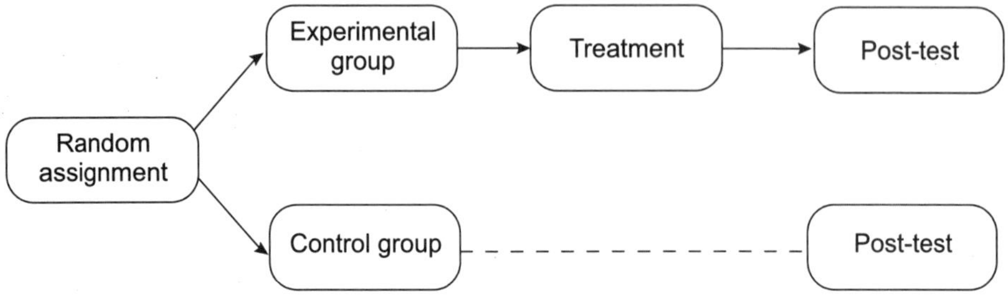

Figure 9.2 Post-test only control group design

In the design, experimental intervention is given only to the experimental group. The control group receives routine or no treatment. Then a post-test evaluation or observation is given. The study is employed when a pre-test cannot be applied or when there is no significance in applying a pre-test.

Merits

1. The threat of reactive effect of pre-test is absent.
2. Easier to carry out than pre-test–post-test group design.
3. The results have more generalizability.
4. There is equitability in number for both experimental and control group.

Demerit

No comparison of pre-test and post-test values possible.

(b) Pre-test–Post-test control group design

This is the most frequently used design. The research design can be symbolically depicted as:

R O_1 X O_2 (Experimental group)

R O_1 O_2 (Control group)

In this design, subjects are randomly assigned to control and experimental groups. A pre-test or observation is given to both groups. Experimental intervention is given to the experimental group whereas control group receives routine care or no intervention. Thereafter, a post-test or observation is made in both groups.

The researcher must ensure that both groups are similar in characteristics. If the groups are not equivalent, the post-test scores must be adjusted statistically.

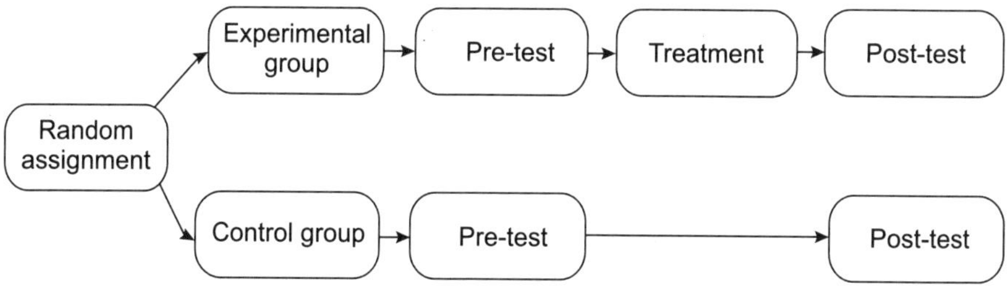

Figure 9.3 Pre-test–Post-test control group design

Merit

The researcher can account for the events that occur between pre-test and post-test through the observation of control group.

Demerits

1. Threat of reactive effects of pre-test may exist in the design.
2. The results can be generalized in situations where a pre-test could be administered.

Pre-test–Post-test control group design can be used in the study of the following topics:

1. "Effect of Exercise Programme on Post-operative Outcome of Women Undergoing Caesarian Section"
2. "Effect of Relaxation Therapy on Level of Stress and Physiological Outcome of Women with Pregnancy-induced Hypertension"
3. "Impact of Prizes on Productivity of Employees in an Institution"

(c) Solomon 4-group design

In Solomon 4-group design, the researcher randomly divides the sample into four groups, namely two experimental groups and two control groups. One experimental and one control group are given pre-test or observed before experiment. For the other control and experimental group, no pre-test is administered. Intervention is applied for only the experimental groups and post-test or second observation is made for all four groups. It is symbolically represented as:

R	O_1	X	O_2	(Experimental group)
R	O_1		O_2	(Control group)
R	X	O_2		(Experimental group)
R		O_2		(Control group)

The Solomon 4-group design is considered to be the most ideal one as it minimizes both internal and external threat to validity.

Advantages *of Solomon 4-group design*

1. Since all four groups are studied at the same time, the effects of events occurring between two observations are controlled.
2. Maturation threat is controlled.

Disadvantages

1. Large sample size is needed.
2. Complicated statistical analysis is required.

(d) Factorial design

This type of design allows the researcher to test multiple hypotheses in a single experiment. It is possible to manipulate two or more variables simultaneously. Here the subjects can be assigned to a combination of conditions, and thus the main interaction effects can be elicited. In factorial design, the major independent variable is known as *factor.* The subdivision of a factor is called *level.*

Merits

1. Able to test multiple independent factors.
2. Used when levels of interventions and specific combinations of interventions are assessed.

Demerit

Large number of subjects is required to obtain statistical significance.

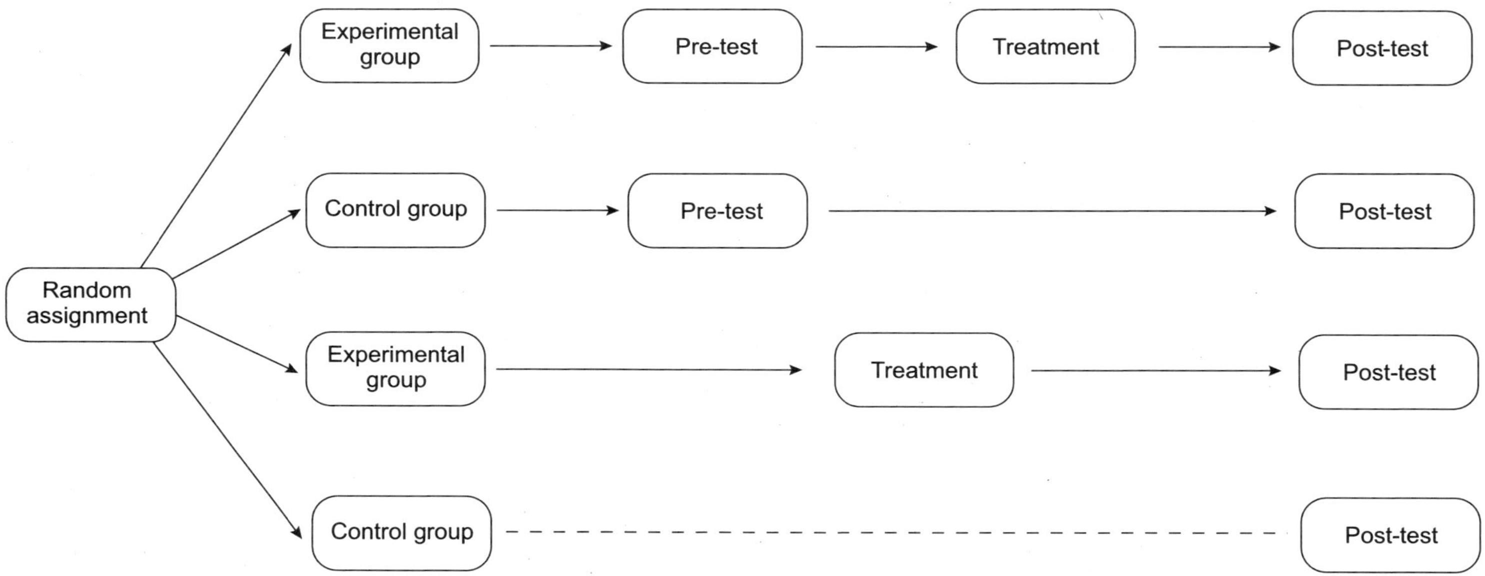

Figure 9.4 Solomon 4-group design

(e) Cross-over design

It is also known as 'repeated measure design'. As the name suggests, it deals with exposing the same subjects to more than one experiment. This design is extremely powerful in yielding a good outcome. The effectiveness of two or more interventions can be clearly found out using this method. A major disadvantage of this method is *carry-over effect*, i.e. the influence of the first intervention may persist when the subjects are exposed to the second intervention.

(f) Randomized block control

It is similar to factorial design. In this type there are two factors, but one cannot be manipulated. Variables such as age, sex, race, geographical location or hospital unit which cannot be manipulated are known as *blocking variables.* The researcher may suspect that these may be confounding variables. So as to control this problem, the researcher can design a study in which the potentially confounding variable is incorporated into the study design as an independent variable; this technique is known as blocking. Subjects are then randomly assigned with each block. For example, a researcher could block by age to test the effectiveness of rehabilitation on stroke patients, if it was assumed that younger subjects would show better recovery than older subjects. Rehabilitation will be easy and quick for these patients. Specific age categories are developed and subjects within each category are assigned to each treatment group.

Merit

Generalization is easy as it uses a large number of samples.

Demerits

1. It is necessary to have an equal number of subjects with the blocking variables.
2. Large number of subjects is required.

(g) Clinical trials

It is one of the most rigorous study designs, and also known as intervention studies. The main focus is on clinical outcomes. It can be either experimental or quasi-experimental depending upon the degree to which randomization is used to select the subjects and assign them to treatment groups. Two major types of clinical trials are therapeutic and preventive. Therapeutic trials determine the effectiveness of treatment in reducing symptoms, preventing relapse, or reducing the risk of death associated with specific illness. Preventive trials determine whether a specific treatment reduces the risk associated with developing a specific disease. The common type of clinical trials is drug studies which are designed to test the efficacy of new types of medications.

Merits

1. The relationship between treatment and outcome is clearly established; hence it provides a strong evidence for inferring causation.
2. When randomization is used in clinical trials, threats to internal and external validity can be reduced and also both known and unknown confounders can be controlled.

Demerits

1. Expensive
2. Ethical consideration is involved in administering treatments in which the risks and benefits of the treatment are not clearly identified.
2. In an experimental study, it may lack generalizability because of the structured and contrived research setting.

Strengths and Weaknesses of True Experimental Design

Advantages

1. Research designs are most superior to other methods and are considered most powerful designs to establish causal relationships between independent and dependent variables.
2. The conditions not found in a natural setting can be created in an experimental setting where an independent variable is manipulated by the researcher.

3. It is beneficial in maximizing systematic variance and in controlling extraneous and error variance.
4. The outcome of a research study gives a greater degree of purity in observation.

Disadvantages

1. The sample selected must be representative and homogenous.
2. Often the population may be unknown.
3. Artificiality in laboratory testing.
4. Threat of Hawthorne effect.
5. Issues related to relevant outcome variables, validity, reliability and systematic bias.

B. Quasi-experimental Design

This design is similar to true experimental design lacking at least one of the other two properties that characterize true experiments. In quasi-experimental designs there are no control groups and subjects are neither randomly assigned to groups.

Quasi-experimental designs are primarily used in social sciences. The term 'quasi' means resembling or likeness. Quasi-experimental designs came about because of the following reasons:

1. Classical experimental method is very difficult to apply in social sciences.
2. Overemphasis on theory testing and development.
3. Classic natural science methods are expensive.
4. Development of new statistical tools that allowed for statistical control.

Many different designs fall into the category of quasi-experimental design. They are:

1. Non-equivalent control group
2. Time series design
3. Multiple time series design

Non-equivalent control group design

Quasi-experimental design is the most frequently used design. It is similar to pre-test, post-test control group design except there is non-random selection of subjects to experimental and control groups.

O_1 X O_2 (Experimental)

O_1 O_2 (Control)

The groups selected are naturally assembled collections such as in a classroom or in a clinic. The researcher selects a more similar group. The similarity can be assessed by pre-test scores. The more similar the score, the more similar is the group.

The experimental group receives the intervention, followed by post-test on second observation of both the groups. Selecting the two groups helps the researcher to determine whether the independent variable actually made a difference in the experiment group.

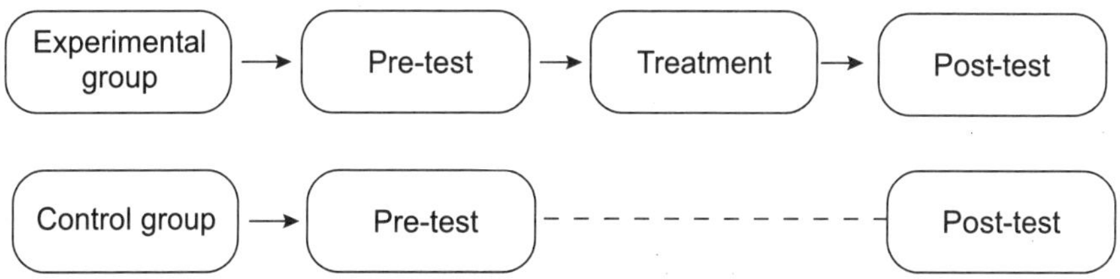

Figure 9.5 Non-equivalent control group design

Non-equivalent post-test design

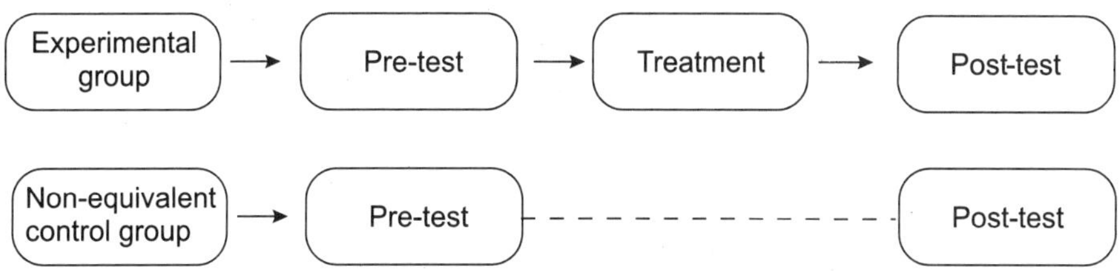

Figure 9.6 Non-equivalent post-test design

This is similar to post-test true experimental design. The design consists of administering an outcome measure to two non-randomly selected groups (experimental and control groups). The effect of the intervention is assessed by a post-test or observation of both groups. Non-equivalent control group design prevents threat to internal validity such as history, testing, maturation, instrumentation, change and selection bias.

Time series design (single group time series design)

In time series design, periodical assessments are obtained from the subjects. The experimental intervention is administered between two of the observations.

	Before	X	After
Experimental group	$O_1O_2O_3O_4O_5$	X	$O_6O_7O_8O_9O_{10}$

These observations are made at periodical intervals (e.g. period of one week).

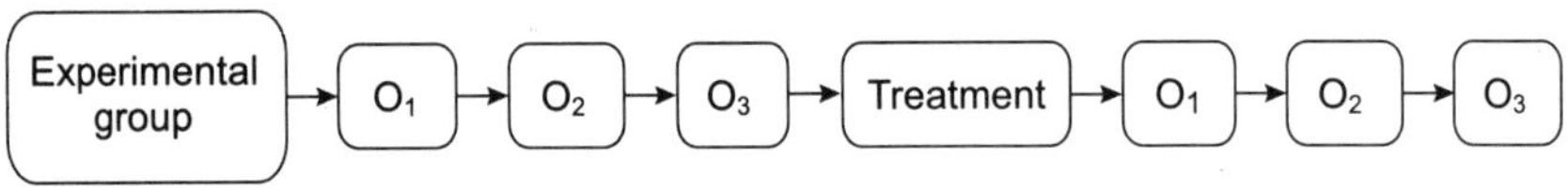

Figure 9.7 Time series design

Multiple time series design

The multiple time series design is similar to that of one-group time series experimental design, except that the control group is added.

	Before	X	After
Experimental	$O_1O_2O_3$	X	$O_4O_5O_6$
Control	$O_1O_2O_3$		$O_4O_5O_6$

The addition of control group and the manipulation of independent variable along with periodical assessment increase the generalizability and validity of the finding. The greatest threats to validity in time series design are history and testing.

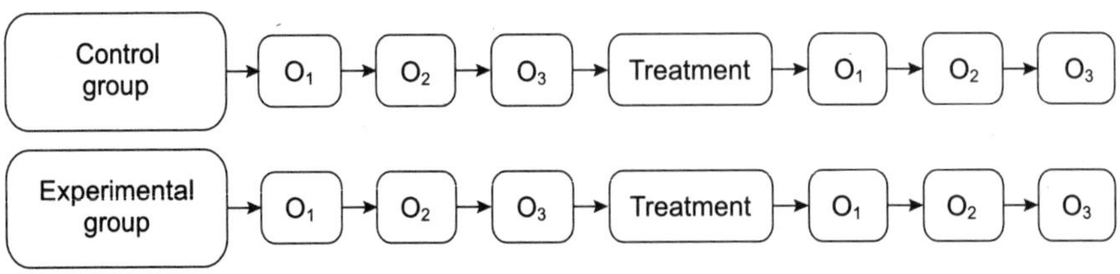

Figure 9.8 Multiple time series design

Merits ***of quasi-experimental design***

1. Compared to true experimental designs, quasi-experimental design is easy to set up.
2. It takes much less effort to study and compare subjects or groups of subjects that are already organized than to have to conduct random assignments of subjects.
3. The design minimizes threat to external validity as natural environments do not suffer the same problems of artificiality as compared to a well-controlled laboratory setting.
4. As quasi-experiments are natural experiments, findings in one may be applied to other subjects and settings, allowing better generalization.
5. The method is effective in longitudinal research that involves longer time periods which can be followed up in different environments.
6. The great strength of quasi-experiments lies in their practicality, feasibility and to a certain extent generalizability.
7. Some control over extraneous variables is possible when full experimental control is lacking.

Demerits ***of quasi-experimental design***

1. The control allowed through the manipulation of quasi-independent variable can lead to unnatural circumstances.
2. This type of design is often opted for field studies where random selection of experimental subjects is impractical, unethical or impossible.
3. Lack of randomization may pose many challenges in terms of internal validity. This makes it even harder to rule out confounding variables.
4. In the absence of randomization, conclusions of causal relationship are difficult to determine due to a variety of extraneous and confounding variables that exist in a social environment.

C. Pre-experimental Designs

Campell and Stanley (1963) coined the term pre-experimental designs to those experimental designs that are considered weak. The researcher has little control over the research.

Types of Pre-experimental Designs

(a) One-shot case study or single case study

In this type of design, a single group is exposed to an experimental treatment and observed after the treatment. It is represented as

X O

A group of patients with diabetic foot ulcer is given a class on self-care and tested for their knowledge level about self-care after the completion of the class. Since no comparison was made, it is difficult to determine whether the level of knowledge exhibited was the result of the class. The design does not control any threats to internal validity. History, maturation and selection bias are the threats to internal validity.

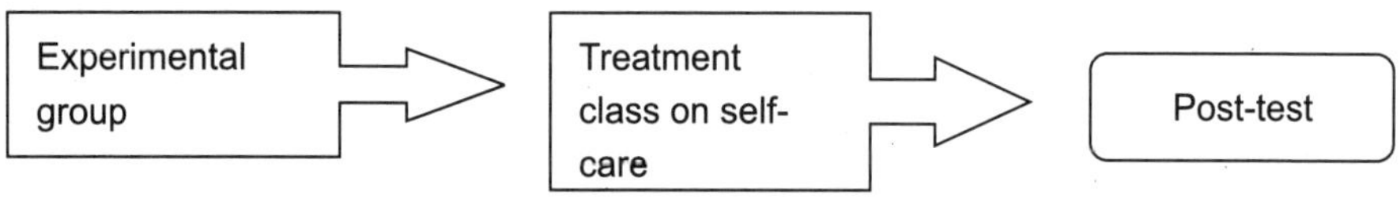

Figure 9.9 One-shot case design

(b) One-group pre-test–post-test design

The one-group pre-test–post-test design provides a pre-test and post-test or observation before and after the experimental intervention. It is represented as

Before After

O_1 X O_2

This design has a threat to internal validity as history, maturation, testing and instrumentation change. This design may be used in situations where it is not possible to have a control group.

Advantages

1. Easy to conduct studies in natural settings, commonly in nursing.
2. This design is appropriate for beginners in the field of experimental designs.

Disadvantages

1. Control over the research is minimal.
2. Threat to internal validity is more and may have a selection bias.

Very weak research design to establish causal relationship between independent and dependent variables.

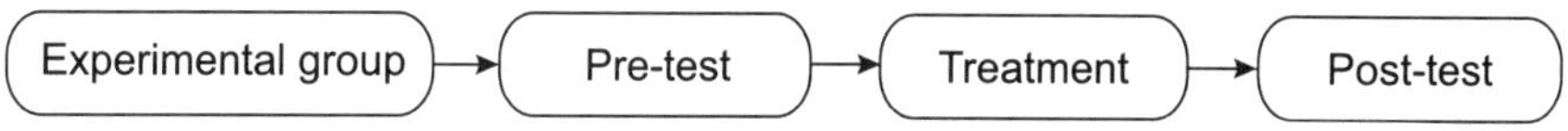

Figure 9.10 One-group pre-test–post-test design

Non-experimental Design

In cases where it is unethical to conduct experimental research on human beings, the study is conducted as a non-experimental design research study. In fact all non-experimental research is descriptive as there is no manipulation and control of variables; the researcher only describes the phenomenon as it exists.

In non-experimental design, measures to control extraneous variables must be taken to obtain valid study results.

Types of Non-experimental Design

There are many types of non-experimental designs. The most common types are the following:

1. Survey design
2. Correlational design/Ex-post-facto design
3. Developmental design
4. Methodological studies
5. Secondary analysis studies

(a) Survey Studies

A survey is assigned to obtain information about the prevalence, distribution and interrelationships of variables. Survey design collects data by means of self-report. This branch of research examines the characteristics, behaviour, attitude and intentions of a group by asking the subjects a series of questions. The data can be collected in a number of ways. The most common methods are personal face to face interview, over telephones or self-administered questions through mail. It enables the investigators to collect current information about what they wish to study.

Surveys, depending upon the objectives, may be descriptive, exploratory, explanatory, comparative and evaluative surveys.

Descriptive survey: The only objective of a descriptive study is to be descriptive. The design describes objectively the nature of situations, behaviour or attitude under study.

Exploratory survey: In this design, the researcher explores regions of a situation or phenomena about which little is known. Through this design, the researcher opens up new boundaries for extensive research rather than mere understanding of the relationship between phenomena.

Explanatory survey: This design is applied in studies to assess the causal relationship between two variables, phenomena or situations. Thcsc studies often involve testing of hypothesis with more significance to the qualitative aspects of the data.

The design needs cause and effect associated with each other in which the causes precede the effect and other explanations for the phenomena present must be ruled out. The researcher in this design needs more sophisticated level of knowledge. The researcher should be familiar with what is so far known about the phenomena under study.

Comparative survey: It compares similar aspects of two distinct groups. It could be knowledge perception or attitude level. A comparative study is different from experimental study in the fact that there is no manipulation of the independent variable.

A comparative study can be used for research studies where the independent variable manipulation is unethical. To study the effect of pelvic floor exercise programme on stress incontinence among antenatal mothers, it could be unethical to select a group that receives pelvic floor exercise programme and a group which does not.

Comparative studies could be prospective or retrospective studies.

In **retrospective studies**, for the dependent variable (effect) identified in the present, an attempt is made to identify the independent variables (cause) that have occurred in the past. Such studies are also termed as **ex-post facto studies** (after-the-fact studies).

In **prospective studies**, the effect (dependent variable) of the present cause (independent variable) is assessed in the future. Prospective studies use an experimental approach. Much of prospective studies are costly and participant dropout rate is also high. So they are less common than retrospective studies. Prospective studies are commonly used by epidemiologists.

Evaluative survey: This survey is characterized by an evaluation judgement that would be made about the respondents. The evaluation would be formative evaluation (which is an ongoing evaluation), summative evaluation (where merits and demerits are evaluated at the end of the development of a programme) or free evaluation (where an external evaluator reviews the findings).

Merits *of survey studies*

1. Data collection is in a natural setting.
2. Variables are assessed as they exist in the social therapeutic environment.
3. The design reaches a large number of subjects and needs less time to administer.
4. A valid result will be obtained if the study is carefully planned.

Demerits

1. Only self-report is assessed.
2. Can involve bias when the response rate is low.
3. Researcher loses the feel of the situation unless he does an interview.

(b) Correlational Studies

In a correlational study, the researcher evaluates the relationship between two or more variables. It measures the strength or to what extent one variable is related to another by determining how changes in one variable are associated with another.

The magnitude and directions of a correlation study is indicated by a correlation coefficient. The correlation coefficient may be positive or negative and range from –1.00 to 1.00. A correlation coefficient of 0.00 indicates no relationship between the variables. These are reported through various statistical analyses such as Pearson's correlation coefficient, Spearman rank correlation coefficient, etc.

A positive relationship indicates a direct relationship; that is, when the value of one variable increases the value of other variable also increases. A negative relationship signifies an indirect relationship; that is, when the value of one variable increases the value of other variable decreases. As the score value increases and reaches up to 1.00, the relationship becomes stronger. The variable that comes first in chronological order is the independent variable and influences the other variable.

Advantages of the *design*

1. Increased flexibility while examining complex relationships.
2. Suitable to collect longer amount of data.
3. Sets the foundation for future studies.
4. To assess relationship between variables that cannot be manipulated.

Disadvantages

1. Investigator is unable to manipulate the variable of interest.
2. Randomization in sampling is not possible which reduces generalizability of the findings.
3. Unable to determine casual relationship between variables due to lack of manipulation, control and randomization.

(c) Developmental Studies

Developmental study design is concerned with changes that take place in a fraction of time. There are two types of study design in developmental studies.

1. Cross-sectional and longitudinal studies
2. Retrospective and prospective studies

Cross-sectional studies

Here, the researcher collects data from subjects at one point of time. The design is appropriate for describing the status of phenomena or relationship among them at a fixed point in time. In an assessment of knowledge and practice regarding infection control measures among nurses working in labour rooms, the assessment from the participants is done at one point of time.

An advantage of cross-sectional studies is that the design is more practical, economical and easy to manage.

Longitudinal studies

In a longitudinal design, data is collected from the same group at different points of time. The basic difference between cross-sectional and longitudinal design is the time factor. Though longitudinal studies are disadvantageous in terms of time, effort and money, increased depth of responses can be obtained through such studies. Longitudinal studies are subjected to bias by confounding variables that interfere with the interpretation of the results. Subjects in such studies respond in a desirable way that is incongruent with investigators' expectations.

Retrospective studies

Here the investigator tries to link present events to that which have occurred in the past. The study begins in the present and connects back to the past and so termed ex-post facts studies.

E.g.: "Assessing Pre-disposing Factors of Peptic Ulcers for the Development of the Illness"

Prospective studies

This study design begins with the cause and then moves forward to determine the effect. The study starts in the present and ends in the future.

(d) Methodological Studies

Methodological studies include those studies aimed at developing, testing and evaluating research instruments and methods. With increased interest in the area of research, these studies are gaining much attention.

(e) Secondary Analysis Studies

This type of design collects a large amount of data, but may not actually analyze the entire data collected. The researcher analyzes data that was collected in the previous study. This type of design is most economical and efficient.

Research Design Based on the Setting of Study

A study is conducted based on the setting; research design is classified as laboratory studies and field studies. Laboratory studies are conducted on subjects in a special environment created by the researcher. In this type of study, the research environment is controlled by the researcher. Field studies are those conducted in the field or in a real-life situation, where not much control is maintained by the researcher.

Simulation studies are also a type of laboratory studies in which the researcher measures subject's response to the description of case studies that represent real-life situations.

Qualitative Research Design

Qualitative research design evolves over the course of the project. It is more flexible and adjusting to the situation of the study. Qualitative studies tend to be holistic and involve intense involvement of the researcher. Qualitative research design requires ongoing analysis of the data to formulate suitable strategies. In short, qualitative research involves merging of various data collection strategies and using a variety of methods. This tendency is termed bricolage, and the qualitative researcher is thus referred as a bricoleur, a person who is adept at performing a large number of diverse tasks managing from interviewing intensive reflections and introspection.

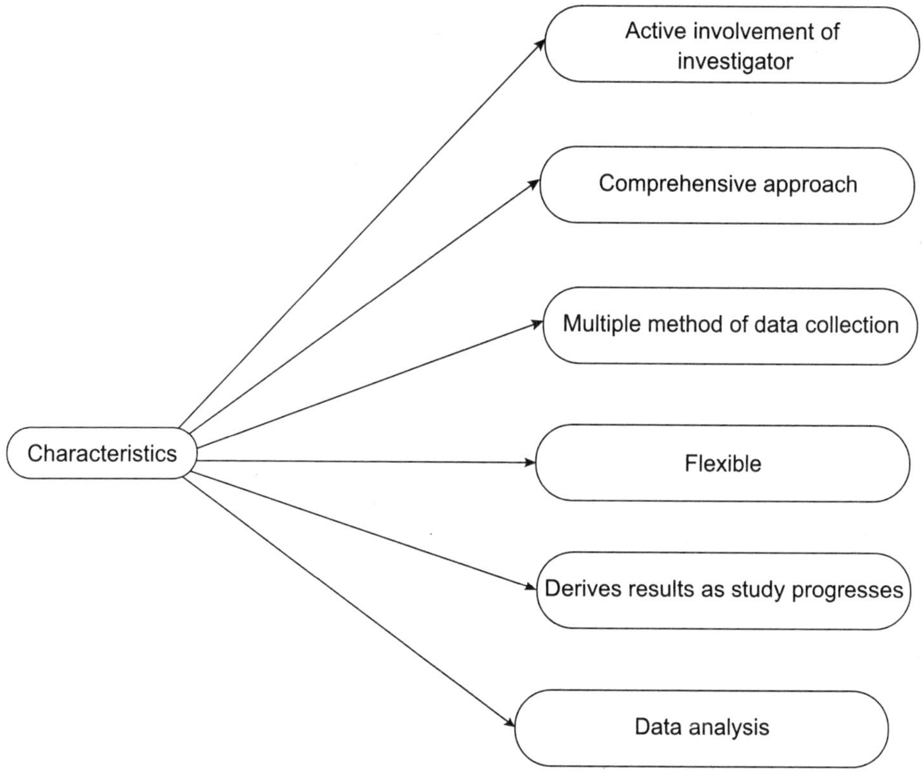

Figure 9.11 Characteristics of qualitative research

Types of Qualitative Research Design

The common types of qualitative design include the following:

1. Phenomenological
2. Ethnographic
3. Grounded theory
4. Historical
5. Case study
6. Action research

Phenomenological Studies

Phenomenological studies assess human experiences through descriptions provided by the people involved. These studies are also called lined experiences. A phenomenological study may focus on a specific health, illness, healing and dying phenomenon or experience. These factors help to gain in-depth understanding of human conditions.

In phenomenological research, the respondents are asked to describe their experience as they perceive them better through an interview. The researcher must first identify what he/she expects to discover and then puts aside those ideas; this process is called bracketing. Only then it is possible to view the experience from the eyes of the person who has lived the experience. Data collection and analysis occur simultaneously.

Donak (2004) wrote that "conducting qualitative research is a challenging, exciting and at times exhaustive process." Phenomenological studies could be difficult to understand especially when the researcher has a little knowledge in psychology.

Ethnographic Studies

Ethnographics is the study of people within their cultured context. It is commonly used in nursing research to study phenomena of health and illness within a cultural, community or environmental context.

Characteristics of ethnic design

It is a holistic combination that provides description about the lifestyle and activities of people in their natural environment. The participants are often considered co-researchers. Identification of cultural themes may lead to the development of theory.

The techniques used by the researcher include participant observations, unstructured or minimally structured interviews, examinations of cultural artifacts, photography, etc. to understand the experience of people within a culture. Ethnographic designs lead to the development of culturally congruent health care interventions and outcomes. The term culture used in ethnographic design specifies, in a broader sense, an entire tribe (e.g. Indians) or in a narrow sense to mean one nursing care unit. Ethnography is in fact the principal method used by anthropologists to study people all over the world.

Grounded Theory Studies

Grounded theory is a qualitative research approach developed by sociologists Glaser and Strauss in 1960's. Grounded theory designs are those studies in which data is collected and analyzed followed by the development of a theory that is grounded in the data. Grounded theory is based on conceptualization of the participant's behaviour.

The fundamental feature of the design is that data collection, data analysis and sampling of the participants occur simultaneously. Method of theoretical sampling, participant observation and in-depth interview and constant comparative analysis form the framework of the design. The data are recorded through handwritten notes and tape recordings.

Diversity rather than similarity is needed in the sample selected. The design assumes that from the diverse data gathered, it is possible to discover fundamental patterns in social life. These patterns are termed basic social processes. The researcher throughout the study makes corrections and adjustments to the theory to allow for the interpretation of new data obtained.

Historical Studies

Historical designs deal with the identification, evaluation and synthesis of data from the past. The historical researcher links the past with present and future. The approach is used when the researcher finds that describing a significant life event facilitates better understanding. The process of historical research is basically the same as in other types of scientific research.

The data are often collected from documents or from relics and artifacts. The data can also be collected through oral reports. The materials can be found in libraries, archives or in personal collections. The sources of historical data can be classified as primary sources and secondary sources. Primary sources provide direct information. Secondary sources provide information from other sources. Oral history, written records, diaries, eyewitnesses, pictorial sources and physical evidences are examples of primary sources.

The data collected is scrutinized for two types of evaluation, namely external and internal criticism. External criticism deals with the authenticity of data collected. An internal criticism refers to the accuracy of data collected.

External criticism analyzes whether the sources obtained are valid and reliable. Internal criticism is much difficult as it evaluates whether an accurate recording of events was made as they happened.

Case Studies

Case studies are in-depth investigations of a single entity or a small number of entities. The entity could be an individual, family, group, institution, community or other social unit. Case studies are meant to explore real clinical situations in-depth.

Case studies may be considered qualitative or quantitative research depending on the purpose of the study. It cannot be used to test hypothesis, but hypotheses may be generated from case studies.

The methods of data collection commonly used in case studies are questionnaires, interviews, observations or written account by the subjects. The data collected are analyzed and interpreted. Content analysis is done in evaluating data from case studies. Case study designs are time-consuming and could be costly. Problems such as dropouts should be considered when the study period exceeds.

There are four basic types of design for case studies.

1. Single case, holistic
2. Single case, embedded
3. Multiple case, holistic
4. Multiple case, embedded

A simple case study deals with a single, unique and a typical case which is often a longitudinal study. A multiple case design involves more than one single case. A holistic design examines the global nature of the case as such.

An embedded design involves analysis of more than one unit. Intrinsic and instrumental case studies are other types of case studies. Evaluation of the process of implementing an innovation is a type of intrinsic case study. In instrumental case study, the researcher identifies a research question and then seeks out a case that offers more information on the research question selected.

Intensive probing often leads to insights concerning previously unexpected relationship. Case study design also helps to clarify concepts or to find ways to capture them.

Action Research Studies

Action research studies are concerned with actions taken to improve practice and study the effect of those actions. Solutions are found to deal with a situation in a particular setting. The findings are not generalized. Implementation of the solution occurs in the course of the research process.

SUMMARY

Different types of designs along with their advantages and disadvantages are discussed. A detailed classification of research designs is elicited, which helps the researcher identify the chief features. Selecting a design for the study demands the consideration of many factors. In the long run, however, a study that is well-designed balances validity and feasibility to answer the research questions. Therefore, a design has to be chosen carefully.

MULTIPLE CHOICE QUESTIONS

1. Retrospective studies are also called __________.
   (a) prospective
   (b) ex-post facto/comparative studies
   (c) descriptive
   (d) longitudinal
2. The most powerful research method for establishing causal relationship is the __________.
   (a) correlational method
   (b) descriptive method
   (c) causal comparative method
   (d) experimental method

3. The type of survey approach appropriate for studying the effectiveness of a particular method useful to meet the criteria stated is __________.
   - (a) comparative
   - (b) cross-sectional
   - (c) evaluative
   - (d) descriptive
4. The research design in which there is either no comparison group or no random assignment of subjects to group is __________.
   - (a) pre-experimental designs
   - (b) quasi-experimental designs
   - (c) Solomon 4-group designs
   - (d) post-test-only control group design
5. When study participants respond in a certain manner knowing that they are being observed is termed __________.
   - (a) reactive effects
   - (b) attrition
   - (c) experimental effect
   - (d) Hawthorne effect
6. The process in which qualitative researchers put aside their own feeling and beliefs about the phenomena under consideration to keep from biasing their observation is __________.
   - (a) inductive reasoning
   - (b) debriefing
   - (c) bracketing
   - (d) internal criticism
7. The term used to indicate the examination of communication message obtained in case studies: __________
   - (a) external criticism
   - (b) historical studies
   - (c) content analysis
   - (d) action research
8. A special kind of action research in which there is collaboration between the study participants and the researcher in all steps of the study: __________
   - (a) participatory action research (PAR)
   - (b) action research
   - (c) case studies
   - (d) content analysis

ANSWER KEY

1. (b) 2. (d) 3. (c) 4. (b) 5. (d) 6. (c) 7. (c) 8. (a)

REVIEW QUESTIONS

1. (a) Define research design.

   (b) Explain the importance of research design.

2. (a) Write the classification of types of research design.

   (b) Discuss the advantages and disadvantages of experimental research.

3. Write short notes on:

   (a) Threats to internal validity

   (b) Threats to external validity

   (c) Survey studies

   (d) Characteristics of experimental research

4. (a) What is historical method of research?

   (b) Explain the advantages and disadvantages of historical method of research.

5. (a) Define experimental research.

   (b) Explain the steps of conducting an experimental study by quoting example from critical area.

6. (a) What is survey method?

   (b) Discuss the different types of survey method.

7. List the elements of experimental research. Explain each one.

8. (a) Define survey method.

   (b) Explain the elements of survey research.

9. What is correlational study design?

10. What are the factors to be considered while selecting research methods?

11. (a) Write the classification of research design.

    (b) Explain the characteristics of qualitative research design.

REFERENCES

Blair, C.E. (1995). Combining behaviour management and mutual goal setting to reduce physical dependency in nursing home residents. *Nursing Research*, 44(3), 160–165.

Campbell, D.T., & Fiske, D.W. (1959). Convergent and discriminant validation by the multitrait-multimethod matrix. *Psychological Bulletin*, 56(2), 81–105.

Clarke, P.N., & Yaros, P.S. (1988). Research blenders: Commentary and response. *Nursing Science Quarterly*, 1(4), 47–149.

Cook, T.D., & Campbell, D.T. (1979). Quasi-experimentation: Design and analysis issues for field settings. Chicago: Rand McNally.

Denzin, N.K. (1989). The research act: A theoretical introduction to sociological methods. (3rd ed.) New York: McGraw-Hill.

Dodd, M., Thomas, M., & Dibble, S. (1991). Self-care for patients experiencing cancer chemotherapy side effects: A concern for home care nurses. *Home Healthcare*, 9(6), 21–26.

________. (1992). Outpatient chemotherapy: Patients' and family members' concerns and coping strategies. *Public Health Nursing*, 9(1), 37–44.

Duffy, M.E. (1987). Methodological triangulation: A vehicle for merging quantitative and qualitative research methods. *Journal of Nursing Scholarship*, 19(3), 130–133.

Fredriksdottir, N., & McCarthy, D.O. (1995). The effect of caloric density of food on energy intake and body weight in tumor-bearing rats. *Research in Nursing and Health*, 18(4), 357–363.

Good, M. (1995). A comparison of the effects of jaw relaxation and music on postoperative pain. *Nursing Research*, 44(1), 52–57.

Goodwin, L.D. (1984). Increasing efficiency and precision of data analysis: Multivariate vs. unvaried statistical techniques. *Nursing Research*, 33(4), 247–249.

Greer, D.S., Mor, V., Sherwood, S., Morris, J.M., & Birnbaum, H. (1983). National hospice study analysis plan. *Journal of Chronic Disease*, 36(11), 737–780.

Hogan, N., & DeSantis, L. (1991). Development of substantive theory in nursing. *Nursing Education Today*, 11(3), 167–171.

Holdich-Davis, D., Barham, L.N., O'Hale, A., & Tucker, B. (1995). Effect of standard rest periods on convalescent preterm infants. *Journal of Gynecologic and Neonatal Nursing*, 24(5), 424–432.

Hyman, L.L., Meininger, J.C., Coates, P.M., & Gallagher, P.R. (1995). Nongenetic influences of obesity on risk factors for cardiovascular disease during two phases of development. *Nursing Research*, 44(5), 277–283.

Kinchi, J., Polivka, B., & Stevenson, J.S. (1991). Triangulation: Operational definitions. *Nursing Research*, 40(6), 364–366.

McGuire, D.B., DeLoney, V.G., Yeager, K.A., Owen, D.C., Peterson, D.E., Lin, L.S., et al. (2000). Maintaining study validity in a changing clinical environment. *Nursing Research*, 49(4), 231–235.

Mitchell, E.S. (1986). Multiple triangulation: A methodology for nursing science. *Advances in Nursing Science*, 8(3), 18–26.

Morse, J.M. (1991). Approaches to qualitative-quantitative methodological triangulation. *Nursing Research*, 40(1), 120–123.

Myers, S.T., & Haase, J.E. (1989). Guidelines for integration of quantitative and qualitative approaches. *Nursing Research*, 38(5), 299–301.

Philips, J.R. (1988). Research issues: Research blenders. *Nursing Science Quarterly*, 1(1), 4–5.

________. (1988). Dialogue or research issues: Diggers of deeper holes. *Nursing Science Quarterly*, 1(4), 149–151.

Porter, P.J. (1989). The qualitative quantitative dualism. *Journal of Nursing Scholarship*, 21(2), 98–102.

Quayhagen, M.P., Quayhagen, M., Corbell, R.R., Roth, P.A., & Rodgers, J.A. (1995). A dyadic remediation programme for care recipients with dementia. *Nursing Research*, 44(3), 153–159.

CHAPTER

10

RESEARCH PROPOSAL

Key terms

★ Research proposal ★ Protocol ★ Work plan

⊙ Outline

- ★ Definition
- ★ Purposes of a research proposal
- ★ Contents of a research proposal
- ★ Work schedule

⊙ Objectives

On completion of this chapter, you will be able to:

- ★ define research proposal
- ★ understand the purposes of writing a research proposal
- ★ explain the contents of a research proposal

Introduction

A research in any discipline starts with a research proposal. A research proposal explains the academic supervisor or funding agency how you conceptualize the research you propose to undertake and justify its suitability and validity. Before starting your study, you must get your proposal approved. Hence it is important for you to understand what constitutes a research proposal.

Concept of Research Proposal

A research proposal is usually a written document prepared prior to the conduct of a study. It communicates the details of the research project to all parties concerned.

The preparation of a research proposal is similar as how an architect makes the sketch of a building. At the time of construction, one may not encourage any deviation from the approved design. Similarly, once a research proposal has been approved by the committee, no modification should be made to it.

Definition

A research proposal is a written document outlining the plan of the research study. It encompasses the overall plan, scheme, structure and strategies designed to obtain answers to the research questions or problems you think to solve through your research project (Ranjith Kumar, 2006).

The suggestions for the design of a research proposal may vary from one university to another and across disciplines. However, any research proposal is expected to be as comprehensive as possible.

Purposes

A research proposal is expected to serve the following purposes:

1. It shows direction to the research work.
2. It helps academic bodies, teachers, funding agencies and the scientific community to understand what the researcher aims to do.
3. Universities always need a formal proposal from students who are about to engage in research for a thesis or dissertation. Such proposals should precisely explain what the investigators intend to do, how they planned to conduct the study and how to monitor the progress of the work.
4. Funding agencies usually allocate funds on competitive basis. They examine the relevance and significance of the study as well as the researcher's competency for conducting such a research project.

Contents of a Research Proposal

A research proposal should contain the following information about the study. However, the institution may set its own guidelines for proposal presentation.

1. Background of the problem
2. Statement of the problem
3. Purposes of the study

4. Objectives
5. Assumption
6. Conceptual framework
7. Operational definitions
8. Hypothesis
9. Research methods
10. Work plan
11. Drafting the research budget
12. Ethical considerations
13. References and appendices

Background of the problem

The background of the problem explains how the proposal builds upon what has already been accomplished in that area. The researcher should use his/her direct personal experience, current clinical statistics and practical reasons for selecting the problem.

Statement of the problem

The problem statement should be presented clearly and briefly, specifying the key variables of the study, the nature of population being studied and the possibility of empirical testing.

Purposes of the study

The researcher should clearly state the purposes of the research. There may be usually two or more purposes to the study.

Objectives

Objectives should be written based on specific questions one expects to find answers through the research. The statement of objectives provides the reader, funding agency, employer or faculty with a comprehensive and coherent understanding of what the researcher hopes to achieve. It spells out the specific aims of the research project. It lists out the criteria for appraisal of research methods used. It is generally not encouraged to write too many objectives or include unrelated objectives.

There are two styles for writing the objectives: one to start with 'to' or directly start with the verb. Consider the following examples:

To identify the factors contributing to wound infection in surgical ward.

OR

Identify the factors contributing to wound infection in surgical ward.

Assumption

The proposal should bring out assumptions that are either self-evident or may have been satisfactorily established by earlier studies. This will act as the basis for accepted knowledge.

Conceptual framework

The research proposal should emphasize the interconnections between concepts/theories and possible outcomes expected through research methods. The entire research project rests upon this conceptual framework.

Operational definitions

Terminologies used in the proposal have to be clearly defined. Moreover, definitions are also important for specific operations the researcher must perform in order to collect the required information.

Hypothesis

The relationships between variables used in the study must be clearly established. A statement giving the prediction of expected outcomes is essential. Hypotheses that need to be tested should be stated clearly on the basis of the objectives of the study.

Research methods

The description of research methods should explain how the objectives would be addressed. This includes a narration of the following:

1. Selection of research methods
2. Selection of research design
3. Research setting
4. Population, sample and sampling technique
5. Selection and development of study instruments including methods to assess their reliability and validity.
6. Result of pilot study
7. Plan for data collection
8. Plan for data analysis

Work plan

A research is always expected to be completed within a desired timeframe. While making a work plan for research, one should list out the different tasks involved and indicate against each task a date to complete it. Make sure the work plan accommodates for unforeseen delays in the project. Develop a chart or table of work plan.

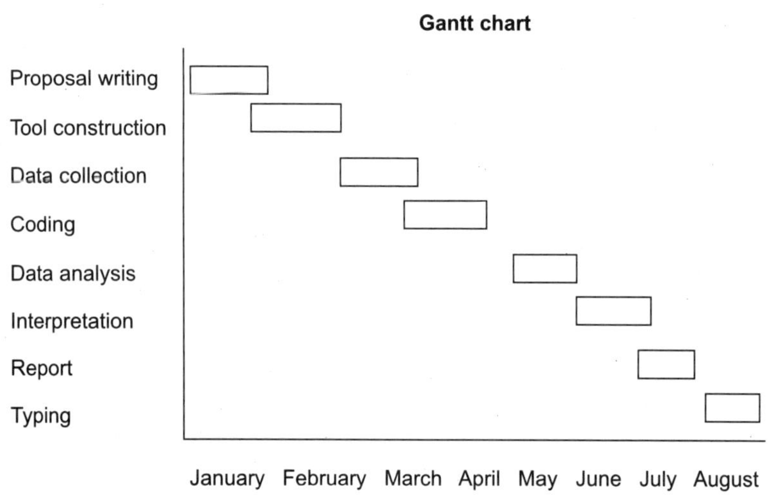

Figure 10.1 Example of a Gantt chart

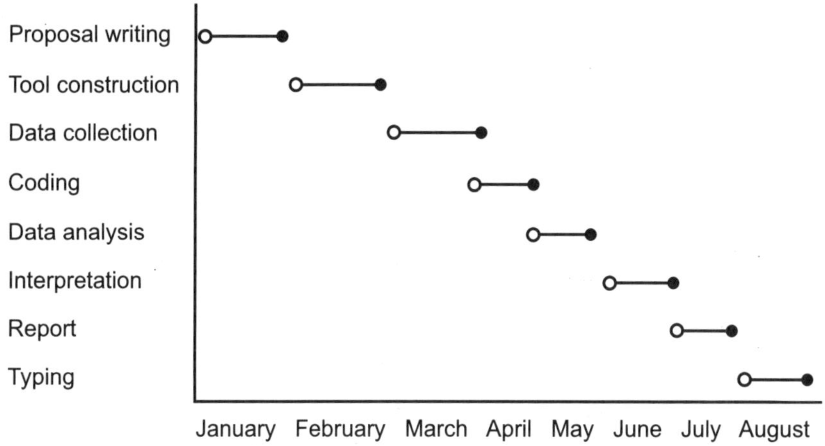

Figure 10.2 Flowchart of work plan

Drafting the research budget

Budgeting will give an account of how much money will need to be earmarked for various tasks. Some important heads of expenditures include staffing costs, transportation, stationery and printing, analysis of results and hired facilities.

Ethical considerations

Ethical considerations applicable for the conduct of the research need to be explained. Codes of ethics for use of human subjects in research have been developed to ensure the protection of subject's dignity and safety and the worthiness of the research.

As per the guidelines of Biomedical Research on Human Subjects 2000, ICMR, New Delhi, any study involving human subjects requires ethical clearance.

References and appendices

Bibliographical cards can be used for this purpose. The card contains the names of authors and other facts of publications.

Submitting a Research Proposal to a Funding Agency

Most researchers submit their research proposals to agencies in anticipation of getting financial support for their research. While drafting a proposal to a funding agency, the following guideline have to be strictly adhered to.

It is critical that the researcher responds cautiously to the priorities of the funding agency.

Guidelines for Preparing Thesis/ Dissertation Protocol

1. Title of the proposed research study: It should carry as much information as possible yet briefly worded.
2. A brief resume of the proposed research (in 1000 words): It includes the following:
   - Introduction
   - Need for the study
   - Review of literature
   - Research problem/question
   - Statement of the problem
   - Objectives of the study
   - Operational definitions
   - Sample and sampling techniques
   - Method of data collection
   - Plan for data analysis
   - List of references

SUMMARY

A research proposal explains the strategies for obtaining answers to the research questions. It shows what you propose to do, how you plan to proceed and why a research method has been chosen.

This chapter explains the framework of a research proposal and assumes that the readers are acquainted well with research methodologies and all academic styles of writing. The contents of a research proposal are background of the study, statement of the problem, purposes and objectives of the study, assumptions, conceptual framework, definitions of terms, hypotheses, research methodology, work plan, budget, ethical considerations, references and appendices. A work schedule provides a timeframe for the study.

MULTIPLE CHOICE QUESTIONS

1. Research in any discipline starts with a __________.
   (a) hypothesis (b) research tool
   (c) research proposal (d) data collection
2. Following are the purposes of writing a research proposal except
   (a) documenting research work
   (b) direction to the research work
   (c) for submitting a funding agency
   (d) for submitting to university
3. Gantt chart is developed for monitoring
   (a) research progress (b) hypothesis
   (c) data collection (d) work plan
4. The following are components of research proposal except
   (a) purpose of the study (b) hypothesis
   (c) ethical consideration (d) review question
5. The relationship between variables used in the study must be clearly stated using
   (a) hypothesis (b) assumption
   (c) operational definition (d) all of the above

ANSWER KEY

1. (c) 2. (a) 3. (d) 4. (d) 5. (a)

REVIEW QUESTIONS

1. (a) Define research proposal.
   (b) Explain the components of a research proposal.
2. Write short note on:
   (a) Significance of a research proposal
   (b) Flowchart of research work schedule
   (c) Bibliography

REFERENCES

Arford, P.H. (2004). Working with human research protections. *Journal of Nursing Scholarship*, 35, 265–271.

Bonifazi, W.L. (2004). Cruelty and courage: Nurses in the Nasi era. *Nurse Week*, 24–26.

Centres for Disease Control and Prevention. (2006). The Tuskgee Timeline. Retrieved May 18, 2006, from http://www.cdc.gov/nchstp/od/tuskegee/time.ht.

Crane, P.B., Letvak, S., Lewallen, L., Hu, J., & Jones, E. (2004). Inclusion of women in nursing research. *Nursing Research*, 53, 227–232.

Erlen, J.A. (2000). "Conflict of Interest". An ethical dilemma for the nurse researcher. *Orthopaedic Nursing*, 19, 74–77.

Grady, P. (2005). Statement Before Congress by Dr. Patricia, A. Grady on the FY 2005 budget. Retrieved August 24, 2005 from http://ninr.gov/ninr/about/legislation.html.

Habel, M. (2005). Can you answer patients' questions about clinical trials? *Nurse Week*, 23–25.

Harden, J.T., & McFarland, G. (2000). Avoiding gender and minority barriers to NIH funding. *Journal of Nursing Scholarship*, 32, 83–86.

Hayter, J. (1979). Issues related to human subjects. In F. Downs & J. Fleming (Eds.). Issues in nursing research (107–147). New York: Appleton-Century-Crofts.

Jacobson, S.F., Chu, N.L., Pascucci, M.A., & Gaskins, S.W. (2004). Characteristics of nursing research on race, ethnicity and culture. *Journal of Multicultural Nursing and Health*, 10(3), 6–12.

Katz, K. (1972). Experimentation with human beings. New York: Russell Sage.

Krugman, S., Giles, J., & Hammond, J. (1971). Viral hepatitis, type B (MS-2 strain): Studies on active immunization. *Journal of the American Medical Association*, 217, 41–45.

Milgram, S. (1963). Behavioural study of obedience. *Journal of Abnormal and Social Psychology*, 67, 371–378.

Olsen, D.P., & Mahrenholz, D. (2000). IRB-identified ethical issues in nursing research. *Journal of Professional Nursing*, 16, 140–148.

Shearer, L. (1982). Now it can be told. Dallas Morning News, 10–11.

Silva, M.C. (1995). Ethical guidelines in the conduct, dissemination, and implementation of nursing research. Washington, D.C.: American Nurses Association.

Solomon, J. (2005). AIDS researchers used foster children who lacked advocates. Dallas Morning News, 12.

Ulrich, B. (2005). Intersecting worlds. Nursing and NASA. *Nurse Week-South Central Edition*, 3.

Williams, S. (2005). The science of care. *Nurse Week-South Central Edition*, 10.

CHAPTER

11

IDENTIFICATION OF PARTICIPANTS AND DATA COLLECTION

Key terms

★ Population and sample ★ Probability sampling ★ Non-probability sampling ★ Power analysis ★ Reliability ★ Validity ★ Research instruments ★ Data collection methods ★ Criteria for selection of tools

⊙ Outline

- ★ Population
- ★ Sampling process
- ★ Types of sampling
- ★ Data collection process & methods
- ★ Data collection instruments
- ★ Criteria for selection of procedures
- ★ Relationship between validity and reliability

⊙ Objectives

On completion of this chapter, you will be able to:

- ★ distinguish between probability and non-probability sampling procedure
- ★ demonstrate skills in selecting appropriate sampling method for a particular study
- ★ recognize different data collection methods
- ★ understand the four sources of error that may occur in data collection

Identification of Participants

Population and sample

Population indicate the aggregate of people, animals and things living together. Sampling refers to the selection of a proportionate population to represent the entire population. Accurate sample exactly represents a population. Precision can be identified by evaluating standard error or derivation of the samples. If the error is small then the precision might be higher. An adequate sample must be in a single term, and must be reliable.

Characteristics of a good sample

1. Representative
2. Free from bias and errors
3. No substitution and incompleteness
4. Appropriate sample size

Sampling theorem

Sampling is the process of collecting a group of individuals or things in order to find out the estimated output through study. The sampling plan indicates the process of selection. The key concepts of sampling theory involve sampling elements, populations, sampling frames and sampling plans.

Elements and population

Elements are referred to as the sole unit of population. It may be a person or thing. Elements relating to persons are known as subjects. The term population is also referred to as target population. The population element consists of characteristics or attributes of the subjects that the researcher wants to study. The population is also a part of the larger group called the universe.

Target population

It consists of the total number of people or objects meeting the designated set of criteria. This is the whole group of individuals to which we are interested in applying our conclusions.

Accessible population

It is the aggregate of cases that confirm to the designated criteria and are also accessible as subjects for a study.

Relationship of sample and population in research process

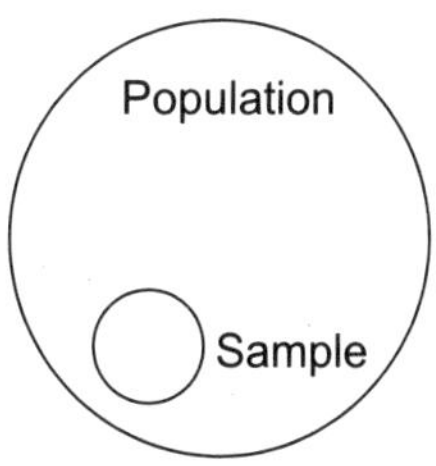

Figure 11.1 Relationship between sample and population in research process

A sample is simply a subset of the population. The concept of sample arises from the inability of researchers to test all the individuals in a given population. The sample must be representative of the population from which it was drawn and it must have good size to warrant statistical analysis. The main function of the sample is to allow researchers to conduct the study on individuals from the population, so that the results of their study can be used to derive conclusions that will apply to the entire population.

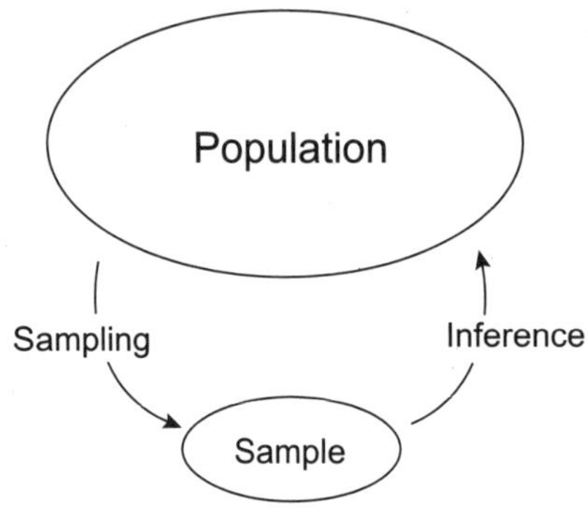

Figure 11.2 Influence of sample on population in research

The relationship between sample and population is like a give-and-take process; the population "gives" a sample and then it "takes" research results obtained from the sample.

Purposes of Sampling

It has already been pointed out that, when the population is too large and spread over a vast region, sampling needs to be done for the economy of time, energy and cost. But, it is also necessary to adopt a method of sampling by which we can generalize about the population. This process of stretching the conclusions from sample findings to describe the total population is called 'generalization'.

Sampling Process

Sampling is a process of selecting a part of the assigned population to represent the entire population. It should be systematically organized to eliminate data bias.

The sampling process includes the formulation of specific criteria for selection.

1. Identify and define the target population
2. Describe the accessible population and ensure sampling frame
3. Specify sample selection methods
4. Determine the sample size
5. Specify sampling plan
6. Selecting a desired sample

Factors influencing sampling process

The factors include:

1. Nature of the researcher
    (a) Inexperienced investigator
    (b) Lack of interest
    (c) Lack of honesty
    (d) Intensive workload
    (e) Inadequate supervision
2. Nature of the sample
    (a) Inappropriate sampling technique
    (b) Sample size
    (c) Defective sampling frame
3. Circumstances
    (a) Lack of time
    (b) Large geographic area
    (c) Lack of cooperation
    (d) Natural calamities

Methods of Sampling

Sampling methods may be of two common types:

1. Probability sampling or random sampling
2. Non-probability sampling or non-random sampling

1. Probability Sampling

Probability means chance. It may be in the value of '0' or '1'. The theories of probability are used in probability sampling. Random sampling is the main feature of this method. When each element in the population has equal chance, then random selection method is adopted. This method results in a representative sample. Here each element has a chance of being selected, and these chances are commonly known as probability. The random selection of elements is an important characteristic of probability sampling.

The common methods of probability sampling are:

(a) Simple random sampling
(b) Systematic random sampling/quasi-random sampling
(c) Stratified random sampling
(d) Cluster random sampling
(e) Random route sampling

(a) Simple random sampling

The basic probability sampling plan is the simple random sampling method. The way of selection depends upon the attitude of the researcher. Under this method, sampling units are selected at random from the entire population and each element has an equal probability and each unit must be independent. The most common method used in this sampling is the use of computer program. In this method, sampling frames are entered into a computer. The subjects are randomly selected by the computer until the ultimate one is detected. Another one is the method of using table of random numbers. The most primitive and mechanical method of simple random sampling is the lottery method. Each member of the population is assigned with a unique number. Each number is placed in a bowl and mixed thoroughly. All individuals bearing the numbers picked by the researcher are the subjects for the study.

Sampling frame: To identify the population by way of sampling, each person must be identified in the population. For this, a list containing details of every individual must be furnished. This is termed as sampling frame. From these, the subjects are selected by sampling plans. It is not a practical method for all types of studies.

Randomization procedures in research: For new researchers, random assignment and random sampling are two areas which need clarification. Random sampling involves the selection of a sample from the population. Random assignment is the process of unbiased assigning of subjects from a sample into groups in an experimental study. It is a necessary condition for a true experimental study. First sample are randomly selected from population. Next subjects are randomly assigned to groups; lastly intervention is randomly assigned to the group.

(b) Systematic/quasi-random sampling

The quasi-random sampling methods are also known as systematic sampling methods. These methods are done when all in the population list are available. In this method, every K^{th} individual is selected on the estimated list by using a starting point which is selected at random. If it is not a random point, then the sample is not a probability sample. For example, if the population size $N = 2000$ and sample size $n = 100$, then $k = 20$. Every 20th person on the list is included in the sample. This is done by the equation

$$k = \frac{\text{Size of population}}{\text{Desired sample size}} \text{ i.e. } \frac{2000}{100} = 20$$

(c) Stratified random sampling

The method of stratified random sampling is adopted when the variables in population are critical for attaining representativeness. Stratification ensures adequate representation of variables in the sample. Stratified sampling may be of two types, i.e. proportionate or disproportionate.

Proportionate stratified sampling: In proportionate stratified sampling, the sample units in distinct strata are of the same proportion in the population. It allows efficient representation to each station. Hence this method is a much established one. This method has the following **merits**:

1. Allows appropriate representation of subgroups in the population.
2. It provides higher statistical efficiency.
3. This method is the easiest one to carry out.

Like every sampling method, these also have some **demerits** such as:

1. This method requires previous knowledge regarding the distribution and composition of population.
2. It has a higher statistical efficiency. This method is more expensive and time-consuming.

Disproportionate stratified random sampling: In this method, the strata are not proportionally represented in the population. The disproportionate state may occur due to the size of state, its internal variance and sampling costs. The stratum elements are mixed or variable; hence it is more sensible to take a larger sample for representing the stratum. Also, the sampling cost per strata may also vary with one another. This method is not usually applicable, but only in the specified circumstances such as:

1. If more important sub-groups are included.
2. When the sub-groups are both homogeneous and heterogeneous.

(d) Cluster sampling

In this method, researchers collect a cluster of sample representing states, cities, institutions, organizations, etc. to identify the population. Randomized samples of these facts are used in research. But in some instances, randomization is done through various stages, and is known as multi-stage sampling. Multi-stage sampling is used where populations are widely dispersed. Under these circumstances, interviews can be concentrated in convenient areas. In cluster sampling, the populations are divided into geographical groups, known as clusters or blocks. This method is less expensive and increases sampling errors. In cluster sampling, we have to:

1. Divide the population into clusters.
2. Randomly sample clusters.
3. Measure all the elements within the sampled clusters.

(e) Random route sampling

It is a probability sampling procedure that is useful in marketing research or other community-based research in which households, business or other such premises need to be sampled. In random route sampling, the interviewer randomly selects an address usually from a sampling frame as a starting point and then identifies subsequent addresses by a predetermined random process and then calls on every *n*th address to conduct the required number of interviews. Although random route sampling is economical in terms of time and money, it can have the disadvantage of precluding the collection of data from a sample that is truly representative.

2. Non-probability Sampling Methods Used in Quantitative Research

In non-probability sampling methods, all elements could not get the chance for representing the sample. This method diminishes the samples' representativeness of population, and is commonly applicable in nursing research studies. The non-probability sampling techniques commonly used in nursing research are convenience sampling, quota sampling, purposive sampling, network sampling and theoretical sampling.

Convenience sampling

In this method, the sample are selected on the basis of convenience of sample. The available subjects are simply entered up to achieve the desired one. This is also known as accidental sampling. These methods are inexpensive, accessible and less time-consuming. The subject of the study cannot be examined with probability sampling. According to Kerlinger and Lee (2000), a convenience is not that bad when it is used with reasonable knowledge and care in implementing a study. These methods are applicable in studies relating to health care. The fact is that the sampling frames are not available for many populations and also it is difficult to find out adequate research subjects; hence the researchers use a sample of convenience.

Quota sampling

This method is similar as convenience sampling method. This is a form of judgement sampling where biases from non-probability methods of selection are controlled to a great extent by stratification, weighing and the setting of quotas for each stratum. This type of sampling is used much by commercial researchers as it is very cost-effective and easy to administer. It has the following advantages:

1. Speed, economy and administrative simplicity.
2. Researcher can obtain sample units without unnecessary travelling.
3. Administratively simple because it is independent of sampling frames.

Quota sampling has the following limitations:

1. A disproportionate number of highly educated people and certain occupations tend to be more highly represented.
2. These problems can cause the data to be invalid.

However, application of random techniques can eliminate these problems.

Purposive sampling

The purposive sampling method may be also known as judgemental or selective sampling because the researcher selects some elements, events and subjects which might be included in the research study. This method also has some limitations such as the accuracy of the judgement of the researcher may not be properly evaluated. In qualitative research, purposive sampling is the best way to obtain a wide understanding among the events.

Network sampling

The network sampling methods are also known as snowball sampling methods. In this method, the subject to be studied should be one which has not been previously studied. When the scholar selects a new unresearched subject, then he collects all the necessary information regarding the subject. These methods are commonly used in qualitative studies. According to Munhall (2001), "In qualitative research, network sampling is an effective strategy for identifying the subjects who can provide the greatest insight and essential information about an experience or event that is being studied."

There are three types of snowball sampling:

1. Linear snow
2. Exponential non-discriminative
3. Exponential discriminative

Theoretical sampling

In theoretical sampling, the theory of research must have great importance. Here, the researcher collects data from one person who provides relevant data regarding theory generation. After the completion of the process, certain codes are dictated by the researcher and he also checks its suitability in the theory. According to Patton (2002), diversity in the sample is encouraged if the theory developed covers a wide range of behaviours in varied situations and settings.

Sample Size

An unavoidable step in a sample study is to determine the size of the sample. This involves both statistical and non-statistical considerations. Among the non-statistical considerations, we can include resources available, nature of the study method of sampling followed, nature of respondents, nature of population, sampling procedure, and statistical test used.

It is always wise to set the sample size larger than what is actually desired to allow for non-response or subject dropout.

Power Analysis

It is a procedure that intents to determine the needed sample size for a research study. The power of statistical test is its ability to detect statistical significance in a study when it is present. When the power is low, the likelihood of making a type II error is high. It is helpful in deciding some other factors necessary for the study in order to make the sample size.

Components of Power Analysis

Power

The experimenter specifies the power that he wishes to achieve. The sample size needed for that level of power can be estimated. For example, if we are trying to assess the popularity of eating pizza among adolescent boys, we feel that 70% of youngsters like to eat pizza.

If we say in this case power is 70%, then out of the data collected from 100 youngsters, it will yield a result 70% of the time and a non-significant result only 30% of the times.

Effect size

It is the size of effect we are looking for and depends on the effect of an independent variable on dependent variable. It can also be just a figure that the investigator intends to arrive at according to their expectations.

Sampling in Qualitative Research

Sampling in qualitative research provides more attention on events, incidents and experiences rather than individuals. The researcher will select the subjects, and be able to provide effective information about the event being researched. Sampling in qualitative research includes methods such as purposive sampling, network/snowball sampling and theoretical sampling. These methods help the researcher find out adequate subjects who give more information regarding the event and situations being studied.

Importance of Sample Size in Qualitative Studies

In qualitative studies, the sample size might have greater importance. It helps to identify the variable relationships and also determines the group differences. Larger sample size ensures higher power relationships. A qualitative study focuses on the quality of information obtained from the person, situation, or event sampled, rather than on the size of the sample (Hubeman Miles, 2002).

The important factors for determining sample size are (1) scope of study, (2) nature of subject, (3) data quality and (4) design of study.

Scope of study

A study with extensive data needs more sampling of events, documents and participants.

Nature of subject

The subject studied must be a clear and easy one. This type of subjects require more participants and makes easy to collect essential data through necessary interviews.

Data quality

The pieces of information obtained from document reviews or interviews might have great importance during sample sizing. The well-informed and communicative participants are able to share data in a clear, positive manner.

Design of study

If more interviews are conducted, then better data quality can be obtained. Interviews done through families produce more data rather than interviewing a particular participant. Proper selection of the design helps for benefits.

1. Economical
2. Improved quality of data
3. Quick study results
4. Precision and accuracy of data

Advantages and Disadvantages of Sampling

Advantages

1. Economy in expenditure
2. Economy in time
3. Greater scope
4. Organization of convenience
5. Intensive and extensive data
6. Suitable in limited resources
7. Better report

Disadvantages

1. Chance of bias
2. Difficult in getting representative supply
3. Need for specialized knowledge
4. Changeability of units
5. Impossibility of sampling

Data Collection

The search for answers to research questions calls for collection of data. Data are facts, figures and other relevant materials (past and present) serving as bases for the study and analysis.

Data collection is an important aspect of research study. Inaccurate data collection can impact the results of a study and ultimately lead to invalid results. Data collection methods for effective evaluation vary along a continuum. At the one end of this continuum are quantitative methods and at the other end are qualitative methods of data collection.

In general, data collection methods can be divided into five types:

1. Physiological
2. Observational
3. Interviews
4. Questionnaires
5. Records

Each of these methods has purposes, separate merits and demerits.

Sources of Data

Information for various research studies depends on their sources. A quality research study requires highly reliable and valid data. Sources of data can be generally classified into two types, viz. primary and secondary sources.

Primary sources

Here information is collected by the researcher directly from the respondents or situations. For collection of data, research methods like interviews, questioning, observation and psychosocial measurement scales are used.

Secondary sources

Secondary data can be collected from internal and external sources.

External sources involve published or unpublished records. Published records include journals, magazines, newspapers, census reports, etc. Unpublished records may include official records, patient records and reports.

Internal secondary sources are also known as private documents which include biographies, personal diaries, letters, etc.

Methods and Tools of Data Collection

Methods of data collection

Research method refers to the way in which the investigator collects data by observation, questioning or other measurements. The various steps used for gathering and analyzing data in a research investigation are known as methods of data collection.

Research tool

It is the instrument used for data collection in a research. It is a device used to measure the concept of interest in a research study, to gather data, e.g. questionnaire, interview schedule.

Table 11.1 Tools and techniques of data collection

Important tools for data collection	Techniques for data collection
Interview schedule	Interview
Questionnaire Opinionnaire Attitude scale Visual analogue scale	Questioning
Rating scales Checklists Anecdotes Videotapes/films	Observation
Biophysiological measurement equipments	Biophysiological methods

Factors Influencing the Selection of Methods of Data Collection

For a good research, appropriate research tool is vital. Several factors must be considered while selecting an instrument. The important factors influencing the selection of methods of data collection are discussed hereunder.

Nature of phenomenon under study

Selection of particular method of data collection is influenced by the nature of phenomenon under study. Each research phenomenon has specific characteristics. For example, for studying the behavioural aspects of a patient, psychological tests can be used whereas observation methods can be used for assessing the incidence of ventilator-associated pneumonia.

Type of research participants

The types of participants under study affect the selection of data collection methods. For example, data collection through questionnaire is possible only if the participants are literate. However, interview schedules can be also used for individuals who are illiterate.

Objectives of the research study

The objectives of the study also influence the selection of methods of data collection.

Type of research study

Different methods of data collection are required for quantitative and qualitative research. For example, in a case study, continuous evaluation of the subject is done by observation method, whereas in quantitative studies like survey method we use interview schedules.

Distribution of the target population

Attention should be given for the geographical area of the population. If the target population is distributed over a large geographical area, mailed questionnaires can be used. From practical point of view, adopting an appropriate data collection method is necessary. Otherwise the researcher will have to spend more money, energy and time.

For example, for a study involving the assessment of knowledge regarding the causes of childhood obesity among school children in four districts of Kerala, mailed questionnaires can be used.

Size of the study sample

Questionnaires are the commonly used method of data collection for large samples. Interviews or direct observations may be possible when a study is conducted on a small sample.

Duration of the study

In short-term research designs, structured methods of data collection can be used whereas in long-term research designs, less structured methods of data collection can be used.

For example, a study to assess the knowledge regarding the predisposing factors of carcinoma cervix can be done for a short-term period (post-graduate nursing studies). Here a structured interview schedule is preferred. A doctoral study on the same topic can take a longer duration (say one-and-a-half years) and it can be done using unstructured interview schedules.

Availability of resources and manpower

Methods of data collection are also influenced by the availability of resources and manpower.

Literary level of the participants

Methods of data collection such as questionnaire cannot be used for illiterate participants. For those participants, other options are available.

Researcher's knowledge, level and competence

The knowledge and competence of the researcher is also very important in deciding the data collection method. Depending on the course of study like GNM, B.Sc. (N), M.Sc. (N) or Ph.D., the method of data collection varies. Thus, before starting the study, the researcher should decide the method of data collection carefully. For example, a true experimental method of study requires a sound understanding of research methodology, psychological knowledge, skills and competence.

Appraisal of Data Collection Methods

The suitability of a method of data collection may be appraised on the basis of following criteria:

1. Efficiency of data collection
2. Anonymity
3. Quality of data and adequacy

4. Ability for controlling variables
5. Accuracy and completeness of data collection

Interview

Interview involves verbal communication between the researcher and the subject during which information is provided to the researcher. Interviews have been described as "conversation with a purpose" (Dexter, 1970; Kahn and Connel, 1937) and a method of data collection in which the interviewer asks questions to a respondent which can be either face-to-face or telephonically.

An interview is a conversation between two or more people where questions are asked by interviewer to obtain information from the interviewee.

Interviewing is an accepted way of gathering information in qualitative research. It is a process of interaction in which the subjects give the needed information verbally in face-to-face situations. Interview requires high-level questioning skills and active participation. In nursing studies, it is a commonly used method; it may be used either as a major method or as a supplementary one in the collection of data. It is a useful method for collecting data from illiterate or less educated respondents.

Characteristics of Interview

1. Researcher and subjects are strangers.
2. Verbal answers are obtained.
3. The relationship between respondent and interviewer is not permanent.
4. The information given by respondent is recorded for future use.
5. It is conversation with a specific purpose.
6. It can be conducted over telephone and does not need face-to-face interaction.
7. It is an interaction process between researcher and subject.
8. Interview is not a standardized process of data collection.

Types of Interviews

Interviews can be classified into the following categories:

Structured interview (directive interview)

In structured interview, the researcher has more control over the content of the interview. The questions are prepared by the researcher before the initiation of data collection.

Structured interview is a type of interview in which the interviewer has a standardized interview schedule. It contains questions in the order in which they are to be answered. These types of interviews are also known as standardized interviews.

It has the following characteristics:

1. The schedule is an organized one and has a set of questions.
2. It increases the reliability and credibility of research data.

Merits

1. Attention is not diverted to irrelevant and time-consuming conversation.
2. Data from one interview can be compared with that of next one.
3. Recording and coding data does not pose any problem.

Demerits

1. Spontaneity of natural conversation is lost.
2. The respondent's views are minimized.
3. The scope of exploration of hidden facts is impossible.

Unstructured interview (Non-directive interview)

It is a type of interview in which the interviewer encourages the respondent to talk freely about a given topic with minimum prompting. These interviews are also known as non-standardized interviews.

In this method, it may include elements of both focused and clinical interview, but these are integrated into a general approach that encourages respondent to explore the topic as long as the respondent wishes.

It is an informal type of interview and consists of the following characteristics:

1. The schedule is not formalized.
2. Questions are open-ended.

Merits

1. Interviewer's bias can be reduced.
2. Increase opportunity to explore the problem in a clear manner.

Demerits

1. The data is not comparable.
2. It may not be an organized interview.
3. Waste of time.

Semi-structured interview

In this type of interview, depending upon the situation new questions are brought up. It is a flexible method. The interviewer prepares an interview guide which is an informal list of topics and questions that the interviewer can ask.

Focused group interview

It is an unstructured interview technique where 8–12 members are brought together under the guidance of a trained interviewer to focus on a specific phenomenon. Here, the interviewer guides the discussion according to a set of written questions or topics to be covered.

The basic characteristics of this type of interviews are:

1. Duration of the interview is 1–2 hours.
2. It has a moderator.
3. The participants can reveal their views.
4. The interviewer chooses the sequence of questions.

Merits

1. New ideas and creative concepts are stimulated.
2. It involves many participants at one time.
3. Wide range of information is collected.
4. Respondents are more active.

Demerits

1. There is chance of bias.
2. It is very difficult to moderate.
3. Coding, analysis and interpretations of data are difficult.

Telephonic interview

This method consists of collecting information by contacting the respondents over telephone. It is used in industrial surveys.

Merits

1. It is more flexible and quick.
2. Respondents can be easily accessed.
3. Cost is less and response is high.
4. Rapid completion of the interview.

Demerits

1. Respondent's characteristics cannot be observed.
2. Rapport is difficult.

In-depth interview

This is an intensive and investigative interview aimed at studying the respondent's opinions and emotions on the basis of interview guide. It requires more training and interpersonal skills.

Merit

Detailed information can be elicited.

Demerits

1. Time-consuming.
2. Interviewer should have in-depth knowledge.

Clinical interview

This is similar to the focused interview. While the focused interview is concerned with the effects of specific experience, clinical interview is concerned with feelings with the course of individual's life experience.

Computer-assisted personal interviewing (CAPI)

It is a form of personal interview in which the interviewer uses a laptop or hand-held computer to collect data. The information is entered directly into the computer-based database instead of using a questionnaire.

Merits

1. The interviewer need not carry questionnaire.
2. Time can be saved.

Demerits

1. This method is expensive.
2. Interviewer needs typing and computer skills.

Process of Interviewing

It includes the following steps:

1. Preparation for interview
2. Introduction
3. Developing rapport
4. Carrying interview forward
5. Recording
6. Closing

Preparation for interview

In this phase, the interviewer should fix up the topic and time of interview. The interviewer should dress in a familiar fashion and should look pleasant. The interviewer must be familiar with the interview schedule.

Introduction

The researcher introduces himself to the respondent and identifies the respondent by name. The purpose and format of the interview is explained thoroughly.

Developing rapport

After the introduction, the researcher starts developing rapport with respondents.

Proceeding with interview

The following guidelines should be used:

1. Start the interview.
2. Ask only one question at a time.
3. Repeat a question if necessary.
4. Listen carefully to the subject's answer.
5. Allow the subject sufficient time to answer the questions.
6. Ask additional questions to seek additional information.

Recording the interview

It is essential to record the information by note-taking.

Closing the interview

After the interview, the interview is closed by thanking the respondent.

Merits

1. People's feelings, perception and opinions can be obtained.
2. More descriptive questions can be asked.
3. Respondent's own words are recorded.
4. High response rate is achieved.

Demerits

1. Interview is time-consuming.
2. There is high degree of chance for interviewer's bias.

Questionnaire

Questionnaires are one of the most popular methods of conducting research. It is a set of questions that may or may not provide with response alternatives which are to be answered by the subjects.

A questionnaire is a printed self-report form designed to elicit information that can be obtained through written responses from the subjects.

A questionnaire is a structured instrument consisting of a series of questions prepared by researcher that a research subject is asked to complete, to gather data from individuals about their knowledge, attitude, beliefs and feelings.

Types of Questions

There are two types of questions.

Open-ended questions

Open-ended questions are those questions in which the respondents express their opinions and answers in their own way. There is no predetermined set of responses.

E.g.: "State your opinion about the need for involvement of nurses in research?"

Close-ended questions

Close-ended questions are those questions which offer respondents a number of alternatives from which they can choose the one that most likely matches the appropriate answer.

In research, close-ended questions facilitate easy statistical calculations of data. It can be asked to different groups at different intervals.

E.g.: "Do you have abdominal pain?"

(a) Yes (b) No

Guidelines for Preparing a Good Questionnaire

1. The questionnaire should be prepared in accordance with the study objectives.
2. Specific instructions should be given to the respondents to give the responses.
3. Each item should be concise, brief and precise.
4. It should be according to the respondent's knowledge.
5. Each question should be clear; confusing and biased questions should be avoided.
6. It should be simple.
7. Open-ended questions are to be avoided as far as possible.
8. Controversial questions are to be avoided.
9. Logical sequence of questions should be maintained.
10. Questions should flow from more general to more specific.

Consideration for question construction

1. Use statements which can be interpreted in the same way by all subjects.
2. Avoid asking double-barreled questions.
3. Ambiguous and long questions should be avoided.
4. Negative and double-negative questions should be avoided.
5. Use positive statements.

Anatomy of Questionnaire

Title: Title of the questionnaire at the top of the first page should indicate the content of items.

Directions: The directions should be explained properly.

Questions: Number the questions consecutively throughout the questionnaire. Even if there are several sections, consecutive numbering lessens confusion.

Transitions: If there are different types of information requested or if the respondent task changes, a transitional statement should be inserted at that place.

Merits

1. Cost effective.
2. Easy to analyze.
3. Requires less time to administer.
4. Reduces bias.
5. Can be used for a large sample size.

Demerits

1. Not suitable for children, blind and illiterate.
2. Low response rate.
3. Only superficial information can be elicited.
4. There are chances of people lying and answering the questions vaguely.
5. These are chances of misinterpretations.

Composite Scales or Attitude Scales

A scale is a device designed to assign a numeric score to people to place them on a continuum with respect to the attributes being measured.

Composite scales are socio-psychological measurements, which are directed towards quantifying the qualitative attributes such as feelings, attitude, etc. The commonly used composite scales include Likert scale and Semantic differential scale.

Likert Scale

Likert scales are the most commonly used self-report measurement. These are designed to measure the attributes. A Likert scale consists of a series of statements of possible responses. It consists of several declarative items which express a topic primarily. This scale was originally developed with a five-point scale. The number of categories may range from four to seven. The choice of response on a Likert scale represents agreement, evaluation and frequency.

1. Agreement responses involve options like 'strongly agree', 'agree', 'uncertain', 'disagree' and 'highly disagree'.
2. Evaluation responses imply a categorical calling such as 'positive' to 'negative' or 'excellent' to 'terrible'.
3. A frequency response includes 'rarely/sometimes/occasionally happens'.

The values from each item are summed to provide a total score.

Statement	Strongly agree	Agree	Uncertain	Disagree	Strongly disagree
Relatives of patients admitted in CCU should be permitted to visit patients at any time					

Characteristics of Likert scale

1. It is basically a psychological measurement tool.
2. It is an illustration of clear judgement about the degree of agreement or disagreement with the particular item on the scale.
3. It contains neutral statements without the bias of researcher.
4. This is composed of alternative positive and negative statements so that response bias can be eliminated.

Scoring of Likert scale

For a positive statement, respondents get higher score if there is agreement with statement. In case of negative statement, the respondent gets higher score if there is disagreement with statement.

Merits

1. It is relatively easy to conduct.
2. It is a reliable and valid tool.
3. It is easy to administer.

Demerit

Feelings of respondents cannot be fully assessed.

Semantic Differential Scale

The semantic differential scale is a type of rating scale designed to measure the respondent's attitude towards objects, events and concepts. These scales consist of two opposite adjectives with a 7-point scale between them. With semantic differential scale, the respondent is asked to rate the concept on a series of "bipolar adjectives" such as good-bad, willing-unwilling, hard-soft, active-passive, strong-weak, etc.

Here also numeric values are assigned to evaluate responses. Values of '1' to '7' are assigned to each response, '1' being the most negative response and '7' being the most positive one.

It is most commonly used in

1. Operational research

2. Patient satisfaction survey
3. Customer satisfaction survey
4. Employee survey
5. Personality measurements
6. Clinical psychology

Merits

1. Easy to administer.
2. Provide valid and reliable quantitative data.
3. Convenient method to assess beliefs, attitudes and values.

Demerits

1. Difficult to select the relevant concepts.
2. Difficult to find the appropriate adjective pairs.

To assess the belief about carcinoma breast

Cure	**1**	**2**	**3**	**4**	**5**	**6**	**7**	**Death**
Social acceptance	1	2	3	4	5	6	7	Social rejection
Affordable treatment	1	2	3	4	5	6	7	Expensive treatment
Normal life	1	2	3	4	5	6	7	Miserable life

Visual Analogue Scale (VAS)

It is a psychomotor response scale used to measure subjective characteristics that cannot be directly measured. It includes pain, discomfort, anxiety, alertness, etc. It consists of 10 centimeter lines, the ends labelled as extreme limits of the response being measured.

E.g.: "VAS for pain is a straight line with 'no pain' at one end and 'worst pain' at the other end."

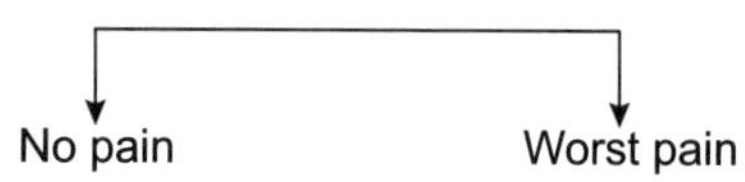

Merits

1. Quantitative assessment of subjective phenomenon is possible.
2. It is reliable and valid in measuring sensations and feelings.

Demerit

This scale cannot be used for comparing results across a group of individuals at the same time.

Observation

Observation is a way of gathering data by watching behaviour, events or physical characteristics in their natural setting. Observation method of data collection is well suited to nursing research.

Observation is a technique for collecting all the data or acquiring information through occurences that can be observed through senses with or without mechanical device.

Types of Observation

Observation may be of different ways:

Structured observation

In structured observation, a structured or semi-structured tool is prepared in advance by the researcher. The researcher observes specific attributes or behaviours in accordance with planned observations. Specific parameters are used for collecting data. It is done by tools like checklists, rating scales, category system, etc. Structured observation evaluates behaviours against these tools that delineate the different roles a participant can assume.

Unstructured observation

It is commonly used in qualitative studies. It is done with minimally structured or researcher-imposed categories. Here unstructured tools like anecdotes, field diary and video recording are used. In unstructured observation, the general observation guidelines address behaviours manifested by participants and how these behaviours are enacted.

Participant observation

In this observation, the observer is a part of the phenomenon which is observed and he acts as both observer and participant. Persons who are observed should not be aware of the researcher's purpose. Here unstructured tools are used to collect data such as logbooks, field notes, field diary, tape and video recording, etc.

Non-participant observation

In this method, the observer is not a participant in the setting. People are observed without their knowledge.

Direct observation

It involves observations of an event personally by the observer when it takes place. This allows the observer to see and record events as they occur.

Indirect observation

In this method, no physical presence of the observer is needed. Recording is done by mechanical, photographic or electronic devices.

Controlled observation

This involves standardization of observational techniques and maximum control over extrinsic and intrinsic variable. The observations are systematically recorded.

Uncontrolled observations

This does not involve control over extrinsic and intrinsic variables.

Planning for Observation

The use of observation method requires proper planning as follows:

1. The researcher should examine the relevance of observation method to the needs of the selected study.
2. The researcher should identify the specific investigative questions.

3. The researcher must decide the observation content, i.e. specific conditions, events and activities that have to be observed for the required data.
4. The research should design a system for data collection. There are three ways of collecting observation data, namely recording sheets and checklists, observation guides and field notes.
5. Select an adequate number of sample representative of the population.
6. Select the observers. They may include staff members, interns, graduate students, etc.
7. The researcher should train observers to high-quality data collection.

Merits

1. It is possible to study behaviour as it occurs.
2. Data are collected to their natural settings.
3. It does not rely on people's willingness.

Demerits

1. Chance for observer bias.
2. People usually perform well when they know they are being observed (Hawthorne effect).
3. Time-consuming.

Rating Scales

Rating scales involve qualitative description of a limited number of aspects of a thing or a person. A rating scale lists an ordered series of categories of a variable that are assumed to be based on an underlying continuum.

Rating scale refers to a scale with a set of opinions which describe varying degrees of the dimensions of an attitude being observed.

In a rating scale one person assesses another person's level of performance. It could be 3-point, 5-point, or 7-point rating scale. A numerical value is assigned to each category.

E.g.: "How many times doctors visit the wards?"

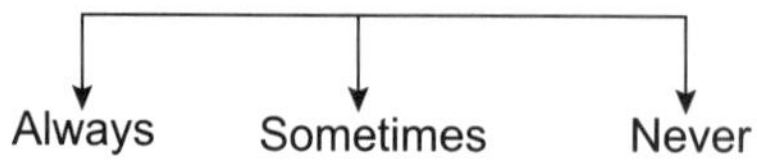

Types of Rating Scales

Graphic rating scale

The performance is marked at various points on a scale. It is anchored by two extremes presented to respondents for evaluation of a concept or object.

E.g.: "How much are you satisfied with the level of performance of staff?"

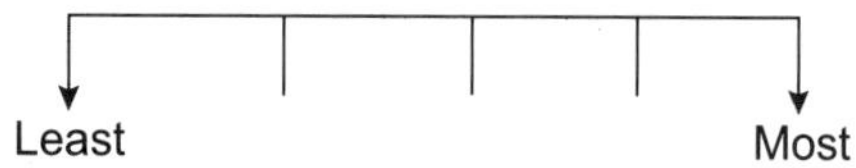

Descriptive rating scale

It includes a series of verbal phrases to indicate the level of performance and does not use numbers.

E.g.: "Level of clinical performance by students"

Numerical rating scale

In these scales, each statement is generally assigned a numerical score ranging from 1 to 10.

E.g.: "Cancer pain assessment scale"

Comparative rating scale

Here the researcher makes a judgement about an attribute of a person by comparing it with that of similar persons.

E.g.: "Mrs. Radha who is a junior staff nurse has health education skills similar to that of Mrs. Anu."

Merits of rating scale

1. Easy to administer and score.
2. Easier to make and less time-consuming.

3. Can be used for a large group.
4. Can be used for interests, attitudes and personal characteristics.
5. It is flexible.
6. Used for quantitative measures.
7. Useful for evaluating performance, skills and product outcome.

Demerit

There is chance of subjective evaluation.

Checklist

It is one of the most commonly used tools for performance evaluation. It consists of a list of steps, activities and behaviours which the observer records when an incident occurs.

Checklist for wound dressing

Sl. No	Steps	Yes	No	Remarks

Guidelines for Preparation of Checklist

1. Express each item in simple language.
2. Avoid negative statements.
3. Ensure that each item has a clear response (Yes/No).
4. It should be complete and comprehensive.

Merits

1. It is a simple method to record observations.
2. Useful in evaluating learning activities.
3. Adaptable to subject areas.
4. It helps in identifying the effectiveness of procedure.
5. Evaluation of processes that can be divided into sets of actions.
6. There is less chance of error in this method.

Demerits

1. Quality of performance cannot be assessed.
2. Accuracy of performance cannot be assessed.
3. Only a limited aspect of clinical performance can be evaluated.

Biophysiological Methods

Psychological and physiological variables need specialized technical instruments, which require specialized training for the interpretation of results. A wide range of instruments are available for measuring physiologic functions. This method is costly when compared to other methods of data collection. It also offers relative precision and sensitivity.

Purposes of biophysiological methods

1. To analyze the basic physiological processes relevant to nursing care.
2. To study the physiological outcomes of nursing care.
3. It can be used to evaluate a new intervention in comparison with standard methods of care.

In-Vivo Biophysiological Methods

In *in-vivo* biophysiological methods, measurements are done on a living organism by using specialized instruments.

E.g.: "Measurement of cardiac activity by ECG machine"

In-vivo measuring systems involve the following components:

Stimulus

Biophysiological measurements need a stimulus to begin them. It can be internal or external.

E.g.: "Doppler Echo for assessing internal structure of heart", where ECG monitoring system needs stimulus from pacemaker of heart.

Participants

Chemical, electrical, mechanical, thermal and other systems of the human body become participants for biophysiological measures.

Sensory equipment

Sensory equipment converts one form of energy into another that can be measured and interpreted. It consists of one or more transducers or electrodes.

Recording equipment

The purpose of recording equipment is to get permanent record of physiological measurements for research purpose.

Signal conditioning

The subject usually produces two types of signals, namely key physiological signals and interference signals. The function of signal conditioning equipment such as amplifiers and signal processors is to amplify the desired physiological signal from the transducers.

In-Vitro Biophysiological Methods

Here measurements are carried out outside the living organism by using specialized equipment. Samples of data related to physical, anatomical or pathological status are collected and sent to laboratory for analysis and interpretation.

E.g.: "Blood sample from patients to assess the liver function (LFT)"

In-vitro biophysiological methods include:

Radiological measurements: Evaluation of body tissues by use of X-rays, CT scan, MRI, PET, etc.

Biochemical measurements: Measuring biochemical attributes such as serum electrolytes, blood sugar levels, LFT, RFT, etc.

Microbiological measurements: These include evaluation of bacterial counts, culture and sensitivity tests of urine, blood, etc.

Cytological measurements: These include detailed examination of cytological attributes of an individual, e.g. Fine needle aspiration of breast tissue, tissue biopsy.

Merits

1. These methods are objective in nature.
2. More accurate and error-less.
3. It is valid measurement.
4. The instruments are easily available.

Demerits

1. Some instruments are costly.
2. The outcome may be affected by environmental conditions.
3. Certain methods have detrimental effect on the organism.
4. It may cause undue anxiety among patients, e.g. Invasive procedures.

Projective Techniques

In direct methods of data collection like personal interview, etc., the respondents may be unwilling to talk about controversial issues or express true feelings. These limitations can be overcome by indirect methods. Projective techniques are indirect methods in which the respondents reveal their inner characteristics.

Individuals are asked to respond to vague and unstructured situations such as sketches, words, pictures or drawings. Types of projective tests are Rorschach ink blot test, word association, sentence completion, construction techniques, etc.

By and large, these techniques are used when direct methods of collecting data are irrelevant. This technique is less popular in nursing research because specific skills in psychology and psychiatry are needed to administer the tests and properly interpret the results.

Merits

1. Information collected is reliable.
2. It is useful in group discussions.
3. These techniques do not necessarily need literary or academic skills.
4. Provides overall functioning of individuals.

Demerits

1. The researcher needs specific skills.
2. There can be subjectivity in the interpretation of responses.
3. It is expensive to administer.

Q-sorts

It is a technique of comparative rating that preserves the subjective point of view of individuals. It is a relatively new technique. Its aim is to inquire into the subjectivity of human mind.

In Q-sort, participants are presented with a set of cards on which words and phrases are written. Participants are asked to sort the cards along a specified bipolar dimension, such as most important/least important. Typically around 50–100 cards are to be sorted.

For example, attitude of mothers towards breastfeeding practice can be studied by writing statements on the cards and asking the participants to sort them on a continuum from totally disagree to totally agree.

Merits

1. It helps in exploratory research.
2. It helps in in-depth study of small sample populations.

Demerits

1. It is not very cost-effective.
2. Only a small sample can be studied.

Vignettes

It is a self-reporting approach which involves a brief description of events or situations to which the respondents are asked to react. The descriptions, which can either be fictitious or based on facts, are structures to elicit information about respondents' perception, opinions or knowledge about some phenomena. The vignettes are usually written narrative descriptions. Questions posed to the respondents after vignettes may be either open-ended or close-ended. Usually 3–5 vignettes are included in an instrument.

Vignettes are an economical means of eliciting information about how people might behave in situations that would be difficult to observe in daily life.

Uses of Vignettes

1. To elicit general attitudes and beliefs.
2. To explore sensitive topics that participants might otherwise find difficult to discuss.
3. It is used in focus group discussions.
4. To analyze different group's interpretations of the same situation.

Merits

1. Allows contact with respondents.
2. Provides detailed data.
3. Detailed analysis and in-depth exploration of topics

Demerits

1. Covers limited sample size
2. Involves response biases

Delphi Technique

The Delphi technique consists of identifying a group of experts or persons concerned with a certain area or programme. Their concerns about their area or programme are elicited and ranked. Then experts are asked to rank the items in the list in order of importance. These are sent back to the same panel and the panel members are then asked to re-rank their responses. The researcher can then focus on those items considered most important by the experts.

Pilot Study

A pilot study is a small-scale methodological test intended to ensure that proposed methods and procedures will work in practice before being applied in a large investigation.

It provides the research worker with ideas, approaches and clues not forcing prior to the pilot study. Such ideas and clues greatly increase the chances of obtaining clear-cut findings in the main study.

A pilot study is a small preliminary investigation of the same general character on the major study, which is designed to acquaint the researcher with problems that can be corrected before preparation for a large research project.

Purposes of a Pilot Study

1. To assess the availability of study subjects.
2. To provide better understanding of the problem under study.
3. To find out the nature of relationship between variables.
4. To provide alternative methods of data collection.
5. To test the adequacy of tools of data collection.
6. To develop appropriate plans for analysis.
7. To estimate the probable cost and duration of main study.
8. To structure the questions.
9. To refuse methodology.
10. To ensure the appropriateness of methods of data collection.
11. To develop a research protocol.

Sociometry

Sociometry is a quantitative method for measuring social relationships. It was developed by psychotherapist Jacob L. Moreno in his studies of the relationship between social structures and psychological well-being.

Sociometry is a way of measuring the degree of relatedness among people. Measurement of relatedness can be useful not only in the assessment of behaviour within groups, but also for interventions to bring about positive change and for determining the extent of change. For a work group, sociometry can be a powerful tool for reducing conflict and improving communication because it allows the group to see itself objectively and to analyze its own dynamics. It is also a powerful tool for assessing dynamics and development in groups devoted to therapy or training.

One of Moreno's innovations in sociometry was the development of the sociogram, a systematic method for graphically representing individuals as points/nodes and the relationships between them as lines/arcs.

There are a variety of classic sociometric assessment techniques. In the peer nomination technique, children in a social group or school classroom anonymously identify social preferences for their classmates. For example, children may be asked to provide a list of the three classmates with whom they would most like to play and the three with whom they would least like to play. Another peer nomination technique is to provide a list of the names of the children in a classroom along with social acceptance items (e.g. "Who do you like to play with?", "Who is most likely to be alone during recess?", "Who gets into trouble the most?"). The children are asked to identify perhaps one to three classmates who they perceive best fit the item description.

Within sociology, sociometry has two main branches: research sociometry and applied sociometry. Research sociometry is action research with groups exploring the socio-emotional networks of relationships using specified criteria, e.g. "Who in this group do you want to sit beside you at work?", "Who in the group do you go to for advice on a work problem?", "Who in the group do you see providing satisfying leadership in the pending project?" Sometimes called network explorations, research sociometry is concerned with relational patterns in small (individual and small group) and larger populations, such as organizations and neighbourhoods.

Reliability

Reliability is the extent to which an experiment, test or any measuring procedure yields the same result on repeated trials. Without the agreement of independent observers able to replicate research procedures, or the ability to use research tools and procedures that yield consistent measurements, researchers would be unable to satisfactorily draw conclusions, formulate theories or make claims about the generalizability of their research.

Reliability is such an important concept that it has been defined in terms of its application to a wide range of activities. For researchers, four key types of reliability are:

1. Equivalency reliability
2. Stability reliability
3. Internal consistency
4. Interrater reliability

Equivalency reliability

Equivalency reliability is the extent to which two items measure identical concepts at an identical level of difficulty. Equivalency reliability is determined by relating two sets of test scores to one another to highlight the degree of relationship or association. In quantitative studies and particularly in experimental studies, a correlation coefficient (statistically referred to as *r*) is used to show the strength of the correlation between a dependent variable (subject under study) and one or more independent variables, which are manipulated to determine the effects on the dependent variable. An important consideration is that equivalency reliability is concerned with correlational, not causal, relationships.

Stability reliability

Test-re test reliability (stability reliability) is the agreement of measuring instruments over time. To determine stability, a measure or test is repeated on the same subject at a future date. Results are compared and correlated with the initial test to give a measure of stability.

An example of stability reliability would be the method of maintaining weights used by the US Bureau of Standards. Platinum objects of fixed weight (one kilogram, one pound, etc.) are kept locked away. Once a year they are taken out and weighed, allowing scales to be reset so they are weighing accurately. Keeping track of how much the scales are off from year to year establishes stability reliability for these instruments. In this instance, platinum weights themselves are assumed to have perfectly fixed stability reliability.

Internal consistency

Internal consistency is the extent to which tests or procedures assess the same characteristic, skill or quality. It is a measure of the precision between the observers or of the measuring instruments used in a study. This type of reliability often helps researchers interpret data and predict the value of scores and the limits of the relationship among variables. For example, a researcher designs a questionnaire to find out about college students' dissatisfaction with a particular textbook. Analyzing the internal consistency of the survey items dealing with dissatisfaction will reveal the extent to which items on the questionnaire focus on the notion of dissatisfaction.

Interrater reliability

Interrater reliability is the extent to which two or more individuals (coders or raters) agree. Interrater reliability addresses the consistency of the implementation of a rating system. A test of Interrater reliability would be the following scenario.

Two or more researchers are observing a first-year B.Sc. nursing classroom. The class is discussing a movie that they have just viewed as a group. The researchers have a sliding rating scale (1 being most positive, 5 being most negative) with which they are rating the student's oral responses. Interrater reliability assesses the consistency of how the rating system is implemented. For example, if one researcher gives a "1" to a student response, while another researcher gives a "5", obviously the Interrater reliability would be inconsistent. Interrater reliability is dependent upon the ability of two or more individuals to be consistent. Training, education and monitoring skills can enhance Interrater reliability.

Validity

For every dimension of interest and specific question or set of questions, there are a vast number of ways to make questions. Although the guiding principle should be the specific purposes of the research, there are better and worse questions for any particular operationalization.

Two of the primary criteria of evaluation in any measurement or observation are:

1. Whether we are measuring what we intend to measure.
2. Whether the same measurement process yields the same results.

These two concepts are validity and reliability. Reliability is concerned with questions of stability and consistency – does the same measurement tool yield stable and consistent results when repeated over time. Think about measurement processes in other contexts – in construction or woodworking, a tape measure is a highly reliable measuring instrument.

Say you have a piece of wood that is 2 1/2 feet long. You measure it once with the tape. Measure it again and you get 2 1/2 feet. Measure it repeatedly and you consistently get a measurement of 2 1/2 feet. The tape measure yields reliable results.

Validity refers to the extent we are measuring what we hope to measure (and what we think we are measuring). To continue with the example of measuring the piece of wood, a tape measure that has been created with accurate spacing for inches, feet, etc. should yield valid results as well. Measuring this piece of wood with a good tape measure should produce a correct measurement of the wood's length.

To apply these concepts to social research, we want to use measurement tools that are both reliable and valid. We want questions that yield consistent responses when asked multiple times – this is reliability. Similarly, we want questions that get accurate responses from respondents – this is validity.

Face validity

This criterion is an assessment of whether a measure appears, on the face of it, to measure the concept it is intended to measure. This is a very minimum assessment; if a measure cannot satisfy this criterion, then the other criteria are inconsequential. We can think about observational measures of behaviour that would have face validity. For example, striking out at another person would have face validity for an indicator of aggression. Similarly, offering assistance to a stranger would meet the criterion of face validity for helping. However, asking people about their favourite movie to measure racial prejudice has little face validity.

Content validity

Content validity concerns the extent to which a measure adequately represents all facets of a concept. Consider a series of questions that serve as indicators of depression (don't feel like eating, lost interest in things usually enjoyed, etc.). If there were other kinds of common behaviours that mark a person as depressed that were not included in the index, then the index would have low content validity since it did not adequately represent all facets of the concept.

Criterion-related validity

Criterion-related validity applies to instruments that have been developed for usefulness as indicator of specific trait or behaviour, either now or in the future. For example, think about the driving test as a social measurement that has pretty good predictive validity. That is to say, an individual's performance on a driving test correlates well with his/her driving ability.

Construct validity

For many things we want to measure, there is not necessarily a pertinent criterion available. In this case, turn to construct validity, which concerns the extent to which a measure is related to other measures as specified by theory or previous research. Does a measure stack up with other variables the way we expect it to? A good example of this form of validity comes from early self-esteem studies; self-esteem refers to a person's sense of self-worth or self-respect. Clinical observations in psychology had shown that people who had low self-esteem often had depression. Therefore, to establish the construct validity of self-esteem measure, the researchers showed that those with higher scores on self-esteem measure had lower depression scores, while those with low self-esteem had higher rates of depression.

Validity and reliability compared

What is the relationship between validity and reliability? The two do not necessarily go hand-in-hand.

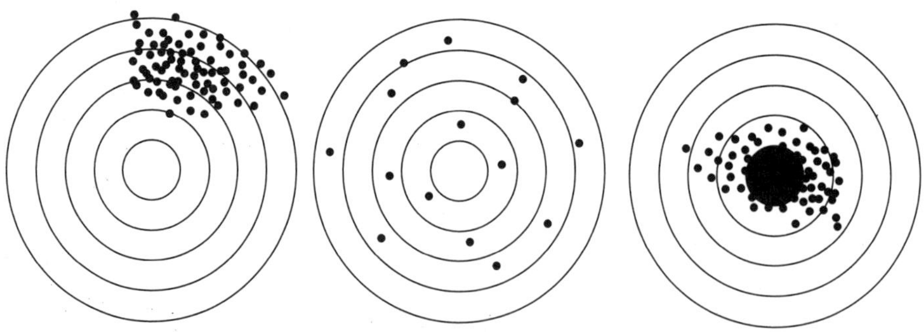

Reliable but not valid — Valid but not reliable — Valid and reliable

At best, we have a measure that has both high validity and high reliability. It yields consistent results in repeated application and it accurately reflects what we hope to represent.

It is possible to have a measure that has high reliability but low validity, one that is consistent in getting bad information or consistent in missing the mark. It is also possible to have one that has low reliability and low validity, inconsistent and not on target.

Finally, it is not possible to have a measure that has low reliability and high validity; you cannot really get at what you want or what you are interested in if your measure fluctuates wildly.

How do you divide on the mode of data collection?

1. Population
2. Characteristics of the sample
3. Types of questions
4. Question topic
5. Response rate
6. Cost
7. Time

Choice of methods of data collection

Which of the above methods of data collection should be selected for proposed research project? This is one of the questions to be considered while designing the research plan. One or more methods have to be chosen. No method is universal. Each method's unique features should be compared with the needs and conditions of the study and thus the choice of the methods should be divided.

The commonly used methods in nursing studies:

1. Knowledge – structured questionnaire, interview schedule
2. Attitude – Likert scale
3. Practice – observation, checklist, rating scale
4. Biophysiological measures – BP, heart rate, pulse rate (anxiety), cortisol levels (stress), ECG changes, SPO_2, pap smear.

Physiological Measurements

Physiological data about patients such as temperature, respiratory rate, pulse rate, blood pressure, etc. are collected by nurses to identify the physiological states of patients. It is also an important criterion for determining the effectiveness of criteria nursing actions. Physiological or biological measurement is suitable to the study of several nursing interventions and is useful to the nurse researchers as well.

Physiological measurements can be

1. Physical methods – weight, temperature
2. Biochemical methods – RBS, electrolytes
3. Microbiological – criteria and sensitivity tests
4. Radiological – CT, X-ray, USG, etc.

Physiological measurements need specialized equipment to make observation and also need specialized training.

Merits

1. It is objective – two readings of the same instrument taken at the same time by two different persons yield the same results.
2. It is precise – mild variations in the variable of interest can be determined.
3. It is sensitive – subjects cannot alter their physiological status.

Demerits

1. Some instruments used may be expensive.
2. The use of instruments requires special knowledge and training.
3. Some instruments are intrusive, i.e. presence of some variables may change the measurement. For example, the presence of BP apparatus itself can make a patient anxious and then increase his blood pressure.
4. Environmental variables may alter the measurements.

SUMMARY

Data collection methods of a study provide the operational definitions of relevant variables. Types of data collection methods include physiological, observational, interviews, questionnaires and available data or records. Each method has merits and demerits.

Physiological measurements are those methods that use technical instruments to collect data about patient's physical, chemical, microbiological or anatomical status.

Observational methods are usually used in research when the variables of interest deal with events or behaviours. Observation necessitates preplanning, systematic recording, controlling the observations, etc. Observers may be passive or active and concealed or obvious.

Interviews and questionnaires are the most commonly used data collection methods in nursing research. Both have the purpose of asking subjects to report data for themselves. Scales provide an estimate of the degree to which the respondents possess some characteristics. Open-ended or close-ended questions may be used when asking questions.

A questionnaire is useful when there is finite number of questions to be asked and the researcher is sure that the questions are clear and specific. Interviews are best used when a large response rate and an unbiased sample are important because the refusal rate for interviews is much less than that for questionnaires. Appropriate use of sampling and research methods are essential ingredients in research work.

MULTIPLE CHOICE QUESTIONS

1. Which of the following is a self-report data collection instrument that asks respondents to report their attitudes or feelings on a continuum?
   - (a) visual analogue scale (VAS)
   - (b) attitude scales
   - (c) Q-sort
   - (d) delphi technique

2. A data collection method in which subjects are asked to sort elements into categories according to their attitudes towards, or rating of, the statements: ________
   (a) observation
   (b) Q-sort method
   (c) delphi technique
   (d) projective technique
3. In which of the following does the researcher describe events or behaviours as they occur with no preconceived ideas of what will be seen?
   (a) unstructured observation
   (b) structured observation
   (c) participant observation
   (d) non-participant observation
4. Additional prompting questions that encourage the respondent to elaborate on a certain topic are called ________.
   (a) contingency questions
   (b) demographic questions
   (c) open-ended questions
   (d) probes
5. A data collection method that uses several rounds of questions to seek a consensus on a particular topic from a group of experts on the topic is ________.
   (a) projective techniques
   (b) Q-sort method
   (c) delphi technique
   (d) personality inventories
6. Likert scale and Semantic differential are commonly used types of ________.
   (a) overt
   (b) covert
   (c) visual analogue scale (VAS)
   (d) attitude scales

7. Name the type of observation method of data collection in the following situations:

   The observer makes no attempt to alter the social setting that is being studied.

   At the same time the observer doesn't make the observation covertly.

   Also the observer is the part of the social setting.

   (a) concealment and participant
   (b) no concealment and participation
   (c) concealment and non-participant
   (d) no concealment and non-participant

8. Which of the following is also called 'Lurking'?

   (a) concealment and non-participant
   (b) no concealment and participation
   (c) concealment and participant
   (d) no concealment and non-participant

ANSWER KEY

1. (b) 2. (b) 3. (a) 4. (d) 5. (c) 6. (d) 7. (b) 8. (a)

REVIEW QUESTIONS

1. Define research tool. Explain the characteristics of research instruments.
2. Discuss the construction of questionnaires and interview schedule.
3. Differentiate between questionnaire and structured interview method of data collection in nursing research.
4. (a) Define questionnaire.
   (b) List the characteristics of a good questionnaire.
   (c) State the advantages and disadvantages of questionnaire.

5. (a) Explain the different types of samples.
   (b) Discuss random sampling with a suitable example.
6. Explain sources of data collection in nursing research.
7. List the criteria in selecting an instrument.
8. (a) Define research tool.
   (b) Explain the different methods of establishing reliability.
   (c) What is observation as a method of data collection?
9. Define pilot study.
10. Explain self-report data collection tool.
    (a) Explain the steps of tool construction.
    (b) Describe questionnaire as a tool for data collection.
11. (a) List the qualities of a research tool.
    (b) Discuss the method of data collection.
    (c) Explain briefly the steps in developing a questionnaire.
12. (a) List the methods of data collection.
    (b) Briefly explain observation as a method of data collection.
13. Differentiate between:
    (a) Probability and non-probability sampling
    (b) Interview schedule and questionnaire
14. Write short notes on:
    (a) Rating scale
    (b) Types of sampling
    (c) Pilot study
    (d) Advantages of interview method of data collection
    (e) Characteristics of a good questionnaire
    (f) Reliability
    (g) Research tool

REFERENCES

Abdullah, F.G., & Levine, A. (1994). Preparing nursing research for the 21st century. New York: Springer.

Burns, N., & Grove, S.K. (2005). The practice of nursing research: Conduct, critique, and utilization. (5th ed.). Philadelphia: Saunders.

Cohen, J. (1988). Statistical power analysis for the behavioural sciences. (2nd ed.). Hillsdale, NJ: Lawrence Erlbaum.

Coyne, I.T. (1997). Sampling in qualitative research. Purposeful and theoretical sampling: Merging or clear boundaries. *Journal of Advanced Nursing*, 26(3), 623–630.

De Von, H.A., Penckofer, S.M., & Zerwic, J.J. (2005). Symptoms of unstable angina in patients with and without diabetics. *Research in Nursing and Health*, 28(2), 136–413.

Deans, C. (2005). Nurses and occupational violence: The role of organizational support in moderating professional competence. *Australian Journal of Advanced Nursing*, 22, 14–18.

Golding, J.M. (1996). Sexual assault history and limitations in physical functioning in two general population samples. *Research in Nursing and Health*, 19(1), 33–44.

Huang, T. (2005). Home environmental hazards among community-dwelling elderly in Taiwan. *Journal of Nursing Research*, 13, 49–56.

Kerlinger, F.N., & Lee, H.B. (2000). Foundations of behavioural research. New York: Harcourt Brace.

Knapp, T.R. (1996). The overemphasis on power analysis. *Nursing Research*, 45, 379–380.

Manojlovich, M. (2005). Predictors of professional nursing practice behaviours in hospital settings. *Nursing Research*, 54, 41–47.

McCain, N.L., Munjas, B.A., Munro, C.L., Elswick, R.K., Jr. Robins, J.L., Ferreira-Gonzalez, A., et al. (2003). Effects of stress management on PNI-based outcomes in persons with HIV disease. *Research in Nursing and Health*, 26(2), 102–117.

McMillian, J., Morgan, S.A., & Ament, P. (2006). Acceptance of male registered nurses by female registered nurse. *Journal of Nursing Scholarship*, 38, 100–106.

Morse, J.M. (1998). Designing funded qualitative research. In N.K., Denzin & Y.S., Lincoln (Eds.). Strategies of qualitative inquiry (56–85). Thousand Oaks, CA: Sage Publications.

Patton, M.Q. (2002). Qualitative evaluation and research methods. (3rd ed.). Thousand Oaks, CA: Sage Publications.

Polit, D.F., & Sherman, R.E. (1990). Statistical power in nursing research. *Nursing Research*, 39, 365–369.

Rew, L. (2003). A theory of taking care of oneself grounded in experiences of homeless youth. *Nursing Research*, 52(4), 234–241.

Roscoe, J. (1975). Fundamental research statistics for the behavioural sciences. (2nd ed.). New York: Holt, Rinehart & Winston.

Simpson, K.R., & James, D.C. (2005). Effects of immediate verses delayed pushing during second-stage labor on fetal well-being. *Nursing Research*, 54, 149–157.

Tsai, J.H. (2006). Use of computer technology to enhance immigrant families' adaptation. *Journal of Nursing Scholarship*, 38, 87–93.

Ulrich, C.M., Soeken, K.L., & Miller, N. (2003). Ethical conflict associated with managed care. *Nursing Research*, 52, 168–175.

Vallerand, A.H., Fouladbakhsh, J., & Templin, T. (2005). Patients' choices for the self-treatment of pain. *Applied Nursing Research*, 18, 90–96.

Wongvatunyu, S., & Porter, E.J. (2005). Mothers' experience of helping young adults with traumatic brain injury. *The Journal of Nursing Scholarship*, 37(1), 48–56.

CHAPTER

12

DATA ANALYSIS AND INTERPRETATION

Key terms

★ Data analysis ★ Interpretation ★ Tabulation ★ Editing data
★ Data transcription ★ Sorting of data ★ Data processing
★ Coding ★ Validation of data

⊙ Outline

★ Data processing and interpretation
★ Plan for data processing and analysis
★ Steps in data processing
★ Summarizing the data
★ Data sorting

⊙ Objectives

On completion of this chapter, you will be able to:

★ define data analysis
★ recognize data processing and interpretation
★ interpret plan for data processing and analysis
★ identify steps in data processing

Introduction

Data analysis and data processing are two different processes. The first step is that of analyzing the data on the basis of objectives, prevailing theories and then dictating appropriate conclusions.

The latter (processing of data) refers to the process of regrouping or rearranging the sorted data which was analyzed previously. Thus, processing depends on analysis.

Data Processing and Interpretation

The collected data must be processed. Processing of data denotes editing, coding, classifying and tabulating the collected data.

For data processing, identifying the variables and its hypothetical relationship is a prerequisite. It involves reduction of data while preparing the data for analysis. It may be either manual or electronic. It is an integral part of research design.

Plan for Data Processing and Analysis

The preparation of a plan helps the researcher to collect information through a standardized way, and to ensure no unnecessary data is collected which will never be analyzed.

Data may be quantitative or qualitative, and hence the procedures for analyzing these can be different.

For quantitative data, the analysis begins usually with a description of data for each variable applicable in the study. Processing of data is done when all the data have been collected.

For qualitative data, the data to be obtained are more likely to be described, summarized and interpreted than to be computed. Hence the researcher may begin the analysis while collecting the data, so that unanswered questions could be identified before completing the process of data collection.

The preparation of plan for data processing and analysis provides better feasibility and also provides an important review of the appropriateness of data collection tools for collecting the data.

Steps in Data Processing

I. Identifying data structures

The data are prepared in a data format, which allows the analyst to use the software such as SAS or SPSS. The primary relationship between variables or between groups of variables has been established by the researcher. Most data structures can be expressed in a graphical format.

II. Editing of the data

The information in a questionnaire should be clear, legible and accurate. Thus, the data needs editing. Editing is for evaluation of the questionnaire for accuracy. It is a process to find out and rectify errors and omissions. Editing is done at two levels, at the time of data recording and at the time of data analysis.

Data editing ensures the following:

Completeness: The researcher should examine whether all schedules in the questionnaire are complete and properly entered. Thus, the first step in editing is to see that each question contains an appropriate answer or variable.

Accuracy: The information in a questionnaire must be accurate and correct. A random checking may help discover errors and omissions.

Uniformity: Lack of uniformity in the interpretation of questions by data recorders must be analyzed. Consistency throughout the questionnaire data set should be ensured.

III. Coding and classification

On completing the editing process, coding and classification is done. Coding refers to the process of translating answers into a form of numbers. It implies data reduction and analysis of data. Coding may be numeric, alphabetic and zero coding. The process of classification is used when open-ended responses have been received.

IV. Data transcription

When the collected observations are simple, they could be easily transferred into a datasheet. The researcher adopts two transcription methods, manual and computerized. Manual transcription needs longer worksheets, sorting cards/strips, etc. Hence it is time consuming. Computerized responses are done through database packages such as spreadsheets (Excel) or text files (Word).

V. Tabulation

Tabulation is a process of summarizing and arranging the data in a compact form for further analysis. Computerized application of tabulation is easier due to the use of software. Tabulation implies tabular representation of data.

A table usually contains:

1. Title clearly indicating a description of the table
2. Heading indicates the table of columns and rows
3. Body of the table containing valuable information
4. Sums of columns and rows
5. Footnotes containing additional information such as the origin of information, level of significance, chi-square values, etc.

Data Sorting

Data processing and analysis need an adequate sorting system. In a comparative study, data sorting is made after collecting the data and placed into two or three groups. These groups are compared by analysis. In a case control study, the cases are compared with the controls. This is possible with coding these categories in a questionnaire distinctly right after sorting. In a cross-sectional survey, it is possible to sort the data into two or more groups for comparison.

Data Processing (Quantitative Data)

Processing and analyzing the data from questionnaires may be either manual or computerized. In the manual method, the data are entered on the master sheets or questionnaires and then compiled. In the computerized method, this is made possible through the use of microcomputers or software programs. Data processing of quantitative data generally involves categorizing, coding and summarizing the data.

Categorizing

It deals with the method of categorizing the responses. Responses may be either categorical variables or numerical variables. Categorical variables are investigated through closed questions and observations. In an open interview, the answers to questions can be pre-categorized depending on the knowledge of possible answers which might be given. There should always be a category called 'others'. All these responses should be treated and placed as logical categories. Unpredictable or difficult answers are put in the category 'others'. These account for only 5% of responses. In the case of numerical variables, the data does not need any pre-categorization. If the data collected should have been a guess (e.g. duration of insomnia for patients with sleep disorder, income for patients attending out-patient clinic), the coded and categorized data might be premature. If the researcher specifies the fact that the category was a wrong one, there is no need of reclassifying the data.

Coding

A coding system must be developed in order to analyze and process the data which we feed into a computer. In computer analysis, each category of variables can be coded as words, letters, numbers or even groups. For example, the answer 'yes' may be coded 'Y' or '1' and answer 'no' may be coded 'N' or '2'. These codes are entered on the questionnaires. For all questions, there should be corresponding boxes for the code in the right margin of the page. If manual analysis is made through master sheets, it is better to code the data.

Coding conventions

Generally, similar codes are applied to reduce mistakes. Some common codes are:

	Code
Yes (positive response)	Y or 1
No (negative response)	N or 2
Don't know	D or 8
Unknown/no response	U or 9

Summarizing the data

Manual analysis of data is done by using **data master sheet**. Master sheets can be made in different methods, e.g. a simple checklist or questionnaire. All answers must be coded and given at the top of the sheet, and answers should be ticked in appropriate columns.

In the below example, we study the use of alcohol/beverages by urban dwellers and its side effects. The straightforward answers from male respondents using alcohol are tabulated as below:

Table 12.1 Master sheet for alcohol consumptions (males)

No.	Q1 Sex	Q2 Age	Q6 No. of peg/ day	Q7 Age on set	Q9 Tried to				Q14 Affects liver prob.	
					Reduce		Stop			
		Yes Cat	No Cat	Yes Cat	Yes	No	Yes	No	Yes	No
1	M	20 (1)	12 (2)	12 (2)	1x					
2	M	38 (3)	30 (4)	20 (4)		NR		1x		
3	M	60 (5)	15 (2)	14 (2)	10x			3x		
Efc.										
Total	31	Av.35	Av. 20	Av.18	26	4 +INR	19	12	11	20

Categories

Age in years	No. of drinks/pegs per day	Age of onset of drinking
15 – 24 = 1	<10 = 1	<10 = 1
25 – 34 = 2	10 – 19 = 2	10 – 14 = 2
35 – 44 = 4	30 – 39 = 4	20 – 24 = 4
55+ = 5	40+ = 5	25+ = 5

Here the categories and corresponding codes are entered, which helps reduce mistakes and calculate averages easily. There were 31 male alcoholics. If there were less than 31 responses, then there arise some non-responders (NR), as happened in Q9, or an error had occurred.

		Education (Q3)									Occupation (Q4)			
No.	None	Highest level reached Years	Type					Still in School		N R	Self 0 1 2 3 4 5 6	Head household 1 2 3 4 5 6	U	NR
			PS	SS	QI	UY	O	Yes	No					
1	*	4												
2	*	9										NA		
3									NA			NA		

Table 12.1 describes the coded answers. However, some answers need more elaborate coding and have more categories. For example, Q4 on education and Q5 on occupation could be summarized as follows:

Categories

Education	Occupation/Income
PS = Primary school	0 = No source of income
SS = Secondary school	1 = Irregular income (seasonal farming)
OT = Occupational training	2 = Unskilled labourers
UY = University level	3 = Farmer (with land)
O = Others	4 = Trade /bear brewer/taxi owner, etc.
U = No response/Unknown	5 = Teacher, nurse, civil servant
NA = Not applicable	6 = Doctor, lawyer, government administrator

For a small-scale study in which groups are compared, a different master sheet should be made for each group, e.g. good and poor compliance to treatment. Gender is also an important cross-cutting theme.

Manual compilation (without using master sheets)

When the sample is small as well as the collected data is limited, manual compilation needs more efficiency. To ensure speed and accuracy, the following procedures should be adopted.

1. If the compilation is done by one person, then use manual sorting. If two persons are doing the compilation, then both manual sorting and tally counting may be used.
2. In manual sorting only one question is taken at a time.

3. One person in the compilation team reads the information and the other one records it in the form of tally. Tally count for no more than two variables at a time shall be resorted to.
4. After using both compilation methods namely manual sorting and tally counting, check out the total response to each question to make sure there has been no omission or duplication.

Compilation by computer

If the sample is larger, then the use of computer will be beneficial. Feeding data into a computer costs time and money. Hence compilation through computer consists of:

1. Choosing an appropriate computer program
2. Data entry
3. Validation/verification of the data
4. Programming
5. Generating outputs/print outs

Choosing an appropriate computer program: A number of computer programs are available for compilation of data. The most widely used among them are Epi Info (ver. 6) (a word processor for creating questionnaire), LOTUS 1-2-3 (a spreadsheet program), dBase III plus/IV (a DBMS program) and SPSS; all of these are user-friendly programs.

Data entry: In data entry, the information relating to each subject in the study is keyed into the computer in the form of a relevant code. Outsourcing the data entry may be fast and less expensive.

Validation/verification: There arises some chance of errors and omissions during the data entry. This step involves giving adequate commands to identify errors.

Programming: If the data is being analyzed with the support of a computer programmer, the researcher should make effective communication with him regarding variable names, its location, subject details, and application of tabulation in the questionnaire. Therefore, a basic knowledge of computer programming is essential to give appropriate commands.

Computer output: A computer can perform different kinds of analysis and validations of the data already fed into it. After analysis, it gives out the results in the form of print outs. The results may contain tables, graphs, and statistical tests which should be applicable in the report.

Analysis of Quantitative Data

Quantitative data analysis implies production and interpretation of tables, frequencies, graphs, etc. that describe the data. A detailed explanation is given in chapter 16.

Frequency counts

Frequency count refers to the enumeration of the influence of a particular measurement or a specific answer to a specific question which occurs. For example,

Alcoholics	–	48
Non-alcoholics	–	86
Total	–	134

In manual data analysis, simple tables can be made with frequency counts for each variable in the data master sheets.

If the numbers are large, then frequency distribution is calculated. For example,

$$\text{Alcoholics} = \frac{48}{134} \times 100 = 35\%$$

$$\text{Non-alcoholics} = \frac{86}{134} \times 100 = 65\%$$

Cross-tabulation

Data analysis through a combination of variables is commonly known as cross-tabulation. Depending upon its objectives and applications, cross-tabulation may be of two types, namely descriptive and analytic. Descriptive cross-tabulation describes the problem under study whereas analytical cross-tabulation compares groups to determine the differences and focuses on the relationship between variables.

Data and its nature

Statistics depends on data and facts. Data relate to population, religion, age, sex, income, etc. Data may be qualitative or quantitative.

Qualitative data are non-numerical and cannot be measurable, e.g. sex, religion, etc. Quantitative data are numerical and can be measurable, e.g. age, income, profit, family members, etc.

Sources of data

Data sources are primary sources and secondary sources. The data collected through primary sources are called primary data and the data collected through secondary sources are called secondary data.

Frequency distribution

Frequency refers to the number of times each variable is repeated in a table. For example, if 10 students in a class get 45 marks in a subject, then the frequency is 10. During frequency distribution, raw data are arranged into classes and frequencies, and are known as grouped data. They may be of discrete or continuous type. Discrete data take certain specific values, whereas continuous data take any numerical value within a specific interval such as profit in rupees, marks in percentage, weight in kilogram, etc.

Data classification

The collected data may be further classified into classes and subclasses depending upon its nature. Hence classification is the process of grouping of related facts into classes.

Types of classification

Classification is of four types:

Geographical classification: Classification of data on geographical basis such as area, place, etc. is known as geographical classification, e.g. number of industrial units manufacturing cloth materials in different states of India.

States	Number of units manufacturing cloth materials
Tamil Nadu	3500
Rajasthan	3700
Karnataka	4200

Geographical classification of manufacturing unit.

Chronological classification: Classification based on periods such as time, months, year, etc. is known as chronological classification, e.g. turnover of a company for 2000–2005.

Profits of a company from 2000–2005

Year	Profit (Rs '000)
2000	65
2001	73
2002	86
2003	91
2004	89
2005	98

Qualitative classification: Categorization of data on the basis of attributes or qualities such as sex, religion, literacy, etc. is known as qualitative classification. These attributes cannot be measured.

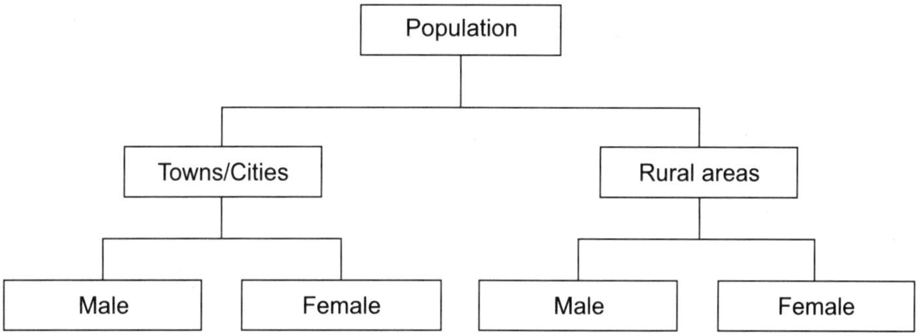

Quantitative classification: Classification on the basis of certain characteristics such as weight, height, income, etc. is known as quantitative classification of data, e.g. marks obtained by the students in a class for a particular subject.

Marks Obtained by Students

Marks	Number of students
Below 10	3
10–20	8
20–30	7

30–40	5
40–50	10
50–60	6
60–70	12
70–80	9
80–90	5
90–100	0
Total	65

Qualitative Data Analysis

Qualitative modes of data analysis provide ways of discussing, examining, comparing, contrasting and interpreting meaningful patterns or themes. Meaningfulness is determined by the goals and objectives of the research project: the same data can be analysed and synthesized from multiple angles depending on the particular research question addressed. The varieties of approach include ethnography, narrative analysis, discourse analysis and textual analysis – each corresponding to different types of data, objectives and philosophical orientation.

Definition

Qualitative data analysis is the range of processes and procedures whereby the collected qualitative data is used to form an explanation, understanding; or interpretation of the people and situations being investigated.

Elements of Qualitative Analysis

According to framework developed by Miles and Huberman (1994) the elements of qualitative data analysis are: data reduction, data display and conclusion drawing and verification.

(i) Data reduction

It refers to the process of selecting, focusing, simplifying, abstracting and transforming the data that appear in written up field notes or transcriptions. Not only do the data need to be condensed for the state of manageability, they also have to be transformed so they can be made intelligible in terms of the issues being addressed.

(ii) Data display

This next element of qualitative data analysis goes a step beyond data reduction to provide an organized, compressed assembly of information that permits conclusion drawing. A display can be an extended piece of text or a diagram, chart or matrix that provides a new way of ranging and thinking about the data. It allows the analyst to discern systematic patterns and interrelationships from the data. At display stage additional higher order categories or themes may emerge that go beyond those discovered during the initial process of data reduction.

(iii) Conclusion drawing and verification

The last element consists of stepping back to consider what the analysed data mean and to access their implications for the questions at hand. Verification integrally linked to conclusion drawing, entails revisiting the data as many times as necessary to cross check or verify these emergent conclusion.

Noticing, Collecting and Thinking Model

Seidel (1998) developed a useful model to explain the basic process of qualitative data analysis. The model consists of 3 parts. Noticing, collecting and thinking about interesting things. These parts are interlinked and cyclical. For example, while thinking about things you notice further things and collect them. Seidel likens the process to solving a jigsaw puzzle. Noticing interesting things in the data and assigning codes to them, based on topic or theme, potentially breaks the data into fragments. Codes which have been applied to the data then act as sorting and collection devices.

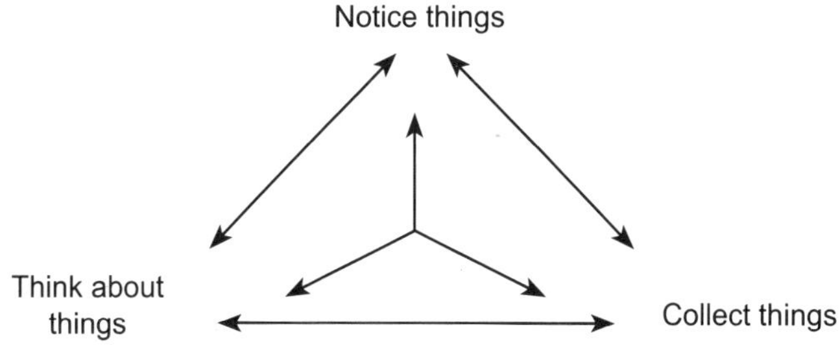

Figure 12.1 The data analysis model (Seidel, 1998)

Qualitative data analysis process

Following are the four processes that play a role in qualitative analysis.

1. *Comprehending*: The researcher tries to comprehend or learn what is going on by reading the topic at hand. By this a thorough and rich description of the phenomenon can be made.
2. *Synthesizing*: It involves 'sifting' of the data and putting pieces together. At this stage the researcher gets a sense of what is typical and what is different about the phenomenon.
3. *Theorizing*: It involves a systemic sorting of the data. The researcher develops alternate explanations of the phenomenon under study and then analyses those explanations to determine their fit with the data.
4. *Recontextualizing*: It involves the further development of the theory such that its applicability to other settings or groups is explored.

Steps of qualitative data analysis

For qualitative data analysis, the researcher will have to carry out the following steps:

1. *Description of study sample characteristics*: A descriptive study sample in terms of age, gender, OCC education; or marital status may be given.
2. *Ordering and coding of data*: During ordering or coding of the qualitative data, research handles two types of data. These include responses acquired through open-ended questions and more elaborate narratives from loosely structured interviews and focus group discussions.
3. *Summarizing data in compilation sheets:* After ordering the data, it has to be summarized like the master sheets for quantitative data, complication sheets for qualitative data consists of a number of columns with topics covered by the study as headings.
4. *Further summarizing of data in narrations, matrices, figures and quasi-statistical tables:* These help in representation of data and qualitative analysis. A matrix is a chart that looks like a cross-table but contains words. A diagram is a figure with boxes containing

variables and arrows indicating relationship between variables. A flow chart is a special diagram expressing the logical sequence of actions or decisions. In quasi-statistical tables, the content of the narrative data is searched for a pre-specified word or theme. The result of the search is information that can be analyzed statistically, hence the name quasi-statistic.

5. *Drawing and verifying conclusions*: It is the essence of data analysis. When we start summarizing our data in compilation sheets, flow charts, matrices or diagrams, we continuously draw conclusions and also make relevant modifications.
6. *Reporting the data*: Qualitative data can be reported in two ways. The first method is to summarize the major qualitative results in a separate section of the findings with examples and quotations along with the objectives that guided the collection of that particular data. The second method is to fully integrated different data sets in the chapter of findings ordered according to the objectives of the entire study.

Data management tips

1. *Check the data*: Make sure everything is together. Decide whether the data are of sufficient quality to analyze, and what level of investment is warranted.
2. *Add identification numbers*: Add an identification number to each instrument, respondent, group or site.
3. Prepare data for analysis.
4. Decide how to format cases.
5. Use a special qualitative data analysis programme.

Minimizing bias

Bias can influence the results. The credibility of the findings can be increased by:

1. Using several sources of data
2. Tracking choices
3. Documenting the process used for data analysis
4. Involving others

Drawback to be avoided

1. Do not generalize results.
2. Choose quotes carefully.
3. Respect confidentiality and anonymity when using quotes.
4. Address limitations.

SUMMARY

Data analysis and interpretation are important elements in a research report. Research results can be presented in the form of narrative presentations, tables and figures. In narrative presentation, the research results will be presented clearly and concisely.

Tables are means of organizing data to present the results more easily to understand and interpret. The vertical entries in a table are columns and the horizontal entries are rows. The point where rows and columns intersect is called a cell.

A figure is used to indicate any visual presentation of data other than a table. Figures include graphs, diagrams, line drawings and photographs.

A discussion of the findings is a more subjective section of a thesis than the presentation of the findings. Hypothesis testing is an important area of findings of the study. The results fall into one of the three types.

(a) Null hypothesis is not rejected and therefore research hypothesis is not supported.
(b) Null hypothesis is rejected and research hypothesis is supported.
(c) Null hypothesis is rejected and the results are in the opposite direction from the prediction of research hypothesis.

Generalization of the research findings is also significant. Conclusions depend upon the findings and take into consideration the study problem, purpose, hypothesis and theoretical framework.

MULTIPLE CHOICE QUESTIONS

1. The term used to indicate any visual presentation of data other than a table __________.
   (a) figure
   (b) graph
   (c) diagram
   (d) all of the above
2. Methods of presenting research findings include __________.
   (a) narrative presentations
   (b) tables
   (c) figures
   (d) all of these
3. Which of the following regarding tables is not true?
   (a) means of organizing data
   (b) vertical entries and columns
   (c) horizontal entries are called rows
   (d) difficult to understand and interpret
4. The recommendations of a study might contain which of the following?
   (a) a means of implementing the study findings
   (b) comparisons of results with previous research findings
   (c) a discussion of study findings
   (d) suggestions for extension of the study

ANSWER KEY

1. (d) 2. (d) 3. (d) 4. (d)

REVIEW QUESTIONS

1. Define data analysis.
2. Describe interpretation of data.
3. Explain the steps in data processing.

REFERENCES

Berinsky, A.J. (2008). Survey non-response. In W. Donsbach, & M.W. Traugott (Eds.). The Sage handbook of public opinion research (309–321). Thousand Oaks, CA: Sage Publications.

Bourke, G.J., & McGilvary, J. (1985). Interpretation and uses of medical statistics. London: Blackwell Scientific Publishers.

David, S. Moore, & George, P. McCabe. "Introduction to the Practice of Statistics".

Dillman, D.A., Eltinge, J.L., Groves, R.M., & Little, R.J.A. (2002). Survey non-response in design, data collection, and analysis. In R.M. Groves, D.A. Dillman, J.L. Eltinge, & R.J.A. Little (Eds.). Survey non-response (3–26). New York: John Wiley & Sons.

Dillman, D.A., Smyth, J.D., & Christian, L.M. (2009). Internet, mail, and mixed-mode surveys: The tailored design method. San Francisco: Jossey-Bass.

Mahajan, B.K., & Khankal, A.B. (2010). Methods in biostatistics for medical students and research worker (7th ed.). New Delhi: Jaypee Brothers Medical Publishers.

Mathew, D.E. (1988). Using and understanding medical statistics. New Delhi: Karger.

Miles, M.B., & Huberman, A.M. (1984). Qualitative data analysis: A sourcebook of new methods. Beverly Hills, CA: Sage Publications.

Negi, K.S. (2010). Biostatistics (2nd ed.). New Delhi: AITBS Publishers.

Patton, M.Q. (1990). Qualitative evaluation and research methods (2nd ed.). Newbury Park, CA: Sage Publications.

Porter, Whitcomb, Weitzer. (2004). Multiple surveys of students and survey fatigue. In S.R. Porter (Ed.). Overcoming survey research problems: Vol. 121. New directions for institutional research (63–74). San Francisco, CA: Jossey Bass.

Rao, S., & Richard, J. (2006). Introduction to biostatistics and research methods (4th ed.). New Delhi: Premier Hall of India.

Reid, N.G. (1987). Research methods and statistics in healthcare. London: Edward Arnold.

Ress, D.G. (1989). Essentials of statistics. London: Chapman and Hall.

Spradly, J.P. (1979). The ethnographic interview. New York: Holt, Rinehart & Winston.

Sprent, P. (1989). Applied non-parametric statistical methods. London: Chapman and Hall.

Vehovar, V., Batagelj, Z., Manfreda, K.L., & Zaletel, M. (2002). Non-response in web surveys. In R.M. Groves, D.A. Dillman, J.L. Eltinge & R.J.A. Little (Eds.). Survey non-response (229–242). New York: John Wiley & Sons.

Walker, R. (Ed.). (1985). Applied qualitative research. Hants, UK: Gower Publishing Company Ltd.

Weller, S., & Romney, A. (1988). Systematic Data Collection (Qualitative Research Methods Series 10). Thousand Oaks, California: Sage Publications, ISBN 0803930747.

Williams, D.G., & Johnson, N.A. (1996). Essentials in qualitative research: A notebook for the field. Hamilton, Canada: McMaster University.

Woolson, R.F. (1987). Statistical methods for the analysis of biomedical data. New York: Wiley & Sons.

Yin, R.K. (1984). Case study research: Design and methods. Beverly Hills, CA: Sage Publications.

CHAPTER

13

COMMUNICATION AND UTILIZATION OF NURSING RESEARCH AND CRITIQUE OF RESEARCH REPORT

Key terms

★ Dissemination ★ Research critique ★ Research utilization

Outline

- ★ Purposes of dissemination
- ★ Guidelines for writing a research report
- ★ Roger's diffusion of innovation model
- ★ Barriers for research utilization
- ★ Significance of research critique
- ★ Guidelines for writing a research critique

Objectives

On completion of this chapter, you will be able to:

- ★ recognize the purposes of research dissemination
- ★ follow guidelines for writing a research report
- ★ utilize nursing research findings
- ★ recognize the purposes of research critique
- ★ list the guidelines for writing research critiques

Communication and Utilization of Nursing Research

Communicating research results is fundamental to the development of nursing knowledge. Nursing research is of little use if the results of investigations are not communicated to other scientists, practitioners and consumers of nursing.

Through communication, new ideas are generated, developed, tested and refined. Thus, it is the responsibility of researchers to propagate the findings among others.

Purposes of Dissemination

Research results are a significant contribution to the society. The main purposes of disseminating research findings are:

Dissemination of knowledge

When researchers submit their work for scrutiny by their peers, it adds to the scientific knowledge base of nursing. It will also help knowledge development in other fields.

Communicating for change

The ultimate aim of research is betterment of the quality of care. This could lead to changes in consumer's health behaviour or changes in public health policy.

Reward

Communicating the results is a type of personal reward, including getting recognition from colleagues, a sense of personal accomplishment, opportunities for job promotion and improved chances of obtaining research findings.

As per UGC and AICTE norms, college teachers need to publish or present research papers in conferences.

Avoid replication

Communication will help in avoiding replication of a research study.

Characteristics of a Good Research Report

Brevity

The research report should be written as concise as possible. It saves reader's time and helps the writers refine their own ideas. Keep sentences short and simple.

'Sell' the Information

Research is worth making if it communicates information in the most effective way. Report writing is to convince and to evolve interest. Too many reports are dry and dull with no spark to encourage interest from the readers.

Clarity

Correct communication will help the readers understand the points being made.

Keep to basic punctuation

The staple diet should be full stops and commas. Semicolons can be tricky except when used to separate phrases which appear as a list. Dashes and brackets can be effective if used only sparingly.

Honesty

The writing should be honest. Maintain respect for the reader and integrity of the author.

Completeness

Present the information completely so that readers can evaluate the study thoroughly.

Accuracy

It is appreciable if the writing is accurate.

Guidelines for Writing a Research Report

1. Develop your thinking
2. Divide your narration into paragraphs
3. Use present tense and active voice
4. Minimize technical language
5. Use visual aids
6. Be objective
7. Revise and rewrite

Factors to be Considered before Dissemination

The following are factors to be considered before starting dissemination of research results.

Choosing a channel for communication

Researchers can communicate results orally or in writing. Oral presentation can be made at professional conferences and written information in a poster session. Written reports, in addition to thesis or dissertation, can take the form of journal articles or in a variety of outlets on the internet.

Plan for dissemination

It can be rewarding to have a plan to facilitate the task of presenting a manuscript.

Knowing the audience

Researchers should be aware of the audience they are hoping to reach. Consumers may be clinical bedside nurses, nursing students, nurse educators, nurse administrators, health care professionals or general public.

Deciding an authorship

If the project has been carried out by a team of researchers, the first author is the chief investigator. To avoid conflict, the order of authors' names should be in the order of their contribution to the work.

Select a journal for publication

The important factors for selecting a journal are the status of a journal, goal, audience, prestige, acceptance and frequency of the publication.

Choosing the contents

Have a clear plan regarding the parts of findings to be presented in a paper. It is unethical to submit the same or similar paper to two journals.

Writing effectively

Prepare a draft entirely, edit it, rewrite and formulate it in a standard and scientific way.

Types of Research Reports

1. Theses and dissertations
2. Journal articles
3. Presentations at professional conferences
   (a) Scientific paper presentation
   (b) Poster presentation

A. Format of a Research Report for Thesis or Dissertation

The following standard format is suggested for preparing a dissertation to be submitted to University.

A. Preliminary section

1. Title Page

(a) Title of the study – concise, indicate the purpose, should be in capital letters

(b) Name of the researcher

(c) Name of the institution to which report is submitted

(d) Date of submission

2. Approval Sheet – Research Guide and Specialty Guide

(a) *Top of page:* Title of the study, then researcher name, space for signature of Guide I (Research Guide) and Guide II (Specialty Guide)

(b) Viva Voice date

(c) Examiner 1

(d) Examiner 2

(e) *Bottom of page:* Mention the degree for which the report is presented, month and year.

3. Certificate by Principal

The Principal certifies the bona-fide work of the student of the particular college submitted in partial fulfillment of the requirements for the *Degree of Master of Science in Nursing/Ph.D.* from the particular University by the researcher.

4. Declaration

The student states that the work is actually done by him/her alone, under the supervision of guides and admits that he/she has not submitted this document to any other University.

5. Acknowledgement

This section expresses courtesy to those who contributed towards the successful completion of the work. The acknowledgement should start with paying gratitude to the institution if sponsored and continues with expressing thanks to the individuals who guided and helped in the successful completion of the study. There is no necessity to praise but specify the purpose for which the person is being acknowledged. Write the acknowledgement in one or two pages.

6. Abstract of the Study

Abstract is a brief description of the study. It should be written in 150–200 words. It includes background of the study, objectives, methodology, results, implication for clinical practice and recommendations.

7. Table of Contents

Listing the various chapters presented in the research report and their respective page number.

(a) Chapter title – capital letters

(b) Subheading – small letters

8. List of Tables and Figures

The titles of tables and figures as they appear in the main body of the chapters with corresponding page number.

B. Main body of the report

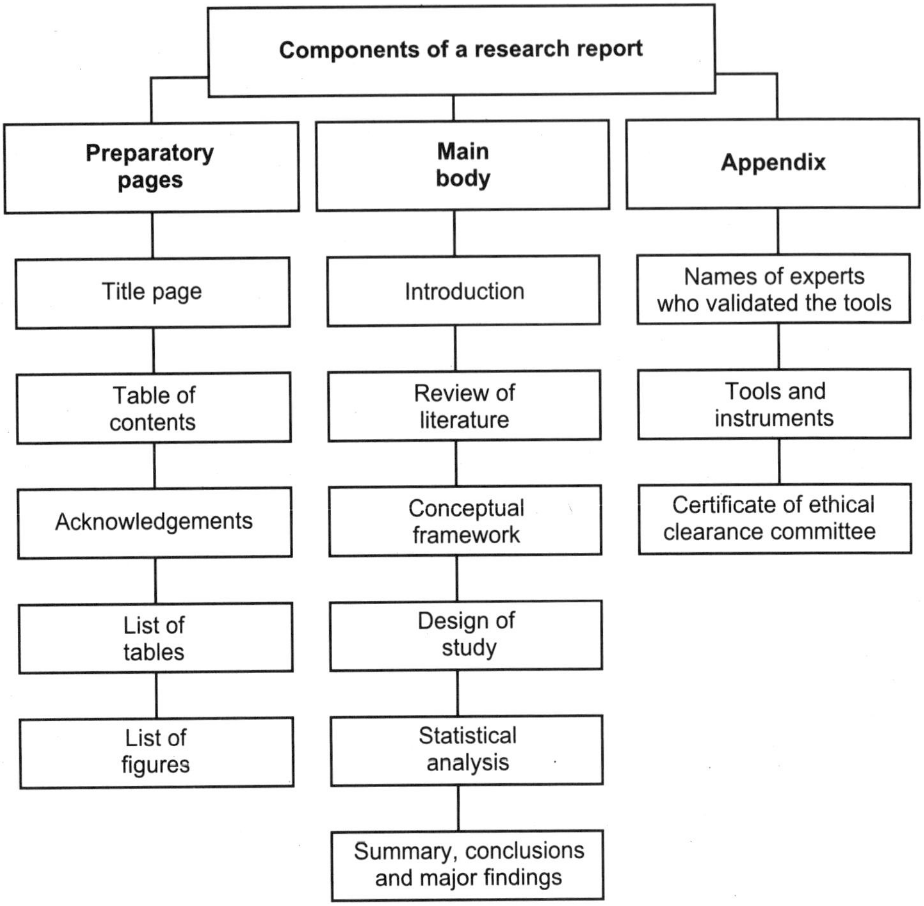

Figure 13.1 The structure of a research report

The main body of a research report includes the following components:

CHAPTER I: INTRODUCTION

(a) Background of the Study

This is the first part of the introduction. This should provide sufficient information to the reader on the topic which allows the reader to understand and evaluate the result of the present study. References should be carefully chosen to provide salient background. It can also include global, national and regional issues pertaining to the topic.

(b) Need for the Study

This should provide the rationale and the purpose for the present study.

It should indicate:

1. How the researcher was interested?
2. Why it is important?
3. What studies have already been done?
4. How this study differs from other study findings?
5. What new knowledge will it bring to nursing knowledge?

(c) Statement of the Problem

This should identify:

1. the problem, issue or phenomenon to be studied.
2. the key study variables and their relationship.
3. nature of population used in the research.

(d) Objectives

It should identify the specific ways in which the problem statement is to be studied. Objectives should be numbered and presented in sequential order. It forms the basis for data analysis, discussion and recommendations.

(e) Operational Definitions

The researcher defines the various terminologies used in research title. Throughout the study, he/she should give the same meaning to the terms used.

(f) Assumption or Hypothesis

Assumptions are statements that are not investigated and which must be taken for granted as truth without proof.

Hypothesis can be stated as working hypothesis or null hypothesis. It should be worded clearly, objectively and written as a stated prediction.

(g) Delimitation

Mention the situations in which the study is restricted. The scope should be to identify the population to which the result of the study can be generalized.

(h) Conceptual Framework/Theoretical Framework

The conceptual framework is adapted from theories and modified by the investigator. It is a brief explanation of theories and how each concept should be framed in such a way that it guides the researcher to develop tools, any intervention, etc.

(i) Outline of the Report

It comprises a brief description of subsequent chapters in the research report.

CHAPTER II: REVIEW OF LITERATURE

The chapter on review of literature should be limited to 15–20 pages. The researcher refers to articles published at least during the last 5 years. It should include the major and recent studies that have been conducted on the topic of interest. It should be directly related to the research problem. Communicating the review of literature involves:

1. Consideration of review content
2. Organization of content and style

Studies relevant to the present study may be discussed in detail with name of author (who has done), when and where the research studies was completed, what approaches were involved in research methodology, tools used, statistical analysis followed and significant results and recommendations.

The sources of literature review include encyclopedia of educational research, books, reports and research articles, and unpublished materials.

Literature relevant to each section should be arranged in a chronological order (older to newer), general to specific, and should be related to the research questions.

CHAPTER III: RESEARCH METHODOLOGY

(a) Overview of the Chapter

(b) Research Design

It can be experimental/non-experimental. Experimental design indicates what variables were manipulated, how subjects were assigned and the type of experimental intervention.

(c) Research Approach

It is an umbrella that covers the basis for conducting research.

(d) Population

It indicates the entire population from which the sample was drawn for the study. The size of the population should be specified in number.

(e) Sample and Sampling Technique

Sample is a group of people selected from the population to participate in the study. Sampling technique is the method of sample selection employed to select a sample. The rationale for choosing a particular sampling technique should be mentioned clearly.

(f) Criteria for Sample Selection

Mention the inclusion and exclusion criteria. Describe the characteristics of subjects like age, gender and other attributes.

(g) Development and Description of the Tool

It should include the type of tools used such as interview schedule, questionnaire, rating scale, structured teaching, SIM (Self-Instructional Module), checklist, etc. Explain how those tools were developed and the methods used for introducing the tools. The scoring procedure should be described in detail.

(h) Validation of the Tool

A brief explanation about how validation was made for tools and number of experts who examined the content validity. Modification may be made according to the expert's opinion.

(i) Reliability

Clear explanation should be given regarding how the reliability of the tool was measured.

(j) Pilot Study

It is a pre-testing of the tool developed and the procedure used to collect data.

(k) Study Setting

Physical location and conditions in which data collections took place in a study.

(l) Procedure for Data Collection

Data are the observable and measurable facts that provide information about the phenomena under the study. A variety of data collection methods are used in nursing studies such as interview, observation, questionnaire, etc.

Interview – Details regarding where, who and when the interview was conducted.

Observation – What was the role of the observer in relation to the subject?

Questionnaire – How and where it was delivered, time taken by the respondent.

Experimental – How much time has lapsed between the intervention and measurement of dependent variables. Document the details of data collection methods. All ethical considerations are to be kept in mind.

(m) Plan for Data Analysis

It summarizes the statistical methods used to analyze the data to meet the objectives of the study.

CHAPTER IV: DATA ANALYSIS, INTERPRETATION AND DISCUSSION

This chapter comprises tables, illustrations for different variables, and objectives stated for the study. The chapter should not exceed 40–50 pages. Illustrations like figures, diagrams or graphs can be shown to highlight the major findings of the study. A graphic representation of a table should immediately follow in the same page or in the next page.

Tables should have precise headings and titles. Tables should be numbered in sequential order. Figures should be numbered and have titles.

Interpretation – Highlight important data only.

Results of statistical tests – The values of calculated statistics, degrees of freedom and significance levels.

Discussion – The findings of the study should be discussed in line with study objectives, hypothesis, review of literature and conceptual framework. Under each objective, data analysis and interpretation should be discussed supporting or contradicting the present study.

If the study findings conflict with earlier research investigations, then explanations should be offered for the same. The integration of conceptual framework should be discussed. The interpretation should be mentioned in percentages and only high, low values are shown.

CHAPTER V: SUMMARY, CONCLUSIONS, IMPLICATIONS AND RECOMMENDATIONS

Summary – Brief report of research steps and major findings.

Conclusion – Conclusion from each finding, test of hypothesis and generalizations. Briefly describe how far the objectives of the study are attained.

Implications – Possible applications of the results in terms of nursing practice, education, administration and research.

Recommendations – Suggestions for improvements and prospect for future research.

C. Bibliography/References

The bibliography should be presented in the alphabetical order of author names. The number referring to a reference should correspond with that of the reference cited within the chapter.

(a) Vancouver style of reference

There are different styles for writing references, including the APA, Campell, and Vancouver styles. However, in medical discipline, the Vancouver style of reference is commonly used. This was introduced by Vancouver in 1978.

This style was based on the American National Standards Institute, and has been adopted by the National Library of Medicine for database such as British Medical Journal and Journal of American Medical Association.

(b) Quotation within the text

Reference in the text – A number enclosed within brackets or parentheses (e.g. (4) or (26)), and placed in the text of the thesis, shows the relevant reference. Each citation corresponds to a numbered reference containing details about the source in the reference list at the end of the publication, thesis or assignment. Note that when a source has been cited, the same number is used for all consequent references. Some examples of references are as below:

Superscript format –

e.g. …anxiety will be more after mastectomy[4]

Bracket format –

1. …complications after craniotomy (13)
2. …self-care theory was first mentioned in (11)
3. Many relevant studies (9, 11, 15, 20)…

Quoting more than one reference at a time – If you are quoting more than one source at a time, each reference number is separated with a comma or dash.

1. (4, 6, 9)
2. (8–10)
3. (12–14, 16, 17)

(c) Tips for writing references

1. **References are numbered** consecutively in the order they are first mentioned. Place each reference number consistently throughout the text, tables and legends.
2. **Direct quotes** are to be used sparingly. If a direct quote is necessary, place quotation marks around the quote and number the reference as usual.
3. **Tables are numbered** consecutively.

4. **Internet sources** may get deleted, changed or moved from time to time; so it is a good idea to keep a hard copy for your records. Also take care to critically evaluate the reliability of the information.
5. **Personal communication** should be avoided as a reference.
6. **Usually write journal title** (abbreviated, if necessary), year; volume, issue number; and page range, e.g. The Nursing Journal of India, 2011; 210(21–23); 50–56
7. **No footnotes** are used.
8. **Authors:** List each author's last name and initials; full first names are not necessary. List all authors, but if the number exceeds six, give the first six followed by "et al". For books with chapters written by individual authors, list the authors of the chapter, then the chapter title, followed by "In:", the editors' names, and the book title.
9. **Book titles, chapter titles:** Capitalize the first letter of the first word in the title. The rest of the title is in lower-case with the exception of proper names. Do not underline the title; do not use italics.
10. **Pages:** For journals, the entire page range of an article or chapter is given, *not* the specific page on which the information was found. For books, no page numbers are given, with two exceptions. The page number of a dictionary entry is included, as well as the page range of a chapter with its own author.

(d) Appendices

Towards the end of report, include various documents and tools utilized for the study to fulfill legal and ethical concerns. Appendices should also include ethical clearance certificate, self instructional modules, etc. Attach important materials used or produced during the study, but those too lengthy have to be included in the body of the report.

General Suggestions for Preparation of Dissertation Report

1. Form and style

The candidate is responsible for the presentation of the content, references, tables, etc. in a form acceptable by the institution.

2. Number of copies

The number of copies to be submitted to the institution should be confirmed with the Head of the Institution. The title must be clearly printed on the front cover and on the spine of the thesis.

3. Paper size and quality

A4 size or executive bond paper is preferred. Same quality of paper must be used throughout for each copy of dissertation. Print on only one side of the paper.

4. Margins

A margin of 1½ inches must be maintained on the left for binding purposes. A ½ inch space on right margin and 1 inch on top and bottom of book are desirable. Diagrams and photographs in any form should fit into standard page size.

5. Photographs

Black and white photographs are preferable for clear reproduction. However, colour photographs are acceptable.

6. Printing

1. Any standard typeface (font) is acceptable if used uniformly throughout the dissertation.
2. Keep a personal floppy/CD for future corrections.
3. Printing should be done only on one side of the paper.
4. The text should be double-spaced throughout. Single space is used in block quotations of three or more lines and bibliography entries.
5. Double space between chapter number and title.
6. Triple space above and below centered headings.
7. Double space below the side heading.
8. Font size:

   Title of chapter – 18 points

   Sub-headings – 14 points, bold and capitals

   Text matter – 12 or 13 points

Figure heading – 14 points, bold, small letters

Figure sub-heading – 12 points, small letters

Table heading – 14 points, bold, small letters

7. Indentation

The first line of each paragraph receives an indentation, which must be uniform throughout the dissertation. An indentation of 5 to 7 spaces is suggested.

8. Pagination

All pages in the dissertation including the graphs, charts, figures, illustrations, bibliography and appendices must be numbered.

9. Length of dissertation

(a) Master's thesis – 100–130 pages

(b) Doctoral thesis – minimum 250 pages

The number of pages in thesis is decided as per the recommendations of the University.

10. Reproduction

Use photocopies.

11. Grammar and spelling

Use of appropriate punctuation is a must. Watch for spelling errors. Editing by an English language expert is recommended before taking the final copies.

B. Journal Articles

Dissertations and final reports are rarely read by more than a handful of individuals. However, publishing scientific findings in a professional journal ensures the broadest possible circulation. A journal article generally follows the same form as the main body of a thesis, but articles are much shorter. A large proportion of a journal report is devoted to the results and discussion sections, because the readers are interested in the findings. A typical research article is only about 10 to 25 pages. Several nursing journals accept research articles for publication. Many publications make an explicit statement concerning the type of manuscripts they are seeking. A prospective author should check information on the circulation of the journal and the number of copies of a manuscript required for submission. When the preparation of manuscript is done, the required number of copies should be sent to the editor with a covering letter. The receipt of the manuscript is acknowledged immediately, but the final decision concerning the paper's acceptance or rejection may require several months.

If the article is suitable for consideration, it will be sent out to the reviewers. Reviewers will read and return it with comments to the journal about its acceptability. Once accepted by the journal, an acceptance letter is sent to the author. After making necessary editorial interventions, the article will be send back to the researcher for proofreading before finally publishing it. At this stage, the researcher reads the article carefully and corrects errors, if any.

If the manuscript was not accepted by the journal, authors are usually provided with copies of the reviewer's comments or reasons for its rejection. This information can be used to revise the manuscript before submitting it to another journal.

C. Presentation at Professional Conferences

Numerous professional organizations sponsor annual national meetings at which research activities are presented either through oral research report or through poster presentation.

Submitting a presentation to a conference

Usually the association sponsoring the conference publishes a 'call for papers' in its newsletter or journal about 6 to 9 months before the meeting date. Each conference has its own guidelines. The notice indicates the requirement and deadlines for submitting papers. Usually an abstract of 500 to 1000 words is submitted rather than a full paper. If the submission was accepted, the researcher is committed to appear at the conference to make a presentation. Research reports presented at professional meetings follow the same format as a journal article. Time prescribed for a presentation ranges from 10 to 20 minutes. Therefore, the content should be concise and include only the most important aspects of the study.

Researchers sometimes present their findings in a poster session. Several researchers simultaneously present visual displays summarizing the highlights of the study. Poster sessions are thus efficient and encourage interactive discussions.

Poster presentation

Research posters are ways to explore the basic elements of a research report in a highly visual format. A poster can be used to present work in progress or a completed study. An effective poster must have a focus and be graphically presented.

Guidelines for preparing a poster

1. Planning

There are several stages in planning a poster presentation:

(a) Gathering information: The process includes a critical examination of the objective of the investigation, approach used and the results obtained. This will give a clear idea of the contributions you have or have not been able to make.

(b) Deciding on the content: Based on the information gathered, the content of the poster is decided.

The decision is based on two factors:

1. What are you trying to achieve by presenting the poster?
2. Who will be attending the presentation?

These define the type of content to include and set a tone for the presentation.

2. Designing

A blueprint must be used so that it draws the attention of people to what you have to communicate.The four main principles of good design are:

(a) Contrast: Use colours sparingly and with taste. Colours should be used only to emphasize, differentiate and to add interest. Choose background and foreground colours that have high contrast and complement each other.

(b) Simplicity

1. Effective use of space, but not to cramp a page with full of information.
2. Be concise. Use only pertinent information to convey the report.
3. Present only the main findings of the project.
4. The poster should not take longer than five minutes to read.

(c) Font type and size

1. Too many font types distract reading.
2. The text should be large enough to be read easily from at least 6 feet away.
3. For section headings, use bold and font size of about 36–42. For text within each section and figure captions, use font sizes of about 24–28 (bold, if appropriate).

In general, use font sizes proportional to importance:

1. largest font size – Title
2. next largest font size – Section headings
3. medium font size – Supporting material
4. smallest font size – Details

Double-space all text, use left-justification; text with even left sides and jagged right sides is easiest to read.

3. Organization

Sound and clear language can strengthen your bond with readers. First organize yourself. Agree on your audience profile, commit to the central message and clarify your purpose. Form the foundation of the document by answering the "**who, what** and **why**". Remember, the reader is a key member of the organizing team. Reader input ensures readability and usability.

(a) Adopt a plain perspective: Every subject can be looked at from different perspectives. Some of the perspectives on a social issue might come from the children, the families, the schools, the neighbourhoods, the police, the court system, the community or the political system.

(b) Organize the information logically

1. Create categories for your information.
2. Divide the information among the categories.
3. Put categories in an appropriate sequence.

Categorize information according to the types of information, the variety of concepts, or their importance or priority. There are three elements to consider when creating information categories:

1. The nature of the subject itself.
2. The reader's objectives and needs.
3. Your guiding purpose or strategy.

Other patterns include:

1. known to new information
2. common to specific
3. frequent to rare occurrences
4. comparison and contrast
5. priority of importance
6. a continuum or measure of value

4. Presentation

Place the elements of the poster in position:

1. The title will appear across the top.
2. A brief introduction will appear at the upper left.
3. The conclusion will appear at the lower right.
4. Methods and results will fill the remaining space.

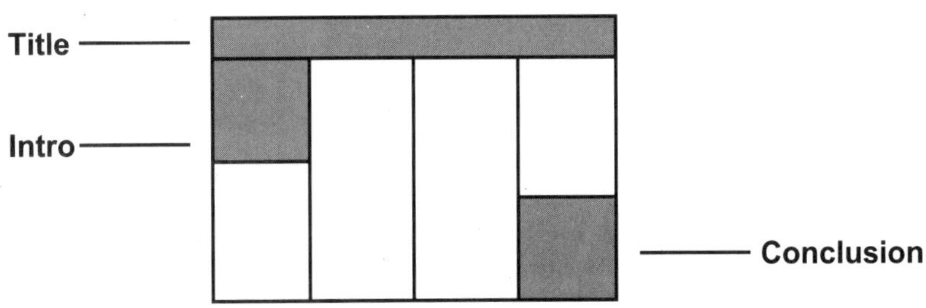

Figure 13.2 A sample poster

The title of the poster includes the title of the work, the author's names and institutional affiliations.

1. The title should be readable from 15–20 feet away.
2. If space permits, use first names for authors to facilitate interactions.
3. Middle initials and titles are seldom necessary.
4. Use abbreviations where possible.

5. Sequencing contents

A poster should use photos, figures, and tables to communicate various aspects of the study. For clarity, present the information in a sequence that is easy to follow:

(a) Determine a logical sequence for the material you will be presenting.

(b) Organize that material into sections, e.g. Introduction, Methods, Results, Discussion and Conclusions.

(c) Arrange the material into columns.

Most poster sessions last at least 90 minutes. Plan to stand up throughout the presentation. Poster presentations are far less formal than paper presentations but are equally demanding. Poster sessions suggest the learner the opportunity to build skills and assurance in making research presentations.

A research poster consists of:

(a) a title page, i.e. the title of the project, people involved in the work and their affiliations;

(b) a summary of the project stating the key findings and the main results;

(c) an introduction that should include clear statements about the problem, aims and objectives;

(d) a theory or methodology section which explains the basis of the technique or the procedure which is adopted for the study;

(e) a results section to show illustrative examples of the main results of the work;

(f) a conclusion section listing the main findings of the study.

Utilization of Research Findings

Research utilization is the process of synthesizing, disseminating and using research generated knowledge to make an impact or change in the existing practices. It is the process by which scientifically produced knowledge is transferred to practice (Brown, 1999).

Purposes

1. Blending of knowledge and practice in nursing.
2. Developing an inquiring mind in researchers.
3. Critiquing and improving the quality of results.
4. Beneficial for cost-effective, quality oriented practice.
5. Enhancing critical thinking and professional growth.

Roger's Diffusion of Innovation Model

Diffusion of innovations

Everett Rogers, a Professor of Rural Sociology, popularized the theory in his book *Diffusion of Innovations* published in 1962. It is a theory which explains how, why, and at what rate new ideas and technology spread through cultures. According to him, diffusion is the process by which an innovation is communicated through certain channels over time among the members of a social system. The origins of diffusion of innovations theory are varied and span across multiple disciplines.

Diffusion of an innovation occurs through a five-step process. This process is a type of decision-making. It occurs through a series of communication channels over a period of time among the members of a similar social system. Ryan and Gross first indicated the identification of adoption as a process in 1943. Rogers categorizes the five stages (steps) as: awareness, interest, evaluation, trial and adoption. An individual might reject an innovation at any time during or after the adoption process. In later editions of the *Diffusion of Innovations*, Rogers changes the terminology of the five stages to knowledge, persuasion, decision, implementation and confirmation. However, the descriptions of the categories have remained similar throughout the editions.

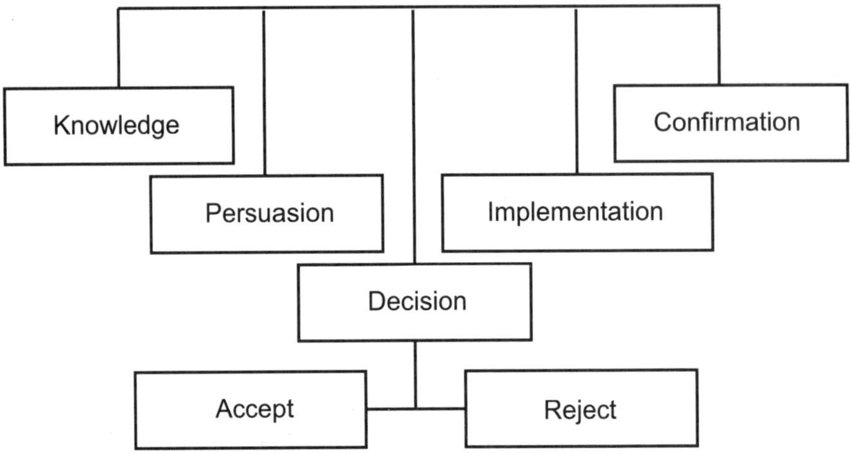

Figure 13.3 Stages of diffusion of innovation process

Five stages of the adoption process

1. Knowledge

In this stage, an individual is first exposed to an innovation but lacks information about the innovation. During this stage, the individual has not yet been inspired to find more information about the innovation.

2. Persuasion

In this stage, the individual is interested in the innovation and he/she actively seeks details of information about the innovation.

3. Decision

In this stage, the individual takes the concept of the innovation and weighs the advantages/disadvantages of using the innovation and decides whether to adopt or reject the innovation. Due to the individualistic nature of this stage, Rogers notes that it is the most difficult stage to acquire empirical evidence (Rogers, 1964).

4. Implementation

In this stage, the individual employs the innovation to a varying degree depending on the situation. The individual determines the usefulness of the innovation and may search for further information about it.

5. Confirmation

In this stage, the individual finalizes his/her decision to continue using the innovation and may use the innovation to its fullest potential.

Barriers for Research Utilization

Research factors

Not publishing the findings

Lack of power to implement

Lack of generalization in population

Accessibility factors

Reduced availability of professional journals

Information overload

Lack of resources to implement results

Personal factors

Inability to comprehend ideas

Time constraints

Lack of self-confidence

Reluctance to change

Lack of perception of value of research

Setting related factors

Lack of cooperation of staff and inadequate facilities

No incentives for conducting research

Accepted tradition

Inadequate facilities

Communication factors

Lack of collaboration between researchers and clinicians

Lack of publications in clinical nursing journals

Implications for practice are not made clear

Research results are not readily available

Difficulty in comprehending statistical analysis

Organizational factors

Other staffs being non-supportive for implementation

Reduced authority for staff nurses

Not allowing implementation of findings

Financial constrains

Enhancing research utilization

Relevant research for profession

Committed administration

Adequate resources

Incentives for clinical researchers

Linking academic and clinical sectors

Interdisciplinary collaboration

Literature access

Critiquing Research Report

A critical appraisal of the research report is an inevitable component of research. The authenticity of research findings needs to be assessed by careful judging to broaden the understanding, to determine evidence for use in practice, and to provide a background for conducting further studies. Research in nursing enriches not only scholarly knowledge but also advanced information for improving nursing practice. Thus critiquing research reports will help for advancement of nursing knowledge.

Definitions

1. A research critique is defined as a critical analysis of a research report on the strengths and weaknesses of the research project and intends to refine the quality of the project.
2. A research critique is a careful, critical appraisal of strengths and limitations of a research report (Polit and Hungler, 2010).

3. Research critique is a careful examination of all aspects of study to judge its strengths, limitations, meaning and significance (Burns, 1995).
4. A research critique reflects a penetrating analysis of a study in which judicious and constructive comments have been made about a piece of work.
5. Research critique is a planned, careful and critical evaluation of a piece of research work against the pre-specified criteria to judge the strengths and weakness of the research study.

Significance of research critique

1. Develops and refines knowledge
2. Helpful for broadening the understanding of the study
3. Improves nursing practice
4. Maintains the standard of study
5. Guarantees the quality of the study

Purposes

Critiquing of research study is done with many purposes. During the course of study, students are given opportunity to critique a research work. This is for checking their mastery of methodological and analytic skills. The overall aim of critiquing a research work is to develop a balanced evaluation of contributing to the knowledge on the subject through the study.

1. To judge the strengths and weaknesses of the study
2. To provide an appraisal of their research work to the researchers
3. To assess the scientific value of investigation
4. To recommend for publication
5. To assess the research findings before applying it to nursing practice
6. To serve as a guide to researchers and practitioners
7. To suggest possibilities for the design of replications
8. To decide how the findings from the study can best be incorporated into practice
9. To identify virtues as well as faults

Elements or Dimensions of a Research Critique

A research report has several important dimensions to be considered in a critical evaluation of the worth of the study.

1. Substantive and theoretical dimension

The reader of a research report needs to determine whether the study was an important one in terms of the significance of the problem studied, the soundness of the conceptualization, the appropriateness of theoretical framework and the creativity and insightfulness of the analysis. The research problem should have obvious relevance to some aspect of the nursing profession.

2. Methodological dimension

The researcher makes a number of important decisions regarding how to go about answering their research questions or testing their research hypothesis. It is the consumer's job to evaluate critically the consequences of those dimensions.

The heart of research critique lies in the appraisal of the methodological decisions adopted in addressing the research question.

1. What design will field the most unambiguous and meaningful results about the relation between independent and dependent variables?
2. Who should participate in the study?
3. What are the characteristics of the population?
4. What sampling approach should be used to select the sample?
5. How should the research data be gathered?
6. How can the variable be operationalized and reliability and validity measured?
7. What statistical analysis will provide the most appropriate answers to the research questions?

In a qualitative study:

1. Where should the study take place?
2. What setting will yield the richest information about the phenomenon?

3. What should the sources of data be and how should the data be gathered?
4. Who should participate in the study?
5. How can participants be selected?
6. How many participants will be needed?
7. What type of evidence can be obtained to support the data, analysis and interpretation?

After evaluating the type of decisions that the researcher made, assess how well the research plan was actually executed.

3. Ethical dimension

In performing a research critique, one should consider whether there is any evidence that the rights of human subjects were violated during the course of investigation. If there is any potential problem, one needs to consider the impact of those problems on the scientific merit of the study on the one hand and the participants' well being on the other.

There may be two types of ethical transgressions. The first one consists of inadvertent actions or activities that the researcher did not interpret as creating an ethical dilemma. In the other one, the researcher may have been aware of having committed some violation of ethical principles, but made a decision that the violation was relatively minor in relation to knowledge that could be gained by doing the study in a certain way.

4. Interpretive dimension

A research report always concludes with a discussion or conclusion section. In this section the researcher attempts to make sense of the analysis, to understand what the findings mean in relation to the research hypothesis, and to consider whether the findings support or fail to support a theoretical framework.

5. Presentation and stylistic dimension

An important consideration is whether the research report has provided sufficient information for a thoughtful critique of the other dimensions. Styles of writing differ for qualitative and quantitative reports. In quantitative research, reports are written in a more formal, impersonal fashion using either the third person or passive voice. In qualitative study, it should be written in a more literary style using the first or second person and active voice to connote proximity and intimacy with the data and phenomenon under study.

Phases in Research Critique Process

Phase I: Comprehension

It is the first step and it involves understanding the terms and concepts of the report as well as identifies the elements of the research process such as the problem, purpose, framework and design.

Phase II: Comparison

It requires knowledge of what each step of research process should be like and then the idea is compared with the real. Here we need to examine the extent to which the researcher followed the rules for an ideal study.

Phase III: Analysis

It involves the critique of logical links connecting one study element with another. The overall logical development of the study must be examined, including variables, study design, instruments used, sample, and analysis techniques needed to provide results that address the purpose of specific objectives. It also means to break down and study the parts.

Evaluation

It becomes a summary of the quality of the study that builds on conclusions reached during the first three phases of the critique. This is usually done at higher levels such as for doctoral students and post-doctoral students by the evaluative committee of experts.

Steps in Critiquing

Beginners often face many practical difficulties in critiquing a research report. From the experience as a research supervisor and a teacher for so many years, the author has seen students making many fundamental mistakes while doing critiquing. Some practical suggestions for conducting effective critiquing process are as follows:

1. Read the abstract of the study carefully.
2. Read the entire study.

3. Examine references.
4. Focus on the presentation, language, style, etc.
5. Read for a second time.
6. Compare with set standards.
7. Analyze the entire study by breaking it down into parts and looking for the links between the components.
8. Evaluate the study.

Guidelines for Writing a Research Critique

1. Maintain an objective attitude. Provide rationale for your critique.
2. Read and understand the research report carefully.
3. Make a critical analysis of all the aspects of the study before documenting the report.
4. Examine the significance of the problems studied for nursing practice.
5. Make a constructive criticism. Make sure that negative comments are made carefully. Never try to ridicule/insult the researcher.
6. Judge the general features, strengths and weaknesses of the study.
7. Make summary, appraisals and recommendations. Solutions and alternatives suggested for problems detected in the study should be practically possible. Suggest modifications for future studies.
8. Avoid vague generalization of praise and fault-findings. Support your positive and negative remarks with examples.

Types of Research Critique

1. Student critique

It helps to strengthen their knowledge and increase their use of research findings in practice.

2. Critiques by the practicing nurse

Incorporation of the generated research findings into practice is possible through critique.

3. Critiques by nursing educators

This type of critiquing is instrumental in refining the curriculum and the contents of instructions.

4. Critiques by nurse researchers

The outcome of critique influences the selection of research problems, development of methodology and interpretation of findings in future studies.

5. Critique after verbal presentation of studies

Researchers can gain increased understanding of the strengths and weaknesses of their studies to generate ideas for further research. This is generally used in journal clubs, paper presentations, etc.

6. Critique after published research report

It increases the reader's understanding of the study. Readers have the opportunity to comment on the strengths and weaknesses of published studies.

7. Critique for abstract selection

This is used for critiquing research abstracts where the focus is on the completeness of the content and expression of ideas.

8. Critique of an article for publication

Only standard articles will be selected for study. It is used by the editorial board in making selection of articles for publication in journals.

9. Critique of research proposals

It is conducted to approve student research projects, to permit data collection, and to select the best studies for finding.

Do's and Don'ts in Critiquing

1. Researchers should not find only mistakes in the study.
2. Some critiques keep only flattering.
3. Do not associate personal prejudice in critiquing.
4. Do not over-estimate or under-estimate the cost, time and ethical considerations of the study.

How to critique a research report

Title

Is the title framed properly?

Has the researcher mentioned the study variables?

Has the researcher mentioned the population?

Is it clear?

Is it concise and informative?

Abstract

Has it been formulated clearly?

Is the word limit within 150–250?

Does it state the problem clearly?

Does it state the hypothesis clearly?

Has the methodology been described clearly?

Are the results summarized?

Are the conclusions stated?

Style of organization

Is the organization of the contents adequate?

Is there clarity in the research report?

Is the project report presented in an acceptable standard style?

Research problem and purpose

Is the problem stated clearly?

Is it a researchable problem?

What is the study purpose?

Is it a significant problem to nursing practice and profession?

Does the statement clearly show the variables, population and place of the study?

Does it meet the criteria?

Is it a feasible problem?

Is the research problem directed to develop or test the nursing theories?

Objectives

Are the objectives specified clearly?

Do the objectives reflect how the result will be useful?

Are the objectives stated in accordance with the research problem?

Are the objectives stated using verbs in a logical manner?

Hypothesis

Are hypotheses properly worded?

Does the hypothesis specify the relationship between variables?

Does it logically relate to the research problem and objectives?

Is it testable?

Operational definitions

Are all the required words clearly defined?

Are operational definitions logical and measurable?

Theoretical and conceptual framework

Does the research report describe theoretical or conceptual framework for the study?

Are the major concepts of the models identified and defined?

Are the types of relationship among concepts within the model described appropriately?

Is the model suitable for the study?

Literature review

Has it been organized properly under each subdivision?

Has the researcher made an indepth review?

How recent is the review?

What are the types of resources the researcher has used for the review?

What concepts are included in the review?

Does the literature review make the relationships among variables explicit?

Does the literature review provide a rationale?

Methodology

The researcher must make a number of important decisions while proceeding with the research process. Evaluate the consequences of decisions taken in this regard.

Research approach

Has the researcher mentioned the research approach?

Is the research approach suitable for the topic of the inquiry?

Research design

Does the researcher clearly depict the design used?

Does it suit the study?

Does the design provide a means to examine all of the objectives, questions, hypothesis?

Are research controls applied in the study?

Is there any evidence of bias?

Are the confounding variables excluded as far as possible?

Setting

Does the candidate mention the setting?

Is it suitable for the study?

Is there any bias in selecting the setting?

Does the setting help in generalization?

Population

Does the researcher mention the population under study?

Is it feasible?

Does it suit the study variables?

Is the target population defined?

Samples

What is the sample size and whether the sample size is adequate?

Is the inclusion or exclusion criterion adequate?

Does it represent the population defined?

Does the researcher use the sampling techniques and follow the criteria?

Is the sample sufficient for generalization?

Data collection methods and tools

Are the research tools suitable for the study?

Have the reliability and validity of the instruments been properly checked?

Are the data collection procedures described clearly?

Are the methods appropriate for gathering data?

Are the instruments explained sufficiently?

Ethical aspects

Are the participants protected from physical harms, risks, psychological and social stress and discomfort?

Is the confidentiality of the information and its anonymity maintained?

Has the written consent for conducting the study been obtained from the subjects/participants?

Data analysis and result presentation

Has the analysis of the data been correctly calculated in terms of its ratio, rates, proportions, inferential statistics, etc.?

Does it provide meaningful information?

Are the results acceptable?

Is the level of probability mentioned?

Is the level of significance reported?

Are results presented with clarity and brevity?

Do the results keep in time with the pre-set objectives?

Are the research findings organized in order?

Were appropriate statistical tests used?

Is there adequate clarity in the presentation of tables and figures in the report?

Discussion

Are the results discussed in terms of research topics?

Are previous research findings compared with the research findings?

Has the researcher addressed the hypothesis properly?

Are the implications and recommendations discussed properly?

Is any practical application possible with the study?

Conclusion and recommendations

Are the results interpreted in the context of the problem, purpose, hypothesis, theoretical framework?

Are the main findings appropriate?

What are the recommendations made for further studies?

Is the description of the study sufficiently clear to allow replication?

Application and utilization in nursing practice

Is direct application of the research findings feasible in terms of time, effort, money and legal/ethical risks?

How and under what circumstances are the findings applicable to nursing practice?

Would it be possible to replicate this study in another clinical practice setting?

References

Are the references relevant and complete?

Have they followed the recommended style?

Are the references from credible sources?

SUMMARY

The research findings of any investigation should be communicated. There are different methods for propagating the research findings, written report and verbal report. Dissemination of research serves scientific, professional and public functions. Through propagating research processes and outcomes, new ideas are generated, developed, tested and refined. Thus, all investigators have the responsibility to contribute to the process by disseminating their research to others for dialogue, debate and evaluation.

Critiquing research report is a systematic method of critically analyzing a research project. It highlights the strengths and weaknesses of a research study, and also recommends alternatives for improvements in future replications. A general research critique utilizes the technique of analysis, validation and replication in the critique process. The research critique gives scope for legitimacy of the information and to analyze the integrity of the findings and to reflect the evidence-base in terms of application possibilities.

MULTIPLE CHOICE QUESTIONS

1. A written or oral summary of a study is called ___________.
   (a) abstract (b) research report
   (c) summary (d) none of these
2. Sheets of paper showing how the article will appear in typeset form is ___________.
   (a) abstract (b) research paper
   (c) galley proofs (d) research poster
3. The review of manuscripts by professional colleagues who are content or methodological experts is called ___________.
   (a) blind review (b) galley proofs
   (c) meta-analysis (d) peer review
4. In which of the following are the reviewers not aware of the author's identity before the manuscript is evaluated?
   (a) peer review (b) presenting research report
   (c) blind review (d) presenting a research poster
5. Brief summaries of research studies generally contain the purpose, methods and major findings of the study are called ___________.
   (a) outcome of research (b) research abstracts
   (c) research papers (d) research utilization

6. The implementation of research findings into practice ________.
   (a) generalization   (b) application of research
   (c) research utilization   (d) triangulation

ANSWER KEY

1. (b) 2. (c) 3. (d) 4. (c) 5. (b) 6. (c)

REVIEW QUESTIONS

1. Write the significance of reporting and publishing the research.
2. Describe research reporting.
3. Explain the precautions for writing a research report.
4. Explain the characteristics of scientific writing.
5. (a) Define research report.
   (b) Explain the major guidelines for a well-written research report.
6. Write short notes on:
   (a) Research report
   (b) References
   (c) Written reports
   (d) Utilization of research findings
   (e) Dissemination of results
   (f) Research critique
   (g) Barriers of research utilization

REFERENCES

Anderson, J., Durston, H., Berry & Poole, Millicent (1985). Thesis and Assignment Writing. Wiley Eastern University Press. New Delhi.

Basavanthappa, B.T. (2007). Nursing Research, (1st ed.). Jaypee Brothers, New Delhi.

Bergman, R. (1994). Are my outcomes better than yours? *Hospital health network*, 68(15).

Bernstein, S. J., & Hill borne, L. (1993). Clinical indicators: The road to quality care? *Joint Commission Journal on Quality Improvement*, 19(11).

Bijlani, R.L. (1983). Teachers. In Bijlani, R.L., Nayar, U. (Eds.). *Teaching physiology-trends and tools.* New Delhi: All India Institute of Medical Sciences.

Campbell,W., Ballou, S., & Slade, C. (1982). Form and style (6th ed.). Boston: Houghtton Mifflin.

Collins, L.M., & Horn, J.L. (1991). *Best methods for the analysis of change: Resent. Advances, unanswered questions, future directions.*Washington, D.C.

Creswell, J.W. (2007). *Designed and conducting mixed methods research.*

Egerton, M.A. (1983). Career preference enquiry among Queen's University medical undergraduates and graduates: As follow up. Med. Educ.

Fink, A. (2009). *How to conduct surveys: A step-by-step guide.* Beverly Hills, J.M. Morse (Ed). *Qualitative nursing research: A contemporary dialogue (Rev. Ed.).*

Kumaraiah, V., Monterio, L., Adiseshiah, W.T.V., Sharma, K.N. (1972). The career aims of medical students. *Ind. J. Med. Educ.*

Lester, J.D., & Lester, J.D. Jr. (2002). Writing research papers: A complete guide. (10th ed.). New York. Longman.

Meloy, J.M. (2001). Writing the qualitative dissertation. (2nd ed.). Mahvah, NJ: Lawrence Erlbaum.

Nancy Burns, *Understanding Nursing Research.* (2nd ed.). Saunder's Publications, 380–389.

Nightingale Nursing Times, "*Communicating Nursing Report*". Vol. 3, Issue 4, July, 2007, 54–56.

Parkshouse, J. (1976.). A follow up of career preferences. *Med. Educ.*

Patton, M.Q. (2002). *Qualitative evaluation of research methods.* (3rd ed.).

Payne, S.L. (1951). *The art of asking questions.* Princeton, NJ: Princeton University Press.

Perera, K.M.H. (1980). Career preferences of doctors qualifying in 1977. A postal survey. *Ind. J. Med. Educ.*

Polit, D.F., & Hungler, B.P. (1991). Denis, *Nursing Research Principles and Methods.* (6th ed.). Lippincott Publications, Philadelphia 624–630.

Roberts, B.L., Srour, M.I., & Winkelman, C. (1996). Videotaping: An important research strategy. *Nursing Research*, 45(6).

Rose Marie, *Foundations of Nursing Research.* (3rd ed.). Appleton and Lange.

Sternberg, David (1981). How to Complete and Survive a Doctoral Dissertation. New York: St. Martin's Press.

Talbot, A. Laura (1995). Principles and practice of nursing research. Mosby, St. Louis.

Veldman, David, J. (1971). Writing a Thesis or Dissertation Proposal in the Behavioural Sciences. Fort Worth, Tex. American Publishing Co.

Williams, M.A. (1980). Editorial: Assumptions in research.

Woods, D.L., Kovach, C.R., Raff, H., Joosse, L., Basmadjian, A., & Hegadoren, K. (2008). Using saliva to measure endogenous cortisol in nursing home resident with advanced dementia. *Research in nursing and health.* 31(3).

CHAPTER

14

EVIDENCE-BASED NURSING

Key terms

★ Evidence-based nursing ★ Research utilization
★ Evidence-based practice ★ Evidence-based medicine

⊙ Outline

- ★ Definitions
- ★ Historical perspective
- ★ Significance
- ★ Competencies required
- ★ Challenges of EBN for nurses
- ★ Barriers in promoting EBN
- ★ Resources to facilitate EBN
- ★ Future of EBN

⊙ Objectives

On completion of this chapter, you will be able to:

- ★ recognize the significance of evidence-based nursing
- ★ differentiate between research utilization and evidence-based practice
- ★ determine the steps of evidence-based nursing
- ★ recognize the challenges of evidence-based nursing for nurses
- ★ interpret the barriers in promoting evidence-based nursing
- ★ identify the resources to facilitate evidence-based nursing

Introduction

In nursing, research is conducted to generate knowledge for use in practice. The ultimate goal of research is equipping one for evidence-based nursing practice. Evidence-based nursing is a new paradigm emerging across the discipline to improve the quality of care. During the last twenty years, improved quality of nursing care resulted in a fall in health care costs. Thus, clients, nurses and health care agencies benefit when care is based on research.

Research Utilization and Evidence-Based Practice

Research utilization (RU) is the process of synthesizing, spreading and using research-generated knowledge to make an impact on existing practice in the society.

Evidence-based nursing is for the profession of nursing and health care. It is a conscious integration of best research evidence with clinical expertise and patient values and is imperative in the delivery of quality-oriented and cost-effective health care (Sackett and Strauss, 2000).

In nursing research, evidence is focused on health promotion, illness prevention, and the assessment, diagnosis and management of chronic patients (American Nurses Association, 2004).

Definition

Evidence-based practice

Evidence-based practice is the conscious use of current base evidence in making clinical decisions about patient-care (Sackett et al. 2000).

Evidence-based medicine

The practice of evidence-based medicine means integrating individual clinical expertise with the best available external clinical evidence from systematic research. It is conscientious, explicit and judicious use of current evidence in making decision about the care of individual patients.

Evidence-based nursing

Evidence-based nursing is the process by which nurses make clinical decisions using the best available research evidence, their clinical expertise and patient's preferences.

Sharma (2011) defines evidence-based nursing as a process of identifying the solid research findings and implementing them in nursing practice, in order to increase the quality of patient-care.

Historical Landmarks of Evidence-Based Practice Movement

Evidence-based practice was founded by Dr. Ardice Cochrane, a British epidemiologist. Cochrane was a strong proponent of using evidence from randomized clinical trials because he believed that this was the strongest evidence on which clinical practice division is to be based. After the demise of

Dr. Ardice Cochrane in 1988, the Cochrane Centre was launched in Oxford, England, in 1992. The major purpose of the centre is to assist individuals in making well-informed decision about health care with international collaboration by developing, maintaining and updating systematic review of health care intervention and ensures that these reviews are accessible to the public.

The rise of evidence-based practice movement in UK was accounted to the following:

1. Increasing cost of health care
2. Glut of research
3. Variation in health care
4. Unnecessary intervention
5. Change in the management of health services

When research results are implemented and sustained, it results in evidence-based practice.

Significance of Evidence-Based Nursing Practice in Research

1. Integration of research evidence into clinical practice is essential for the delivery of high-quality nursing care.
2. Cost of health care is ever increasing, while resources are shrinking and people are more health-conscious. The best available evidence added by patient's circumstances and performance improves the quality of clinical judgements and facilitates cost-effective health care.
3. Use of research findings may not be enough to answer all clinical questions for promoting quality care. Hence other forms of evidence may be required to obtain answers. So evidence-based practice sounds much more significant to nursing and health care.
4. It will enable to bridge the gap in utilization of research findings and theoretical application in practice, because enough research evidence in a particular area is the base for evidence-based practice.

5. It conveys and demonstrates the importance and usefulness of research in nursing practice, continues to develop research awareness and shares the high and low areas of research.
6. It reduces individual workload and improves efficiency, competency, intellectual skills, and refines practice skills as well as research skills.
7. It encourages critical thinking and reflective practice.
8. It continues to develop research awareness and promotes research acceptance in nurses.
9. It helps to standardize the nursing language.

Persons/Agencies Involved in Implementing Evidence-Based Nursing Practice

1. Individual nurses, nursing administrators and nurse leaders
2. Professional regulatory associations
3. Nurse educators, nursing institutions
4. Organizations that employ nurses
5. Accrediting agencies and government
6. Users of evidence-based nursing practice

What Competencies are Required?

1. Intellectual skills
2. Critical and reflective thinking skills
3. Analytical skills
4. Problem-solving skills
5. Empowering skills
6. Communication skills
7. Interviewing skills
8. Linguistic, computer and documenting skills

Evidence-based Nursing is a Five-step Process

The five A's will help one understand the evidence-based nursing process.

Ask: Specific clinical problems are converted into focused, structured questions.

Acquire: The questions identified are used as a basis for collecting the most relevant and best evidence.

Appraise: The research evidence is critically appraised for validity.

Apply: The best available evidence is used alongside clinical expertise and patient's preferences and values to plan care.

Assess: Performance is evaluated through a process of self-reflection, audit or peer assessment.

Steps in Evidence-based Nursing

Evidence-based nursing involves a series of five steps (Fig. 14.1).

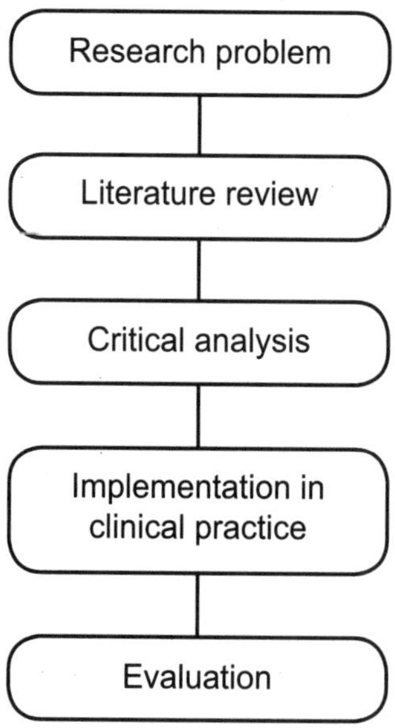

Figure 14.1 Process of evidence-based practice

Step 1: Identify the research problem clearly

Do a detailed assessment in the practice area and identify the pertinent research problem. It can be guided by health care personnel.

E.g.:

1. "Increased Incidence of Infections in Intensive Care Units"
2. "Sensory Overload of Post-Operative Patients in Cardiothoracic ICU"
3. "Identification of Risk Factors of Diabetic Foot Ulcer"

More research studies can be conducted to add to evidence-based nursing.

In step 1, a clinical question should be asked in **PICO** format to yield the most relevant and best evidence.

P – Patient population
I – Intervention of interest
C – Comparison intervention
O – Outcome

Step 2: Literature review

A detailed search of literature related to the problem is to be done. A researcher can perform a thorough search through integrative literature reviews, meta-analysis and care guidelines. A literature review can be done through a careful process. Standard reviews and latest study results should be incorporated.

The meta-analysis often needs an overall summary, and statistics that represents the effects of interventions across multiple studies. A systematic review and meta-analysis yield the strongest level of evidence on which a practice decision is based upon.

Step 3: Critical analysis of the evidence

A critical analysis of the evidence obtained from the search process is important. Critical appraisal is a hallmark of evidence-based practice. Choose interventions with most valid evidence. A critical analysis of the evidence can be accomplished by *three cardinal questions.*

- What are the research findings?
- Are the findings valid?
- Will the results help in caring patients?

Step 4: Implementation in clinical practice

Implementing useful findings in clinical practice based on research evidence is crucial. It is useful in addressing the research problem. Integrate the evidence found from literature search with the health care provider's experience, clinical assessment of the patient and available health resources to implement a decision. Although the concept of applying "best evidence" in a clinical decision seems clear, it is actually very complex. Skillful critical thinking is needed to evaluate the evidence.

Step 5: Evaluating the evidence-based intervention

Evidence-based practice is evaluating evidence-based intervention in terms of how the intervention worked or how effective the critical decision was with a particular patient. This type of appraisal is essential in determining whether the change based on intervention resulted in the expected outcome.

Three P's of Proficient Questioning: Practice, Practice, Practice

The key to proficiency in formulating searchable, answerable questions is practice. Many textbooks present established, accepted ideas of diagnostic and therapeutic techniques. However, these are not the best resource for finding current evidence to answer clinical questions because textbooks often took several years to complete.

For current information in health care, a review of full-text databases that hold the latest studies reported in journals is the best choice for finding relevant evidence to answer compelling clinical questions. Journals are useful for identifying information about recent advances and new methods of treatment. These may have limitations in that studies which have positive outcomes are more likely to be published than those where no effects are shown.

Often the source of evidence will be a database of published studies. Databases that contain references to medical literature often refer to physical objects such as books or journal publications. Choosing the right database and being familiar with its language are essential to be successful, and it expedites the search for answers to a clinical question.

Table 14.1 Example of searchable databases

No.	Database	Description
1.	CINAHL – Cumulative Index of Nursing and Allied Health Literature (1982 to present)	Studies in nursing, allied health and biomedicine. Individual subscription varies with time you expect to use.
2.	MEDLINE (1966 to present) http://www.ncbi.nlm.give/entrez/query.fegi	Studies in medicine, nursing, dentistry, psychiatry and veterinary.
3.	Psyc INFO (1887 to present) http://www/apa.org/psycinfo/	Psychology and related healthcare disciplines.
4.	Cochrane Database of Systematic Review http://www.cochrane.org/	Full text of regularly-updated systematic reviews prepared by the Cochrane Collaboration Completed Reviews and Protocols; available via internet or CD-ROM.

Internet can be an excellent source of evidence. Randomized controlled trials (RCTs) would be the strongest study design that would provide best answers.

Evidence-based practice

1. The transformation of scientific evidence from research results through the stages of:
   (a) evidence summary
   (b) translation into clinical recommendation
   (c) implementation as best clinical practice
   (d) evaluation of outcome
2. It is the "integration of best research evidence with clinical expertise and patient values". (Sackett, Straus, Richardson, Rosemberg & Haynes, 2000)
   (a) Is best available evidence with clinical expertise and judgement
   (b) Emphasizes pivotal role for patient-centered care

Evidence-based nursing

1. Evidence-based nursing is the process by which nurses make clinical decisions using the best available research evidence, their clinical expertise and patient's preferences.
2. Sigma Hecta Tau International Honour Society for Nurses recently identified evidence-based nursing practice as international priority.
3. Evidence-based nursing practice is the integration of the best evidence available, nursing expertise and values and the preferences of the individuals, families and communities who are served.

Research findings are paramount. So evidence-based practice is a process of:

1. synthesizing research evidence
2. designing clinical practice guidelines
3. implementing practice changes
4. evaluating outcomes

In carrying out evidence-based nursing, the following factors must be considered:

1. Sufficient data of research must have been published on the specific topic.
2. The nurse must have the skill in accessing to and critically analyzing research.
3. The nurse's practice must allow her/him to implement changes based on evidence-based nursing.

Evidence-based nursing practice solves problems encountered by nurses by carrying out four steps:

1. Clearly identify the issue or problem based on accurate analysis of current nursing knowledge and practice.
2. Search the literature for relevant research.
3. Evaluate the research evidence using established criteria regarding scientific merit.
4. Choose interventions and justify the selection with the most valid evidence.

Evidence-based teaching is conscientious, explicit and judicious use of current best evidence in making decision about the education of professional nurses.

Evidence-based health promotion

It means that one should practice medical activities that have evidence for successful work. For example, those who believe that decisions about health care interventions should be based on evidence would argue that one may not undertake operations that research has shown no benefit to patients.

The most distinguishing factor of evidence-based practice is that a new scientific base for practice is built through a summary of studies on a topic. These summaries are called evidence syntheses. An evidence-based approach to health promotion implies a rigorous approach in collecting and analyzing data as to whether the study in question is qualitative or quantitative.

An evidence-based approach to health promotion develops an attitude of mind that constantly questions what one is doing. Evidence-based approach provides a defense against indiscriminate use of practice in situations which have no research-based legitimacy. It implies a willingness to write and publish one's work for the benefit of others. It is about building a culture where criticism is constructive and health promoters openly share their experience.

Where is evidence-based practice found?

1. Published research
2. Systematic review
3. Special collection of evidence-based practice resources

Evidence-based practice for public health

It involves using the best available evidence to take public health practice decisions. Many websites provide free access to evidence-based public health resources, knowledge domains and public health journals and databases. These resources are arranged along a pathway of evidence to allow public health practitioners to easily find and use the best evidence to develop and implement effective interventions, programmes and policies.

Research Utilization through Clinical Guidelines

One of the many ways to facilitate the instrumental use of research in practice is through clinical guidelines. This is an important tool to promote evidence-based practice. Clinical guidelines have been defined as systematically developed statements to assist practitioner and patient decision about appropriate health care for specific clinical circumstances (Field and Lohr, 1990).

Research-practice gap is assumed to exist when there is sufficient research knowledge about a particular practice which is not used by practitioners. Rigorously developed clinical practice guidelines can be tools to help bridge the research-practice gap. The current emphasis on evidence-based guideline development, implementation and evaluation activities is a positive step towards evidence-based decision-making at the bedside.

The Royal College of Nursing (1995) explains that national clinical guidelines can provide a way for health professionals, patients and service-users to work together to make decisions about appropriate care.

Challenges of evidence-based nursing

1. To update themselves in constantly changing background.
2. To establish creative approaches to old and new health problems and beginning new and innovative programmes.
3. To empower themselves for social relevance.
4. To evaluate and change one's practice methods constantly and voluntarily.
5. To learn and operate various skills.

Barriers in promoting evidence-based nursing

Nurses are faced with many barriers for implementing evidence-based nursing practice.

1. Lack of accessibility to journals and library.
2. Lack of habit of reading research findings.
3. Lack of conduct of research.
4. Inability of nurse practitioners for critical appraisal of research.

5. Resistance in the practice environment to changes.
6. Inadequate continuing education programmes.
7. Inability to transform information into a sense of significant relationships through inductive and deductive processes.

Resources to facilitate evidence-based nursing practice guideline

1. Systematic reviews
2. Centre for evidence-based nursing practice
3. Evidence-based nursing practice guidelines
4. Evidence-based journals

Future of evidence-based nursing practice

1. Better base of evidence expected through more researches.
2. Evidence-based centres may facilitate further development.
3. More nurses at all levels may come for research activities.
4. Promote reflective thinking.
5. Become mandatory standards of practice.

SUMMARY

The movement of evidence-based practice began in medicine with the work of Ardice Cochrane, who is known as the father of evidence-based practice. Evidence-based medicine is defined as conscientious, explicit and judicious use of current best evidence in making decisions about the care of individual patients (Sackett, 1992).

MULTIPLE CHOICE QUESTIONS

1. The meaning of word evidence in research is __________.
   (a) proof of thing
   (b) substitute for nursing care
   (c) clear document
   (d) research findings

2. Who was the founder of evidence-based practice movement?
   (a) Ardice Cochrane
   (b) Polit
   (c) Sackett
   (d) Liolya E. Hall
3. Which level of evidence is most often placed at the top of the hierarchy of evidence for practice decisions?
   (a) meta-analysis of multiple randomized clinical trials
   (b) results from true experimental study
   (c) case control studies
   (d) a consensus of opinion from a group of experts
4. More emphasis to be placed on what type of evidence on which to base practice decisions?
   (a) results from qualitative research studies
   (b) except opinions
   (c) cost-containment data
   (d) nurse's preferences for type of care they provide
5. The ultimate goal of nursing research is __________.
   (a) evidence-based nursing
   (b) comprehensive nursing care
   (c) sharpening of nursing skills
   (d) health promotion of patients

ANSWER KEY

1. (d) 2. (a) 3. (b) 4. (a) 5. (b)

REVIEW QUESTIONS

1. (a) Define evidence-based nursing.
   (b) Explain the significance of evidence-based nursing.
   (c) Explain the steps of evidence-based nursing.

2. Write short notes on:
   (a) Significance of evidence-based nursing
   (b) Challenges of evidence-based nursing
   (c) Barriers in promoting evidence-based nursing
   (d) Future of evidence-based nursing

REFERENCES

Clinical Pharmacy, 7(11), 832–836. Marwick, C. (1997). Aspirin's role in prevention now official. JAMA: *The Journal of the American Medical Association*, 277(9), 701–702.

Coyle, L.A., & Sokop, A.G. (1990). Innovation adoption behaviour among nurses. *Nursing Research*, 39, 176–180.

Craig, J.V., & Smyth, R.L. (2002). The evidence-based practice manual for nurses. Edinburgh: Churchill Livingstone. CURN Project. (1981, 1982).

Cyganski, J.M., Donahue, J.M., & Heaton, J.S. (1987). New York: Grune & Stratton.

Donham, J., & Denning, V. (1987). Heparin vs. saline in maintaining patency, intermittent infusion devices: Pilot study. The Kansas Nurse, 62(11), 6–7.

Dracup, K.A., & Breu, C.S. (1978). Using nursing research findings to meet the needs of grieving spouses.

Dunn, D.L., & Lenihan, S.F. (1987). The case for the saline flush. *American Journal of Nursing*, 87(6), 798–799.

Epperson, E.L. (1984). Efficacy of 0.9% sodium chloride injection with and without heparin for maintaining indwelling intermittent injection sites. Clinical Pharmacy, 3(6), 626–629.

Fitzpatrick, R., & Roberts, K. (2001). Including qualitative research in systematic reviews: Opportunities and problems. *Journal of Evaluation in American Journal of Nursing*, 87(6), 796–797.

Forbes, D.A. (2003). An example of the use of systematic reviews to answer an effective question. *Western Journal of Nursing Research*, 25(2), 179–192.

Forrest, J.L., & Miller, S.A. (2004). The anatomy of evidence-based publications: Article summaries and systematic reviews. Part 1: *Journal of Dental Hygiene*, 78(2), 343–348.

Garrelts, J., LaRocca, J., Ast, D., Smith, D.E., & Sweet, D.E. (1989). Comparison of heparin and 0.9% sodium chloride injection in the maintenance of indwelling intermittent I.V. devices. Clinical Pharmacy, 8(1), 34–39.

Geritz, M.A. (1992). Saline vs. heparin in intermittent infuser patency maintenance. *Western Journal of Nursing Research*, 14(2), 131–141.

Germantown, M.D., Aspen Kruszewski, A., Lang, S., & Johnson, J. (1979). Effect of positioning on discomfort from intramuscular injections in the dorsogluteal site. *Nursing Research*, 28(2), 103–105.

Glaser, E.M., Abelson, H.H., & Garrison, K.N. (1983). Putting knowledge to use. San Francisco, CA.

Goode, C.J., Titler, M., Rakel, B., Ones, D.S., Kleiber, C., Small, S., & Triolo, P.K. (1991). A meta-analysis of effects of heparin flush and saline flush: Quality and cost implications. *Nursing Research*, 40(6), 324–330.

Greenway, K. (2004). Using die ventrogluteal site for intramuscular injection. Nursing Standard, 18(25), 39–42.

Haller, K.B., Reynolds, M.A., & Horsley, J.A. (1979). Developing research-based innovation protocols: Process, criteria, and issues. *Research in Nursing and Health*, 2(2), 45–51.

Hamer, S., & Collinson, G. (1999). Achieving evidence-based practice: A handbook for practitioners. Edinburgh: Bailliere Tindall.

Hamilton, R.A., Plis, J.M., Clay, C., & Sylvan, L. (1988). Heparin sodium vs. 0.9% sodium chloride injection for maintaining patency of indwelling intermittent infusion devices. Clinical Pharmacy, 7(6), 439–443.

Holford, N.H., Vozeh, S., Coates, P., Porvell, J.R., Thiercelin, J.E., & Upton, R. (1977). More on heparin lock. *The New England Journal of Medicine*, 29(22), 1300–1301.

Horsley, J.A., Crane, J., & Bingle, J.D. (1978). Research utilization as an organizational process. *Journal of Nursing Administration*, 8(7), 4–6.

Horsley, J.A., Crane, J., Crabtree, M.K., & Wood, D.J. (1983). Using research to improve nursing practice: A guide. New York: Grune & Stratton.

Jossey-Bass, Goode, C.J. (2000). What constitutes die "evidence" in evidence-based practice? *Applied Nursing Research*, 13(4), 222–225.

Kasparek, A., Wenger, J., & Feldt, R. (1988). Comparison of normal vs. beparinized saline for flushing of intermittent intravenous infusion devices. Unpublished manuscript.

Keen, M.F. (1986). Comparison of intramuscular injection techniques to reduce site discomfort and lesions. *Nursing Research*, 35(4), 207–210.

Krueger, J. C. (1978). Utilization of nursing research: The planning process. *Journal of Nursing Administration*, 8(1), 6–9.

Krueger, J.C., Nelson, A.H., & Wolanin, M.O. (1978). Nursing research: Development, collaboration, and utilization.

Lombardi, T.P., Gunderson, B., Zammett, L.O., Walters, J.K., & Morris, B.A. (1988). Efficacy of 0.9% sodium chloride injection with or without heparin sodium for maintaining patency of intravenous catheters in children.

Melnyk, B.M., & Fineout-Overholt, E. (2005). Evidence-based practice in nursing & healthcare: A guide to best practice. Philadelphia: Lippincott Williams & Wilkins.

Mercy Medical Centre, Cedar Rapids, IA, 1–18.

Miracle, V., Fangman, B., Kayrouz, P., Kederis, K., & Pursell, L. (1989). Normal saline vs. heparin lock flush solution: One institution's findings. The Kentucky Nurse, 57(3), 1, 6–7.

Pelz, D., & Horsley, J. (1981). Measuring utilization of nursing research. In J. Ciarlo (Ed.). Utilizing evaluation. Beverly Hills, CA: Sage.

Peterson, F.Y., & Kirchhoff, K.T. (1991). Analysis of the research about heparinized vs. nonheparinized intravascular lines. Heart and Lung, 20(6), 631–640.

Randolph, A.G., Cook, D.J., Gonzales, C.A., & Andrew, M. (1998). Benefit of heparin in peripheral venous and arterial catheters: Systematic review and meta-analysis of randomized controlled trials. *British Medical Journal*, 316(7136), 969–977.

CHAPTER

15

QUALITY IMPROVEMENT IN NURSING RESEARCH

Key terms

- Quality improvement
- Research centre
- Research scholars
- Research map

⊙ Outline

- Importance of quality improvement in research work
- Factors affecting quality of research work
- Measures to improve quality of research work

⊙ Objectives

On completion of this chapter, you will be able to:

- recognize the importance of quality improvement in research work
- identify the factors affecting quality of research work
- understand the steps to improve quality of nursing research

Introduction

Research is much harder than clinical work, more exact with less opportunity to cover up mistakes.

—James Calnan

Research is a process of creation of knowledge through investigations, recording and analysis of evidence. It is the quest for new knowledge. The decline in the standard of research is a problem of concern in academic circles. A large number of studies are being undertaken in colleges without any practical utility. Sometimes research guides and scholars are not performing their duty as guides and scholars in a true sense. This will affect the quality of research work.

In the new National Policy on Education, it is observed, "in the context of unprecedented explosion of knowledge, higher education has to become dynamic as never before, constantly entering unspecified areas. The need for quality research is stressed in these disciplines."

It is important for the nursing community to examine this problem with due regard in all spheres in all its aspects and undertake appropriate measures to rectify this trend of decline in the quality of research and make impeccable.

Check Points... *Major drawbacks in research in nursing are summarized as follows:*	
1	Lack of proper theoretical background
2	Lack of understanding of research methodology
3	Using tools of western origin without considering its adaptability
4	Inadequate supervision of research activities
5	Lack of commitment from researchers
6	Slackness in scheduling for research work
7	Irrelevant and substandard topics selected for study
8	A number of research studies in different areas under one supervisor
9	Paucity of qualified/experienced research guides in nursing

Factors Influencing the Quality of Research

The major factors influencing the quality of research are:

(a) Quality of research centres
(b) Quality of research scholars
(c) Quality of research guides

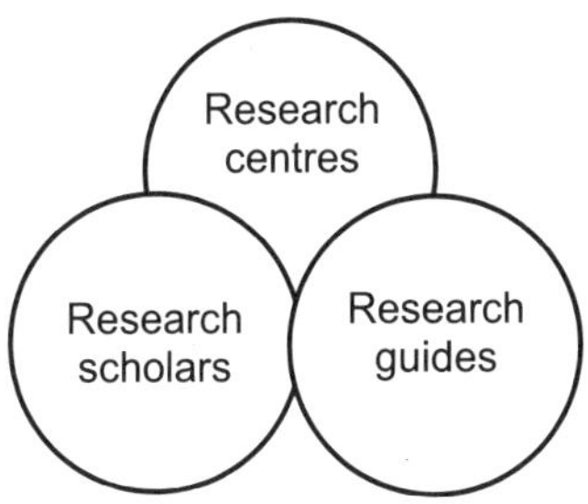

Figure 15.1 Factors influencing quality of research

Research centres: Research centres are where research facilities are provided to research scholars. Most research centres have inadequate facilities like equipment, materials, books and periodicals. Information required for research work is not optimally available from here.

***Research scholars*:** Scholars with no genuine interest in research shall show poor commitment, dedication and hard work towards the assigned work.

***Research guides*:** Qualified and experienced faculty members should be appointed as research supervisors. Research guides shall maintain their intellectual curiosity and academic alertness in their area of specialization. An essential requirement of a research guide is updating oneself on the current knowledge and research methodologies in their areas of specialization.

Steps to Improve the Quality of Nursing Research

1. Help research scholars develop competence and aptitude for research studies. The selection of a research problem has great importance for the research process. The choice of topics needs the careful attention of the candidate as well as the supervising teacher. The role of a guide in this regard is limited to offering necessary advice.
2. Avoid duplication of research. Many of the cases reported are a replication of research problems. To avoid duplication of studies, colleges and universities might prepare a database on research problems to be addressed in order of priority to maintain the quality of research.
3. The guide has a significant role in ensuring quality research. It is rewarding to guide students who belong to a similar specialty. Guides must frequently interact with their students and render all help and assistance to them. The guide must also encourage them to keep a research diary for writing the daily details of research work.
4. A research proposal should be prepared by the candidate. The proposal should be complete and precise; a research map is useful for the proper conduct of research. A research guide should make a periodical assessment to check the progress of research. This will enable the guide to give timely intervention as needed.
5. Library use is another important skill. Literature search, rules of bibliographic citation and research methodology are areas that need improvement. Each college should conduct regular training programmes in these areas for all research students.

6. Colleges should provide facilities of computer lab to researchers. Specific guidelines should be prescribed for the presentation of data tables, figures and writing of the dissertation.
7. The written content of the thesis should be simple, straightforward and free from mistakes, and presentation of the matter must be lucid, logical and coherent. For editing the content, seek the help of a language expert.
8. The research committee in each college should prepare a list of research topics (thrust areas) in the different fields of study. A selection of topic from this list will avoid repetitive research.
9. Update programmes may be conducted for research students and research guides. Strictly adhere to the guidelines of the respective university or institution for presenting the PG thesis and Ph.D. thesis. Consider research as a higher level of learning. Be serious in carrying out the research activities.
10. Evaluation of the thesis should be bias-free and objective. The remuneration for examiners should justify the competency of the experts handling the evaluation of theses.
11. Research findings should be properly documented by the institution and provided in the internet for indexing by search engines and for global access.
12. Awards may be announced to research guides and researchers in order to encourage qualitative and productive research.

SUMMARY

Maintaining the quality of research work is of utmost important. Quality research work contributes to practical utility. Quality of research centre, research scholar and research guide are factors that influence the outcomes of scientific research.

Selection of a research problem, avoiding duplication of research, good supervision, skilled utilization of library, application of information technology, editing, attending research conferences, efficient evaluation of the theses, and proper dissemination of research findings are key factors for improving the quality of research.

MULTIPLE CHOICE QUESTIONS

1. Major drawbacks which influence quality of Nursing research are __________.
   (a) lack of commitment from researchers
   (b) inadequate supervision of research activities
   (c) inadequate knowledge of research methodology
   (d) all of the above
2. Quality of research centre influencing quality of research __________.
   (a) availability of equipments, materials and books
   (b) dedication and hard work
   (c) intellectual curiosity
   (d) commitment to work
3. Factors influencing quality of research are __________.
   (a) quality of research centre
   (b) quality of research scholar
   (c) quality of research guide
   (d) (a), (b) and (c)
4. Research scholars with no genuine interest in research shall show poor commitment and hard work towards the assigned work
   (a) yes
   (b) no
5. To avoid duplication of research studies universities might prepare a data base on research problems to be addressed to maintain the quality of research.
   (a) no
   (b) yes

ANSWER KEY

1. (d) 2. (a) 3. (d) 4. (a) 5. (b)

REVIEW QUESTIONS

1. Write the significance of quality improvement in research work.
2. List the factors affecting the quality of research investigations.
3. Explain the various steps for the improvement of quality of a research work.

REFERENCES

Beck, C.T. (2004). Post-traumatic stress disorder due to childbirth. *Nursing Research*, 53, 216–224.

Burns, N., & Grove, S.K. (2005). The practice of nursing research: Conduct, critique and utilization. (5th ed.). St. Louis, MO: Elsevier Saunders.

Cobb, A.K. (2000). Acculturation and accommodation in qualitative and quantitative research. *Journal of Professional Nursing*, 16, 188.

Connelly, L.M., & Yoder, L.K. (2000). Improving qualitative proposals. Common problem areas. *Clinical Nurse Specialist*, 14, 69–74.

Daly, P. (2005). Mothers living with suicidal adolescents: A Phenomenological study of their experiences. *Journal of Psychosocial Nursing and Mental Health Services*, 43(3), 22–28.

DeSantis, L., & Ugarriza, D.N. (2000). The concept of theme as used in qualitative nursing research. *Western Journal of Nursing Research*, 22, 351–372.

Donalek, J.G. (2005). The interview in qualitative research. *Urologic Nursing*, 25, 124–125.

Field, P.A., & Morse, J.M. (1985). Nursing research: The application of qualitative approaches. Rockville, MD: Aspen.

Ford-Gilboe, M., Campbell, J., & Berman, H. (1995). Stories and numbers: Coexistence without compromise. *Advances in Nursing Science*, 18, 14–26.

Gance-Cleveland, B. (2004). Qualitative evaluation of a school-based support group for adolescents with an addicted parent. *Nursing Research*, 53, 379–386.

Haase, J.E., & Myers, S.T. (1988). Reconciling paradigm assumptions of qualitative and quantitative research. *Western Journal of Nursing Research*, 10, 128–136.

Harmon, R.B. (2005). Nursing care in a state hospital before and during the introduction of antipsychotics: 1950–1963. *Issues in Mental Health Nursing*, 26, 257–279.

CHAPTER

16

INTRODUCTION TO STATISTICS

Key terms

★ Normal distribution ★ Percentile ★ Frequency distribution ★ Positively skewed ★ Frequency polygon ★ Range ★ Histogram ★ Scatter diagram ★ Inferential statistics ★ Standard deviation ★ Central tendency ★ Symmetrical distribution ★ Measures of relationships ★ Measures of condensed data ★ Variance

⊙ Outline

★ Definitions
★ Scales of measurement
★ Descriptive statistics
★ Inferential statistics
★ Test of significance
★ Statistical packages and applications

⊙ Objectives

On completion of this chapter, you will be able to:

★ define statistics
★ list the purposes of descriptive statistics
★ identify the level of measurement in a research study
★ describe central tendency
★ identify the purposes of inferential statistics
★ explain probability as it applies to the analysis of sample data
★ distinguish between parametric and non-parametric tests
★ list the commonly used statistical tests and their purposes

Introduction

Statistics is a set of mathematical techniques used to organize and manipulate data for answering questions and testing theories. If one does not understand the basics of a language, they will have problems in their conversation. The root of the word 'statistics' comes from the Italian word 'statista' (statesman) and German word 'statistik'(political state). It was used for the first time by Professor Gottfried Achenwall in Marlborough in 1949. It refers to the subject matter as a whole. Statistics is the language of the researcher.

Nurse researchers use statistics as a means of communication. Statistics is the study of techniques and procedures for collecting, classifying, summarizing, analyzing and interpreting numerical data.

The success in research work is possible only with a proper knowledge of statistics, interpretation and a proper use of the results of the study.

Definitions

"From here on, as far ahead as one can see medicine must be building, as a central part of its scientific base, a solid underpinning of statistical knowledge. Intuitive impressions are essential for getting the work started, but it is only through the quality of the numbers at the end that the truth can be hold." (Lewis Thomas, 1982)

Best and Kahn define statistics as a "body of mathematical techniques or process for gathering, organizing, analyzing and interpreting numerical data."

According to Kendall, "A quantitative data affected to marked extent by multiplicity of causes and that the methods used to elucidate such multiplicity of causes are called statistical methods."

Biostatistics is the application of statistics in the field of health sciences such as biology, medicine, nursing, public health, dentistry, pharmacy and physical therapy.

Reviewing Basic Terminologies

Data: It is the factual information collected during the data collection period of the research study. The singular is datum.

Discrete data: When the collected data is in whole number then it is called discrete data, e.g. pulse rate, blood pressure.

Continuous data: When the collected data is assessed in fractional values, then it is continuous data, e.g. height, weight, body temperature.

Qualitative data: When the observed variables can be categorized according to certain characteristics or qualities, those are referred to as qualitative data. They are non-numerical in nature and cannot be measured, e.g. gender, marital status, religion, etc.

Quantitative data: When the collected data can be measured quantitatively, it is called quantitative data, e.g. height, weight, serum cholesterol, SGOT, SGPT.

Parameters: These refer to the characteristics of a population, e.g. average height of children of age 3 to 6 in Trivandrum district.

Parametric test: Statistical test that involves assumption about the distribution of variables and estimation of a parameter.

Non-parametric test: Statistical test that does not involve any assumption about the distribution of the population.

Central tendency: Suppose a teacher counts the scores of his students; he wishes to inspect the data to see "centre" or "middle area" of central distribution. There are three ways to measure this central tendency, and each of these averages has a different meaning.

Mean: The mean is simply the arithmetic average. It is a very common measure of central tendency.

Median: It is the next measure of central tendency; median is the midpoint of distribution or 50th percentile. In other words, median is the value below which half of the values in the sample fall.

Mode: The most frequently occurring score or number value. In statistics, mode is the measure of central tendency that merely identifies the value that occurs most often.

Standard deviation: A general indicator of dispersion or spread of scores from the mean. The standard deviation is a quantitative index of a distributive spread or variability. It is the square root of variance.

Correlation: The strength of quantifiable relationship between two or more variables.

Correlation coefficient: The number that represents the strength of quantifiable relationship between two or more variables.

Characteristics of Statistics

1. They are collection of facts.
2. Statistics is influenced by multiplicity of causes.
3. Statistical data need to be collected in an organized manner.
4. Statistical data are collected for a predetermined purpose.
5. Accuracy in collection of data is maintained carefully.

Uses and Applications of Statistics

The main uses of statistics are:

1. To describe a particular set of data.
2. To use data to draw conclusions about a population.

The practical uses are:

1. To use data to draw conclusion about a population.
2. Formulate hypothesis of the study.
3. Test the hypothesis of the project.
4. Make comparisons between groups and assessments.
5. Summarize data for analysis and interpretation and to draw results in a meaningful and convenient form.
6. Make predictions of relationships of variables.
7. Generalize the study findings.

Statistics is an integral part of biological researches. Some of the important aspects are detailed below:

1. Research involves precise observations and accurate description as well as comparisons. Statistical methods help the researcher to suitably plan for the collection through suitable statistical design.
2. Inherent features of all biological observations are their variability. In order to define the normal value and also to compare those from one group to the other, statistical methodologies have an important application.
3. Statistical quantities serve as indices for the measurement of health of a community in terms of rates and ratios of fatalities, morbidities, mortalities and health facilities.
4. These methods are useful in the evaluation of health care delivery system or various control measures in an objective manner.
5. Records of health care activities help to assess the effectiveness of these programmes.
6. Statistics plays a vital role in planning and interpretation of epidemiological studies.

7. Sophisticated statistical methodologies help in evolving suitable models for the delivery of health care activities. These statistical methodologies are essential tools for planning various research studies and interpretation of results of the studies.

Applications of Biostatistics

Biostatistics has many vital applications.

1. Normal and deviation from normal in various aspects of health and illness.
2. Experiment planning and its result analysis.
3. Accuracy of the diagnostic procedures can be established.
4. Signs, symptoms, course, variation, etc. which are included in the natural history of illness, can be observed.
5. Treatment protocol and different interventions used for care and treatment of the patients can be assessed.
6. Collection, analysis and dissemination of various population health statistics.

Measurement of Statistical Data/Scales of Measurements

Measurement is defined as the use of the rules or standard procedures to allocate numerical values to the properties or characteristics of individuals, objects or events. There are four levels of measurement (Figure 16.1).

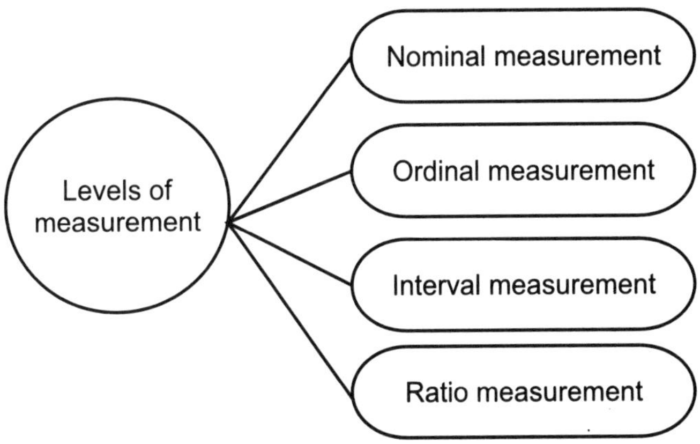

Figure 16.1 Levels of measurement

Nominal measurement

The lowest level of measurement is nominal measurement, which involves assigning numbers to classify characteristics into categories. Categorical data and numbers that are simply used as identifiers or names represent a nominal scale of measurement. The word nominal derives from a Latin word meaning "name". Individuals might be grouped as male or female, healthy or unhealthy, rich or poor. Here there are two or more named groups into which objects, individuals, and responses are grouped. It is possible to distinguish two or more categories relating to the specified attribute. Grouping people based on gender is a common application of nominal scale. For example, number 1 is assigned to male and number 2 is assigned to female. We can also assign number 1 to female and 2 to male.

Ordinal measurement

Ordinal measurement involves sorting objects on the basis of attributes. The word ordinal derives from a Latin word meaning "for order". The order of position will be measured. Numbers are assigned to indicate only the relative position. In this, observations are placed into a set of categories on a scale which has a rule of order. It gives rank to the objects based on their relative standing. The level implies ranking, but there is no equal distance between groups on scale. For example, for grading students in 10th standard exams, the grades might be recorded as A+, A, B+, B and so on.

Interval measurement

This is the third level of measurement. It possesses the characteristics of ordinal measurement especially the rank order and it also mentions the distance between objects, e.g. temperature 10–20 degrees. In this measurement, the position of zero is arbitrary.

Ratio measurement

This is the highest level of measurement. The ratio scales have a meaningful zero. Measurement scales having a constant interval size and a true zero point are said to be ratio scales of measurement. Here there is not only an order and equal intervals but there is also a meaningful zero point, e.g. height, weight.

The ratio scale of measurement is similar to the interval scale in that it also represents quantity and has equality of units. However, this scale has an absolute zero; no numbers exist below zero.

Statistics can be broadly classified as:

1. Descriptive statistics and
2. Inferential statistics

A. Descriptive Statistics

Descriptive statistics deals with the enumeration, organization and graphical representation of the data. It helps the investigator to interpret the data meaningfully in order to answer the research questions appropriately.

Descriptive statistics includes the following:

1. Frequency distribution, percentages, proportion, rates and graphical representation
2. Measures of central tendency: mean, median and mode
3. Measures of variability/dispersion: range, standard deviation and variance
4. Measures of relationship between two or more variables: correlation coefficient

Frequency Distribution

The process of condensing total data into a concise form in order to answer the research questions is important. One such technique that concise the data with minimal loss of information is frequency distribution.

Quantitative data are usually condensed and frequency distribution is presented through tables, charts, graphs and diagrams.

Tables

A table helps to present data in concise form. Tabulation is the process of systematic presentation of data in rows and columns in relation to some characteristics.

Construction of a Frequency Distribution Table

A frequency distribution table is an arrangement of the range of values that are expected to take a variable along with respective frequencies of occurrence of each variable represented in a tabular form.

Steps for constructing a frequency distribution table

1. Spot the smallest and largest observations.
2. Subtract the smallest from the largest to obtain the range of data.
3. Find out the number of classes. An ideal class interval is between 6 and 14 to provide information without being overly detailed.
4. There should be enough classes to exhibit the shape of the curve.
5. Divide the range of observations by the number of classes to obtain the width of the class. It is better to have consistent width for all classes.
6. Class limits must not overlap. If possible avoid open-ended classes at the upper and lower end because this does not accurately communicate the range of observations.
7. If possible, class limit should be so chosen that most of the observations in the class are closer to the midpoint of the class than to either end of the class.
8. Finally, find the number of observations in each class.
9. Percentages are calculated by dividing the number of observations in a given class by the total number of observations and then multiply it by 100.

Types of Tables

Frequency distribution table

Tabulation refers to the orderly arrangement of data in a table or other summary format. Counting the number of responses to a question and putting them in a frequency distribution is simple or marginal tabulation. These tables present the frequency and percentage distribution of the data collected from samples. The following is an example of frequency distribution table.

Table 16.1 Frequency distribution of income

Income	Frequency (number of people with income in each range)
Less than Rs. 5000	811
Rs. 5000–9999	530
Rs. 10000–14999	562
Rs. 15000–19999	718
Rs. 20,000 or more	499
Total	3120

Contingency table

These tables present the frequency distribution of two nominal/ordinal variables simultaneously. These are also called cross tables or bivariate tables. The tables may be 2 × 2, 2 × 3, 3 × 3, depending upon the number of categories of variables being studied. The following is an example of 2 × 2 contingency table.

Table 16.2 Example of a 2 × 2 contingency table

Irritation to eyes	Exposure to hazardous chemical spill		Total
	Yes	No	
Present	80	60	140
Absent	140	350	490
Total	220	410	630

Multiple responses table

The following is an example of multiple responses table where many variables are being observed by the researcher.

Table 16.3 Contingency table showing distribution of subjects according to type of institution, sex and place of residence

Place of residence	Hospital A		Hospital B		Total
	Male	Female	Male	Female	
Rural	99	130	106	122	457
Urban	73	99	70	100	342
Total	172	229	176	222	799

Graphical Presentation of Data

Some practical advantages of using graphs are:

1. Easy to understand the comparisons.
2. Useful to get overall view of entire data.
3. Most convenient way of presenting the data.
4. Is visually attractive.

In graphical presentation of data, the following are commonly used:

1. Bar diagram
2. Pie diagram
3. Histogram
4. Frequency polygon
5. Cumulative frequency curve
6. Line graphs
7. Scattered diagram
8. Pictogram

Bar Diagram

It is an easy method of presenting nominal or ordinal data. The bars can be drawn either vertically or horizontally.

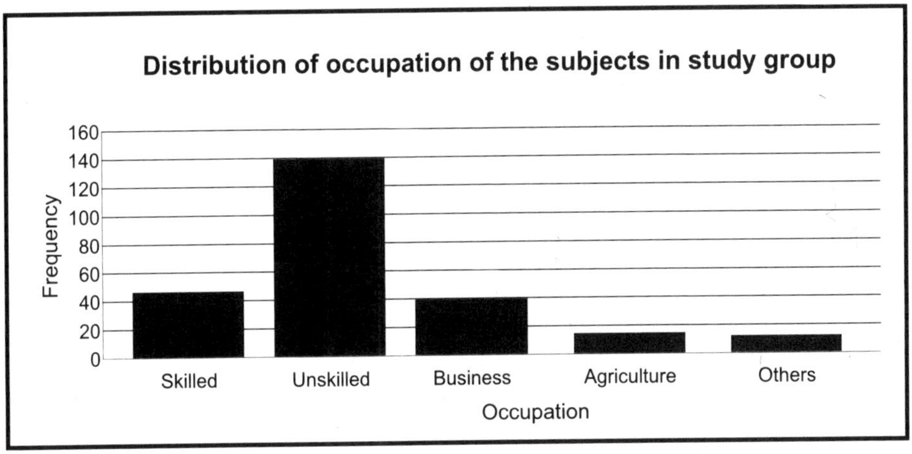

Figure 16.2 Bar diagram showing the distribution of patients based on occupation

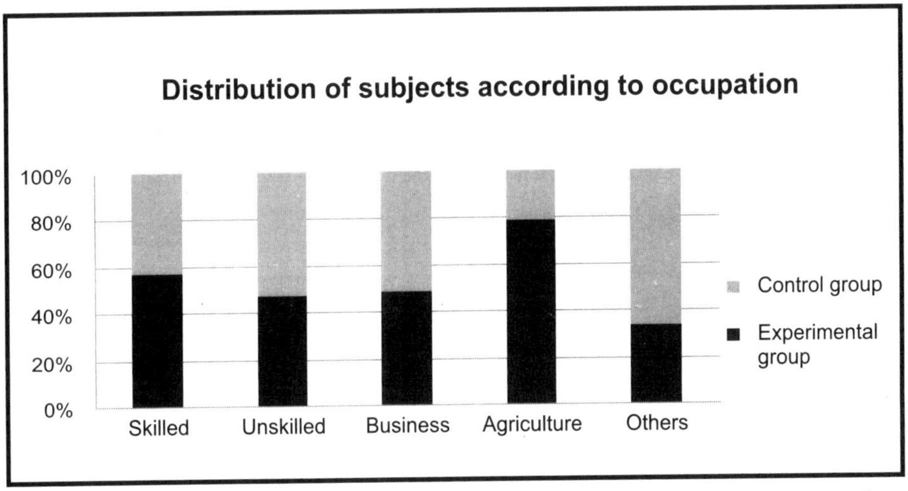

Figure 16.3 Percentage bar diagram based on occupation

Pie Diagram

A pie diagram is useful in presenting discrete data of qualitative characteristics such as gender. Percentage data is shown only in a pie diagram.

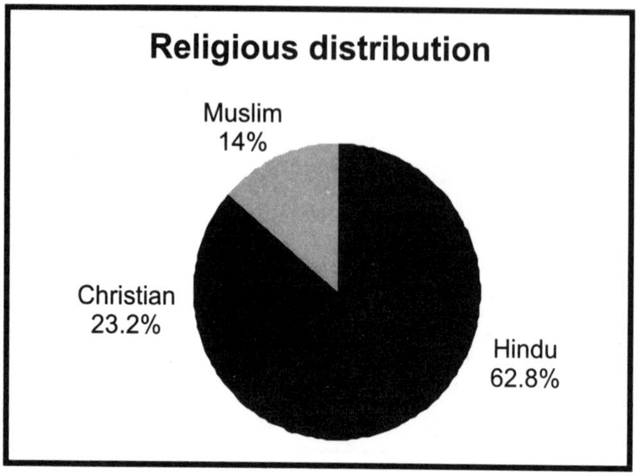

Figure 16.4 A pie diagram showing the distribution of patients with carcinoma cervix according to religion

Histogram

In this representation, the class intervals are presented on X-axis and the frequency is plotted on Y-axis. The frequency of each group forms a column. It is commonly used for grouped frequency distribution. It is ideal when the level of measurement is interval/ratio.

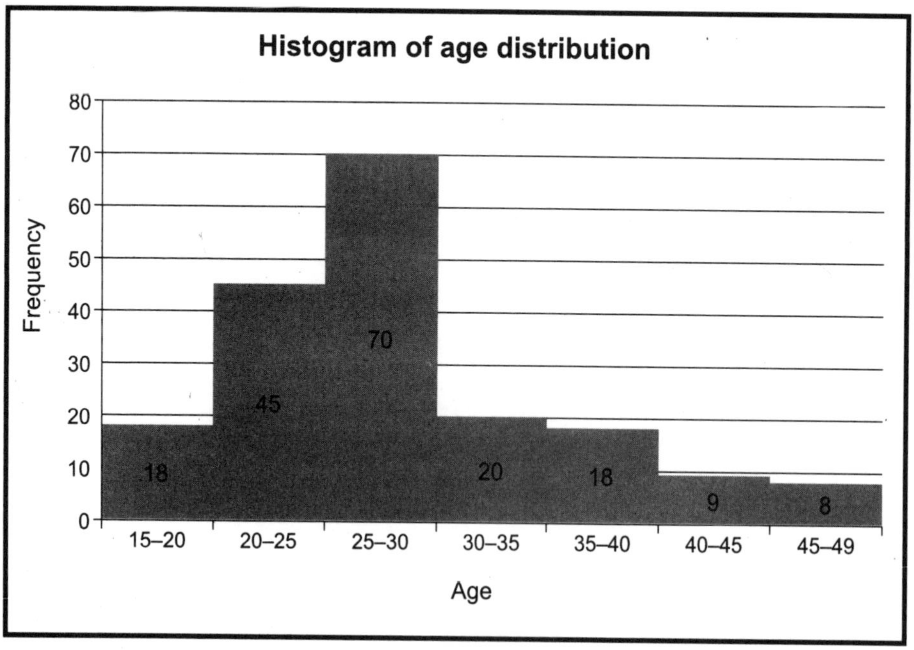

Figure 16.5 Histogram showing age distribution

Analysts rarely exhibit frequency data by means of graphs. The most widely used graphs for displaying interval and ratio level data are histograms and frequency polygons. Both are constructed similarly. Initially score values are arrayed on a horizontal dimension, lowest value on the left sloping upwards and highest value on the right side. Frequencies or percentages are displayed upright. A histogram is made by drawing adjacent bars above the score class.

Frequency Polygon

When the midpoints of the tops of rectangles in a histogram are joined by straight lines, then it becomes a frequency polygon, and the points are usually joined to the horizontal axis.

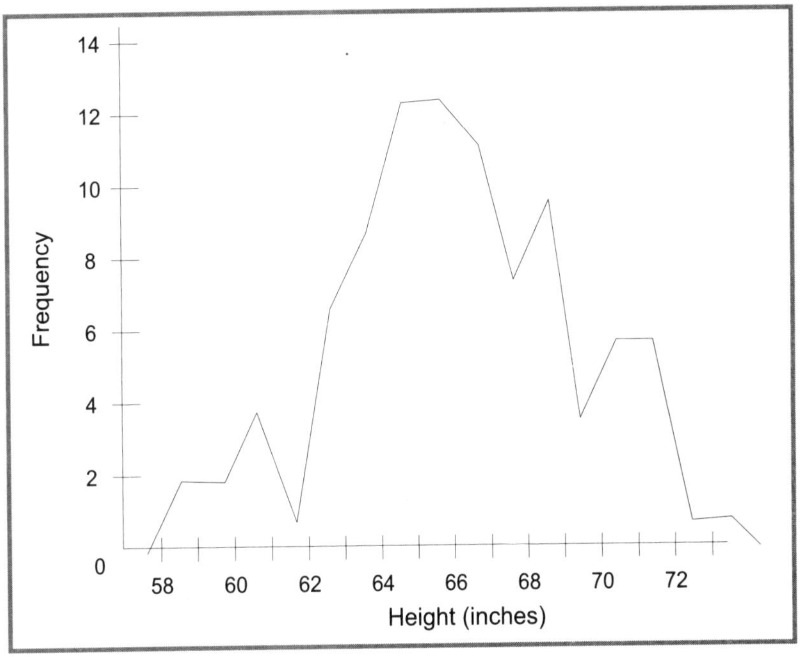

Figure 16.6 Frequency polygon of height distribution

In the case of frequency polygons, dots are used instead of vertical bars to connect straight lines for showing frequencies. A dot is placed corresponding to the frequency above each score. Normally a connection is made with a line to the base at the score below the minimum value and above the maximum. If the plotted points are joined by a smooth free-hand curve, it is called "frequency curve".

Cumulative Frequency Curve

This is for representing a frequency distribution by means of a diagram. Similar to a frequency polygon curve, the scores are plotted on X-axis and cumulative frequency on Y-axis. The plotted points are joined to give the s-shaped curve called cumulative frequency curve.

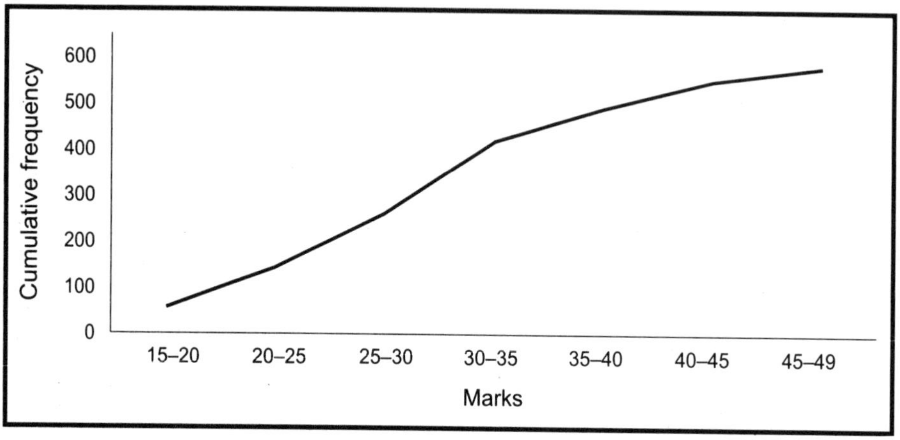

Figure 16.7 Cumulative frequency curve showing marks secured

Line Graphs

In line graphs, the independent variable or time is plotted as X-axis and the dependent variables on Y-axis. The given data are plotted and joined by straight lines.

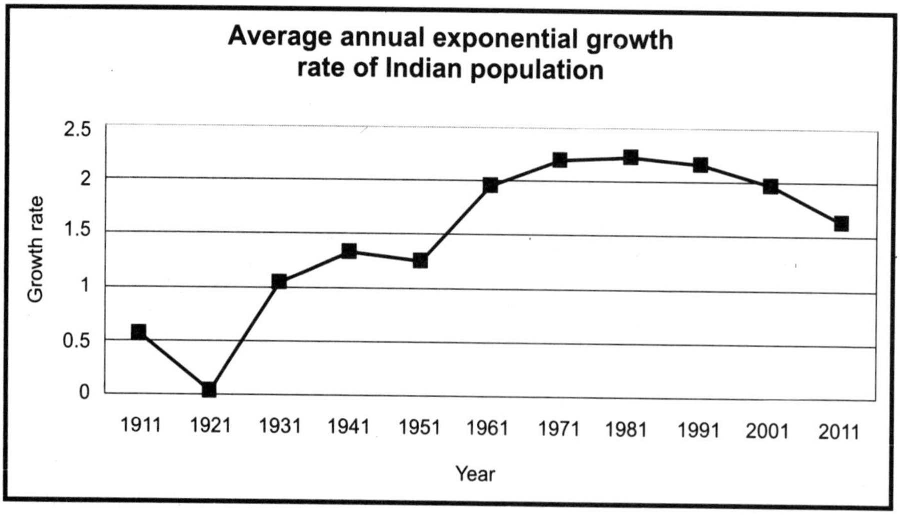

Figure 16.8 Line graph showing the annual exponential growth rate

Scattered Diagram

It is otherwise called correlation diagram as it shows the nature of correlation between two variables.

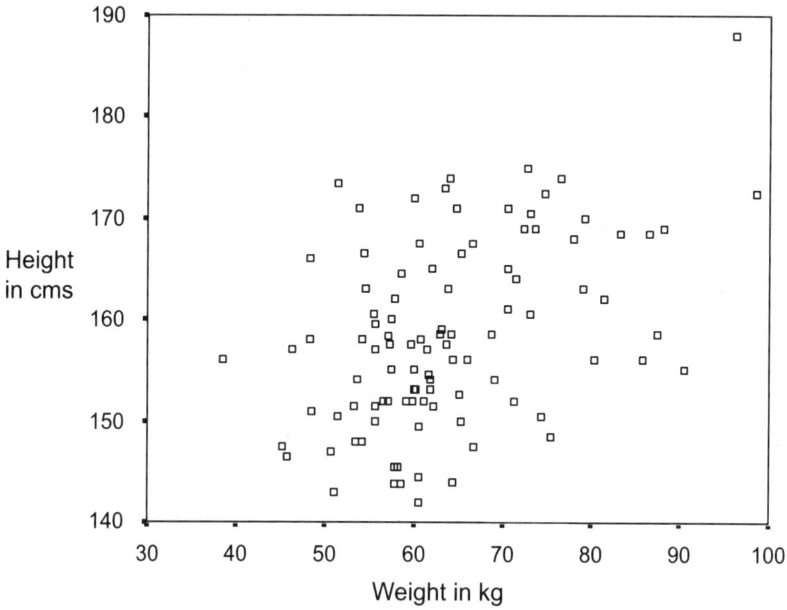

Figure 16.9 Scatter diagram for height and weight

Pictogram

This method may be used to represent the events like accidents in a given population, number of inpatients, number of surgeries, etc.

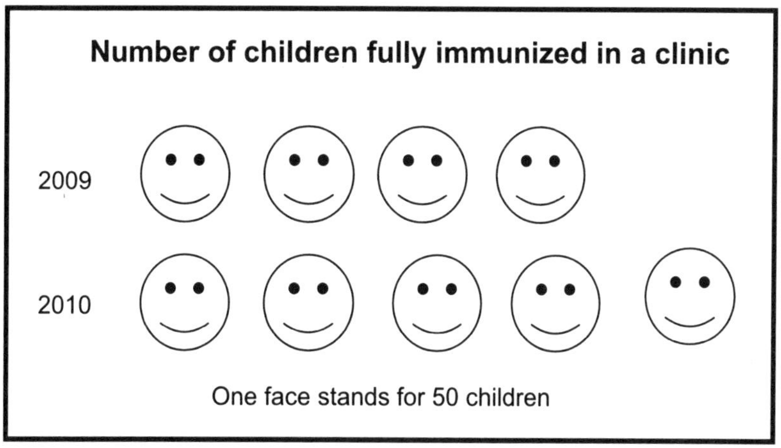

Figure 16.10 A pictogram

We know that a frequency distribution consists of two parts: first one is observed values (X-axis), the second is frequency of cases of each value (Y-axis). The values are listed in numerical order. Here the score value must be mutually exclusive and collectively exhaustive. Here the total sum of frequencies will be equal to the sample size.

Distribution Shapes

Frequency polygons can assume different shapes. A frequency distribution is said to be symmetric when it is folded over and the two halves are superimposed on each other. Thus, it consists of two halves that are mirror images of each other.

Example of symmetric distribution

Most biological variables follow symmetrical distribution when collected in large numbers.

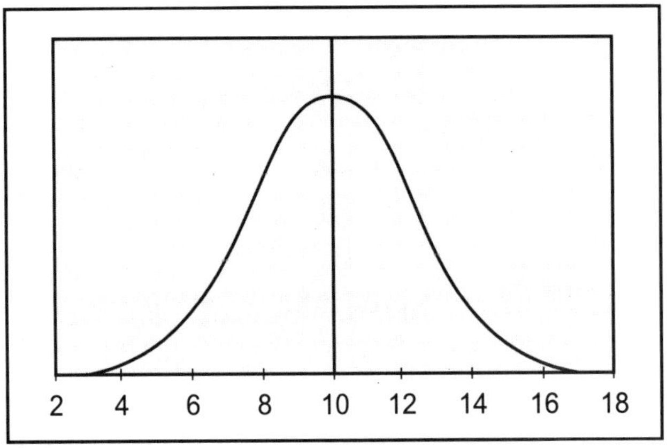

Figure 16.11 Symmetric distribution

Skewness and kurtosis

A frequency curve reveals the nature of distribution. It provides answers to questions about the location of observations, whether they are centrally located or in any of the infinity in values or in a unimodel or bimodel. Thus, the degree of peakness is measured by the terms 'skewness' and kurtosis.

In a normal distribution, the mean, median and mode are of the same value. The values are changeable during symmetrical distribution. As the symmetry of a distribution increases, the measures of central tendency such as mean, median and mode converge on the same value. The lack of symmetry or degree of asymmetry is probably known as skewness. The probability curve has a tail that is either on the left or right side. There may be two types of skewed curves.

Positively skewed: A positive skew indicates that the *tail* on the right side is *longer* than that of the left side and the bulk of values lies to the left of the mean. For a positively skewed distribution, the mean will always be the highest estimate of central tendency and the mean lies to the right of the median.

Negatively skewed: A negative skew indicates that the *tail* on the left side of the probability density function is *longer* than that of the right side, and the bulk of values (possibly including the median) lies to the right of the mean. For negatively skewed distributions, the mean will always be the lowest estimate of central tendency and the mean lies left of the median.

The formula to find the degree of skewness (Pearson's skewness coefficient) is:

$$S_k = \frac{3\,(\text{mean} - \text{median})}{\sigma}$$

$S_k = 0$ = No skewness/Normal curve

$S_k > 0$ = Positive skewness

$S_k < 0$ = Negative skewness

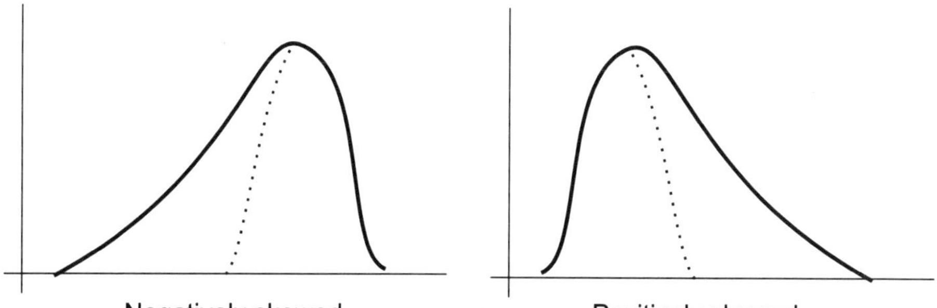

Figure 16.12 Skewness

Kurtosis

The lack of curvicity is probably known as kurtosis. There will be three types of curves. The curve which is more peaked than a normal curve is known as **leptokurtic**. The curve which is more flattened than normal is known as **platykurtic**. The curve which is similar to normal curve is known as **mesokurtic**. A normal distribution will have kurtosis value zero. In case of asymmetric distributions, the peak will be off centre; one tail will be longer than the other.

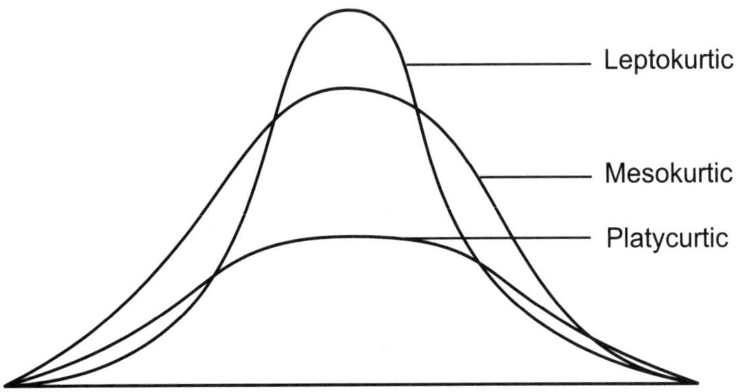

Figure 16.13 Kurtosis

For a sample of n values, kurtosis is

$$g_2 = \frac{m_4}{m_2^2} - 3 = \frac{\frac{1}{n}\sum_{i=1}^{n}\left(x_i - \bar{x}\right)^4}{\left(\frac{1}{n}\sum_{i=1}^{n}\left(x_i - \bar{x}\right)^2\right)^2} - 3$$

where m_4 is the fourth sample moment about mean, m_2 is the second sample moment about mean (i.e. the sample variance), x_i is the ith value, and $\bar{x}$ is the sample mean.

Central tendency

A measurement that is used to describe the tendency of all individual observations to be in the centre is termed as measures of central tendency or statistical averages. The measures of central tendency reduce or cut down a group of observations into a single number of indexes.

Measures of central tendency refer to a central position with reference to a group's performance. It is an "average" and represents all the scores obtained from the group. It describes the performance of a group as well as enables the researcher to compare two or more groups in terms of their averages.

Characteristics of a good average

1. It should be easy to realize.
2. Rigorously defined.
3. Simple to calculate.
4. Average should be based on all items in series.
5. It should be capable of further algebraic treatment.
6. It should haxve sampling stability.

Arithmetic mean

Mean is the most common measure of central tendency represented by $\bar{X}$ which is calculated by summing all values and dividing by the number of values.

For individual observations, $\bar{X} = \frac{\sum x}{n}$,where x stands for individual scores and n being the number of scores.

For frequency distribution, $\bar{X} = \frac{\sum xf}{\sum f}$, where f stands for frequency of each class interval and x stands for the midpoint of class intervals.

Example: The marks of 75 students of medical nursing are tabulated.

Table 16.4 Marks of nursing students

Marks awarded (x)	No. of students (f)	xf
10	10	100
20	30	600
30	20	600
40	15	600
Total number of students	75	$\sum xf = 1900$

The arithmetic mean of marks = 1900/75 = 25.33

Advantages

1. It is defined by a rigid formulae and use for further algebraic treatment.
2. It is based on all observation.

Disadvantages

1. In cases of skewed distribution, mean may not provide a representative value.
2. It is influenced by extreme values.

Median

A point in a distribution above which and below which 50% of cases fall is called median. Thus, median is the middle most observation, when the values are arranged in ascending order or descending order. Therefore, median divides the total value into two, 50% above median and 50% below median. Hence median is also known as 50th percentile value. An important characteristic of median is that, here, quantitative value of scores is not taken into account.

For frequency distribution, median is calculated by using the formula:

$$M = l + \frac{\left(\frac{N}{2} - m\right)}{f} \times C$$

where l is lower boundary of median class, N is total frequency, m is cumulative frequency up to the median class, c is class interval and f is frequency of the class interval containing N/2.

First, the frequencies have to be cumulated from top to bottom. By inspecting the cumulated frequencies, locate the class interval containing the N/2 value. This is the median class.

Generally, median is not a good measure of central tendency because it has no desirable properties except easiness to understand and a well-defined formula.

Advantages

1. Appropriate for ordinal level measurements.
2. Unaffected by extreme scores.

Disadvantages

1. Its value is not based on each and every observation.
2. Value of median is affected by sampling fluctuations.

Example: Following data give the heights of nine individuals in cm: 165, 168, 170, 162, 163, 164, 172, 150, 152.

Solution:

The median of given data is calculated as follows:

1. Arrange the data in ascending order: 150, 152, 162, 163, 164, 165, 168, 170, 172.
2. Use the formula $m = \frac{(n+1)}{2} = \frac{9+1}{2} = 5.$
3. Therefore, the 5th observation is the median. In our example, the 5th value is 164.

Example: Calculate median for the following frequency table data.

Table 16.5

Cholesterol	200	220	230	250	260	300
No. of individuals	5	12	8	4	10	4
Cumulative frequency	5	17	25	29	39	43

Solution:

1. Here from the discrete frequency table we have to calculate cumulative frequency first.
2. Then consider the final cumulative frequency (n) and calculate median using the formula:

$$m = \frac{(n+1)}{2} = \frac{43+1}{2}$$

By inspecting the cumulative frequency array we can see that this quantity is contained in the 25th observation in the array, and the value corresponding to it is 230. Thus median value will be 230.

In case the exact calculated array value does not match the cumulative frequency in the table, the next higher cumulative frequency closer to the calculated value is considered in the observation for median.

Example: Calculate median for the following frequency table.

Table 16.6

S. Cholesterol	200–220	220–240	240–260	260–280	280–300	300–320
No. of individuals	6	3	4	5	1	2
Cumulative frequency	6	9	13	18	19	21

Solution:

In case of continuous frequency table,

$$M = \ell + \frac{\left(\frac{N}{2} - m\right)}{f} \times C$$

Class interval, C = 20

$$m = \frac{(n+1)}{2} = \frac{43+1}{2}$$

Frequency of the median class, f = 4

Previous cumulative frequency of the median class, M = 9

Lower limit, $\ell = 240$

$N = \Sigma f = 21$

$$M = 240 + \frac{\left(\frac{21}{2} - 9\right)}{4} \times 20$$

$$= 240 + \frac{(10.5 - 9)}{4} \times 20$$

$$= 240 + 7.5$$

$$= 247.5$$

Mode

The most frequently occurring score value in a distribution frequency is termed as mode. Mode is widely used to fix up the incubation period of diseases, duration of infection, recovery period, etc. in medical field also, i.e. typical nominal level measures.

Mode is calculated using the formula

$$\text{Mode} = \ell + \frac{cf_2}{f_1 + f_2}$$

where

ℓ is the lower boundary of the mode class;

C is class interval; class interval having the highest frequency is called the mode class;

f_1 is frequency in the class, just preceding mode class;

f_2 is frequency in the class succeeding mode class.

Suppose the scores are as follows: 6, 3, 5, 6, 7, 8, 9, 4, 3, 3, 6, 6, 8, 9, 6.

Out of 15 scores, 6 is observed 5 times, 8 twice, 9 twice and 3 thrice. The most occurring observation is 6.Therefore, mode is 6.

In the case of ungrouped data, mode can be located easily by observation. Modes are a quick way to determine a standard score. However, these are unstable, which means modes tend to fluctuate widely from sample to sample drawn from the identical population. Still, mode is the best measurement in cases where priority is the location of the most popular observation.

Advantages

1. Mode gives a quick and fairly accurate measure of central tendency.
2. It is used to portray the qualitative phenomenon.

Disadvantages

1. It is not capable of algebraic manipulation.
2. This value of mode cannot always be calculated.

Measures of Dispersion

The measures of central tendency are not sufficient to compare the data or to draw conclusions. Hence, the variability, scattering or nature of dispersing the observations from central value is also being measured. Such measures are called 'measures of variability' or dispersion.

Characteristics of a good measure of dispersion

1. Rigorously defined.
2. Should be based on all observations.
3. It should increase in values as the scores become heterogenous.
4. It should have sampling stability.
5. It should be capable of further algebraic treatment.

The important measures of dispersion are:

1. Range
2. Mean deviation
3. Variance
4. Standard deviation and standard error
5. Quartile deviation
6. Coefficient of variation

Range

Range (R) is a simple measure of dispersion that will provide quick and easy deduction of data. Range is the difference between the highest (H) and lowest (L) observation in a given set of data. In health research, instead of finding the difference, the lowest and highest values itself will be provided and are useful in some way.

Range is the simplest measurement of dispersion, yet it will provide only a rough estimate about the variability since it considers only two observations, the highest and the lowest. It also provides a quick and easy inference about variability of a given set of observations and, therefore, is generally used for pre-test–post-test evaluation.

The chief advantage of range is its computational advantage, since it is only based on two scores; the range is highly unstable. Range also tends to fluctuate when different samples are being drawn from the same population. There is also another limitation of range; it ignores variations upon scores among two extremes.

Mean Deviation

It is also called absolute deviation. Mean deviation is defined as mean of the absolute deviation of observations from one measure among several measures of central tendency. There is no particular rule for choosing the measure. It can be taken from anywhere. When deviation is taken from arithmetic mean, it is called 'mean deviation about the mean', and when taken from mode it is called 'mean deviation about the mode'. Mean deviation is not considered as a good measure of dispersion because it lacks most of the desirable properties.

$$\text{Mean deviation about mean} = \frac{\text{Sum of absolute deviation from the mean}}{\text{Number of observations}}$$

Variance

The square of standard deviation is known as variance. It is also referred to as measure of variability. Variance provides a measure for average variability of the scores about the mean expressed as squared deviation. It is mostly used in inferential statistics.

Standard Deviation

The most extensively used measure of variability is standard deviation. It indicates the average of deviation of values from the mean and is calculated using every score. Standard deviation is defined as 'root mean square deviation' or it is square root of average of sum of squares of deviation taken from arithmetic mean. It is considered as the best measure of dispersion. It is considered as the 'gold standard' for measuring deviation from mean if the data is quantitative. Standard deviation is used to calculate variability and to generalize sample estimates, to fix up the confidence intervals, to define probability distributions, and to test hypothesis.

It is calculated using the formula for ungrouped data:

$$SD = \sqrt{\frac{\Sigma(x-\bar{x})^2}{n-1}}$$

The reason for taking n – 1 in the denominator is that it produces a more accurate estimate of the true proportion standard deviation and has desirable mathematical properties.

$$SD = \sqrt{\frac{\sum f(x-\bar{x})^2}{\sum f}}$$

where $\sum f$ is the total frequency.

Coefficient of Variation

It is also a useful measure of the relative spread of data. It produces a measure of relation variations relative to the size of the mean. Coefficient of variation (CV) is defined as the ratio of standard deviation to mean. It is computed as:

$$CV = \frac{SD}{\text{mean}}$$

CV is defined only for non-zero mean and the absolute value is taken for the mean to ensure it is always positive. It is sometimes expressed as a per cent, in which case the CV is multiplied by 100.

A frequent application of CV is in laboratory testing and quality procedures. It is also used for testing the reliability of the data.

Example: The diastolic BP of 10 individuals is as follows: 83, 75, 81, 79, 71, 95, 75, 77, 84 and 9. Calculate mean, range, MD, SD, variance and coefficient of variance.

Solution:

x	$x - \bar{x}$	$(x - \bar{x})^2$
83	2	4
75	−6	36
81	0	0
79	−2	4
71	−10	100
95	14	196
75	−6	36
77	−4	16
84	3	9
90	9	81
$\sum x = 810$	$\sum\lvert x-\bar{x}\rvert = 56$	$\sum(x-\bar{x})^2 = 482$

Mean deviation,

$$MD = \left|\frac{\Sigma(x-\bar{x})}{n}\right| = \frac{56}{10} = 5.6$$

Variance,

$$V = \frac{\Sigma(x-\bar{x})^2}{n-1} = \frac{482}{10-1} = 53.56$$

Standard deviation,

$$SD = \sqrt{\frac{\Sigma(x-\bar{x})^2}{n-1}} = \sqrt{\frac{482}{9}} = 7.3$$

Coefficient of variance,

$$CV = \frac{SD}{\bar{x}} \times 100 = \frac{7.3}{81} \times 100 = 9\%$$

Example (grouped data): Ages of patients admitted in a hospital are given. Find mean, variance, mean deviation, standard deviation and coefficient of variance.

Age in years	No. of patients
5–15	12
15–25	5
25–35	2
35–45	1
Total	20

Solution:

Age	Mid value (x)	No. of patients (f)	$x \cdot f$	$x - \bar{x}$	$(x - \bar{x})^2$	$(x - \bar{x})^2 f$	$\lvert x - \bar{x}\rvert f$
5–15	10	12	120	–6	36	432	72
15–25	20	5	100	4	16	80	20
25–35	30	2	60	14	196	392	28
35–45	40	1	40	24	576	576	24
				48		1480	144

$$\text{Mean} = \frac{\sum xf}{n} = \frac{320}{20} = 16$$

$$\text{Variance} = \frac{\sum (x - \bar{x})^2 f}{20} = \frac{1480}{20} = 74$$

$$\text{Mean deviation} = \frac{\sum \lvert x - \bar{x} \rvert f}{N}$$

$$= \frac{144}{20}$$

$$= 7.2$$

$$\text{Standard deviation} = \sqrt{\text{Variance}} = \sqrt{74} = 8.6$$

$$\text{Coefficient of variance} = \frac{SD}{\bar{x}} \times 100 = \frac{8.6}{16} \times 100 = 53.75$$

Sampling distribution

To generate a sampling distribution, draw several parallel samples of same size from the parent population and calculate the mean values for all samples. Now the distribution of means of these samples is called sampling distribution of the means. The mean of sampling distribution is equal to the population mean, and standard deviation is equal to a quantity $\frac{\sigma}{\sqrt{n}}$.

Standard error

Standard error is simply the standard deviation of sample means or sample proportions or standard deviation of sampling distribution. The term error stands for 'difference' and not to indicate some kind of mistake. Standard error is a vital component in the estimation of parameters and hypothesis testing. The following standard errors are more frequently used in inferential statistics.

$$\text{Standard error of mean} = \frac{\sigma}{\sqrt{n}}$$

$$\text{Standard error of proportion} = \sqrt{\frac{pq}{n}}$$

where p is proportion having a given characteristic;

q = 1 – p, proportion not having the characteristic.

Quartile deviation

Median is the value of variate which divides the total frequency of distribution into two equal parts. Quartiles may be defined as those values of the variate which divide the total frequency into four equal parts. Quartiles are denoted by Q_1, Q_2 and Q_3. Q_2 is the same as median. The value of variate which divides the lower half below the median into two equal parts on the basis of frequency is called the lower quartile, denoted by Q_1. Similarly when the upper half which is above the median is divided on the basis of frequency into two equal parts, the value of variate is called the upper quartile, denoted by Q_3. The difference between the two quartiles, $Q_3 - Q_1$, represents the inter-quartile range. Half of this difference, which is semi-interquartile range, is called the quartile deviation.

Thus, quartile deviation is given by $\frac{Q_3 - Q_1}{2}$.

Before computing quartiles, data must be arranged in ascending order. The procedure to obtain Q_1 and Q_3 is same as that for the median.

$$\text{where } Q_1 = \ell + \frac{\left(\frac{N}{4} - m\right)}{f} C;$$

$$Q_3 = \ell + \frac{\left(\frac{3N}{4} m\right)}{f};$$

ℓ is the exact lower limit of the interval in which the quartile falls;

c is class interval;

m is cumulative frequency up to the interval which contains the quartile;

f is the frequency of interval containing the quartile.

Measures of Relationship

Correlation (Linear correlation)

Correlation may be defined as the relationship or association between two quantitatively measured or continuous variables. It is a statistical measure of determining the degree of association between two variables. Correlation may be negative or positive according to the movement of variables 'X' and 'Y'.

Correlation coefficient

Correlation coefficient (r) indicates the relationship between two random variables. Commonly, it is a line relationship. In statistical terms, correlation determines the departure of two random variables from independent one.

In mathematical terms, correlation can be measured by computing the correlation coefficient 'r'. It is commonly known as Karl Pearson's correlation coefficient. The method or formula for computing the correlation coefficient 'r' is as follows:

Formula 1:

Correlation coefficient, $r = \frac{p}{(\text{SD of x}) \times (\text{SD of y})}$

where p = covariance of (x, y)

$$r_{xy} = \frac{\sum_{i=1}^{n}(x_i - \bar{x})(y_i - \bar{y})}{(n-1)s_x s_y} = \frac{\sum_{i=1}^{n}(x_i - \bar{x})(y_i - \bar{y})}{\sqrt{\sum_{i=1}^{n}(x_i - \bar{x})^2 \sum_{i=1}^{n}(y_i - \bar{y})^2}}$$

If the correlation coefficient 'r' = +1, then the correlation is a perfect one.

If the correlation coefficient 'r'= –1, then the correlation is a perfect negative one.

If the correlation coefficient 'r' = 0, then there is no correlation/or no linear correlation.

From this point, it can be noted that the correlation value lies between –1 and +1; i.e. negative correlation lies between –1 and 0, and positive correlation lies between 0 and +1. To measure the statistical significance of correlation coefficient, statistical tables are also available. Then referring the statistical table for correlation coefficient *r*, degree of freedom can be calculated with the formula:

$$\text{d.f.} = (\text{no. of pairs of observations}) - 1 = n - 1$$

Example: In a study, to assess the hours of study per day for second year B.Sc. Nursing exams and the marks obtained in the exams, the following data were obtained. Calculate the correlation coefficient.

Hours of study: 2, 8, 10, 6, 3

Marks obtained: 20, 40, 42, 24, 36

x	y	$(x_i - \bar{x})$	$(x_i - \bar{x})^2$	$(y_i - \bar{y})$	$(y_i - \bar{y})^2$	$(x_i - \bar{x})(y_i - \bar{y})$
2	20	–3.8	14.44	–12.5	156.25	47.5
8	40	2.2	4.84	7.5	56.25	16.5
10	42	4.2	17.64	9.5	90.25	39.9
6	24	0.2	0.04	–8.5	72.25	–1.7
3	36	–2.8	7.84	3.5	12.25	–9.8
$\sum x = 29$	$\sum y = 162$		44.8		387.25	92.4

$$r = \frac{92.4}{\sqrt{(44.8)(387.25)}} = +0.70$$

The value of correlation coefficient is positive indicating a positive relationship between two variables. For each hour of study, marks will increase by 0.7.

Formula 2:

$$r = \frac{\sum xy - \frac{\sum x \sum y}{N}}{\sqrt{\left(\sum x^2 - \frac{(\sum x)^2}{N}\right)\left(\sum y^2 - \frac{(\sum y)^2}{N}\right)}}$$

where x is the first variable, y the second variable and n the number of pairs.

Schematic representation for calculation of 'r'

Subjects	Score on one variable X	Score of second variable Y	XY	X^2	Y^2
1					
2					
n					
Total	ΣX	ΣY	ΣXY	ΣX^2	ΣY^2

The previous problem has been worked out using the second formula and given below:

Hours of study (x)	Marks obtained in the university exam (y)	xy	x^2	y^2
2	20	40	4	400
8	40	320	64	1600
10	42	420	100	1764
6	24	144	36	576
3	36	108	9	1296
$\sum x = 29$	$\sum y = 162$	$\sum xy = 1032$	$\sum x^2 = 213$	$\sum y^2 = 5636$

$$\text{Correlation coefficient, } r = \frac{\sum xy - \frac{\sum x \sum y}{N}}{\sqrt{\left(\sum x^2 - \frac{(\sum x)^2}{N}\right)\left(\sum y^2 - \frac{(\sum y)^2}{N}\right)}}$$

$$= \frac{1032 - \frac{29 \times 162}{5}}{\sqrt{\left(213 - \frac{29^2}{5}\right)\left(5636 - \frac{162^2}{5}\right)}}$$

$$= \frac{92.4}{\sqrt{17346.56}}$$

$$= +0.70$$

Rank correlation

When evaluating a candidate in a competition by two judges, the measurements of variables are not available and hence Karl Pearson's correlation coefficient cannot be calculated. Then the investigator is focused to go for a distribution-free correlation coefficient called 'rank correlation'. It was introduced by Spearman and hence popularly known as 'Spearman Rank Correlation', which is denoted by 'R' (r_s). Rank correlation 'R' can take the values from −1 to +1, and if it takes the value '+1', there is a perfect positive correlation, if it is '−1', there is perfect negative correlation.

Schematic representation for calculation of r_s

Subject	Score on one variable (x)	Score on second variable (y)	Rank of scores in x	Rank of scores in y	Difference between ranking (d)	d^2
1						
2						
n						
Total						$\sum d^2$

Spearman's rank correlation is computed by the formula:

$$R = 1 - \frac{6\sum d^2}{n(n^2 - 1)}$$

where d is the difference between ranks assigned independently and n is the number of pairs.

When two sets of observations are available, firstly the scores are arranged in the two sets in terms of magnitude and ranks are given.

The procedure of computing r_s with ranking of X and Y scores is as follows. The smallest of X is assigned a rank of 1, the next smallest a rank of 2, and so on. The same is done with Y scores. Once the X and Y scores are ranked separately, find the difference between X rank and Y rank for each individual. This is represented by letter 'd'. Now square the d values and sum it. Substituting this value in the equation, r_s can be calculated.

Ranking tied scores

There are instances the researcher has to deal with two (or more) identical scores. Whenever two (or more) scores have exactly the same value, they should have the same ranks. The procedure is outlined here.

List the X scores (including the tied values) from the lowest to the highest. Allocate a rank (first, second, etc.) to each position in the ordered list. When two or more scores are tied, obtain the mean of their ranked positions, and assign this mean value as the final rank for each score. The procedure is repeated for the Y scores.

Example: Information on IQ and personality scores of 6 students is given below. Study the relationship between these two variable using Spearman correlation.

Sl. No.	**IQ index (x)**	**Rank of x**	**Personality score (y)**	**Rank of y**	**Difference in ranks**	**d^2**
1.	10	6	9	5.5	0.5	0.25
2.	9	4.5	9	5.5	−1	1
3.	6	2	7	3	−1	1
4.	9	4.5	5	1.5	3	9
5.	8	3	8	4	−1	1
6.	4	1	5	1.5	−0.5	0.25

Spearman's rank correlation,

$$R = 1 - \frac{6\times12.5}{6\times35} = 1 - \frac{75}{210} = 0.64$$

The two variables are positively correlated. For each unit increase in IQ, personality score will be increased by a value 0.64.

Linear regression

The word regression means prediction. In bivariate correlation, one variable is known as independent or principal variable, and the other is called dependent or auxiliary variable. Sometimes, one of the variables may be easily measurable but the other may not. Then the prediction of unknown variable is possible with the help of a mathematical relationship. Then the relationship might express in a mathematical expression or equation by predicting the known variable from the unknown variable. Such an equation is known as "regression equation".

Regression is measured by computing the regression coefficient. It makes change in the dependent variables for every unit change in the independent variable. As there are two variables X and Y, there are two regression coefficients which can be calculated if (1) variable 'X' is known or (2) variable 'Y' is known. There are two equations applicable, such as

1. Regression equation Y on X, if X is known.
2. Regression equation X on Y, if Y is known.

Regression Y on X:

$$Y = a + b_{yx}X$$

where b_{yx} is the regression coefficient Y on X, which is calculated by the formula

$$b_{yx} = \frac{\Sigma xy - \frac{\Sigma x \Sigma y}{N}}{\Sigma x^2 - \frac{(\Sigma x)^2}{N}}$$

and

$$X = a + b_{xy}Y$$

where

$$b_{xy} = \frac{\sum xy - \frac{\sum x \sum y}{N}}{\sum y^2 - \frac{(\sum y)^2}{N}}$$

Regression equations can be fitted to a regression line which indicates a number of points. There are two regression lines: one indicates the regression of Y on X and the other indicates regression of X on Y. In the first case, the value of a is obtained as $a = \bar{y} - b\bar{x}$ and for the second line $a = \bar{x} - b\bar{y}$.

The concept of regression can be illustrated with the problem of hours of study and marks obtained in the university exams. The independent variable is the hours of study and is denoted by letter x and the dependent variable is marks obtained and denoted by y. Now two equations can be constructed: one to predict the y values and the other one to predict x values. The same table can be used to calculate Pearson's correlation.

1. To construct regression equation of Y on X:

$$Y = a + b_{yx}X$$

To use the equation two values, b shall be known.

$$b_{yx} = \frac{\sum xy - \frac{\sum x \sum y}{N}}{\sum x^2 - \frac{(\sum x)^2}{N}}$$

$$= \frac{1032 - \frac{29 \times 162}{5}}{213 - \frac{29^2}{5}}$$

$$= 2.06$$

$$a = \bar{Y} - b\bar{X}$$

$$= 32.4 - (2.06)(5.8)$$

$$= 20.45$$

$\bar{X}$ and $\bar{Y}$ can be obtained by dividing ΣX and ΣY by n.

The regression equation is $Y = 20.45 + 2.06X$. By substituting different values for X, Y values (marks) can be predicted.

2. To construct regression equation of X on Y.

$$X = a + b_{xy} Y$$

To find the value of b_{xy} the above expression can be used. The numerator remains unchanged and the denominator of b_{xy} is

$$\Sigma y^2 - \frac{(\Sigma y)^2}{N}.$$

Similarly, $a = \bar{X} - b\bar{Y}$. The readers may work it out as an exercise.

The equation will be $X = -1.98 + (0.24)Y$.

By substituting different values for Y, X values (hours of study) can be predicted.

B. Inferential Statistics

This part of statistics helps the researcher to make inferences about the population using information from a sample. This can be achieved by two ways:

1. Estimation of parameters
2. Testing of hypotheses

Concepts in Inferential Statistics

1. Type-I and type-II errors
2. Level of significance
3. Confidence interval
4. Testing of hypothesis
5. Degree of freedom

Type-I and type-II errors

Hypothesis testing is based on probability theory. Because we cannot make any statement about a sample with complete certainty, there is always a chance that an error can be made. A researcher runs the risk of committing two types of errors. Table 16.7 summarizes the state of affairs in the population and the nature of type-I and type-II errors.

Table 16.7 Type-I and type-II errors in hypothesis

State of null hypothesis in the population	Decision	
	Accept Ho	Reject Ho
Ho is true	Correct – No error	Type-I error (α error)
Ho is false	Type-II error (β error)	Correct – No error

Type-I error is an error caused by rejecting the null hypothesis when it is true. Type-II error is an error caused by failing to reject the null hypothesis when the alternative hypothesis is true.

If the decision has been made to reject the null hypothesis and in fact the null hypothesis is true, we have made a type-I error. Type-I error occurs when the researcher concludes that there is a statistically significant difference; when in reality, it does not exist. Type-I and type-II errors are inversely related. When the probability of type-II error reduces, the probability of type-I error increases.

A type-I error has the probability of alpha (α), the level of statistical significance that the researcher has set up.

If the alternative hypothesis is, in fact, true and the null hypothesis is actually false but the decision-maker concludes that we should not reject a null hypothesis, then we have made what is called a type-II error. The probability of making this incorrect decision is called beta (β). The quantity (1 – β) is called the power of a test.

No error is made if the null hypothesis is true and the decision is made to accept it. A correct decision is also made if the null hypothesis is false and the decision is made to reject the null hypothesis.

Level of significance

Level of significance is defined as probability of making a type-I error. In medical research, usually this is used in statistical analysis while interpreting the results of a study. We consider the level of significance as 1% (0.01) or 5% (0.05). If the significance level is 0.05, it means that the investigator is ready to take risk of being wrong in 5% of the times or 5 out of 100 when rejecting the null hypothesis.

The significance may be set at 0.01 or even 0.001. With a 0.01 level of significance, the researcher stands the risk of being wrong 1 time out of 100 when rejecting the null hypothesis; but for 0.001 level of significance, the risk is 1 time out of 1000. Practically, in our clinical studies, we consider 0.05 level of significance to take a decision regarding whether to accept or reject a null hypothesis.

Confidence interval

Confidence interval estimation is one way to make inference about the parameter. After drawing a random sample of adequate size, a sample statistic, either sample mean or sample proportion, is calculated. This value is called point estimate. Then the researcher defines an interval around this value within which the population value is likely to lie. Since the researcher uses a sample, the first step in constructing an interval estimate is to decide on the risk the researcher is willing to take of being wrong. An interval estimate is wrong if it does not contain the population parameter. This probability of error is called α (alpha).

The exact value of α will depend on the nature of research question, but a 5% (.05) probability is commonly used. Setting α to .05, also called 95% confidence level, means that over the long run the researcher is willing to be wrong only 5% of the times. In other words, if the researcher draws 100 random samples of same size and if the limits are calculated every time, then it may not contain the parameter in five times.

From the table of normal distribution, it is known that mean ± 1.96 SD will contain 95% of the cases and only 5% of the cases will lie outside it. Similarly, mean ± 2.58 SD will contain 99% of the cases and only 1% of the cases will lie outside. These properties can be used in the estimation procedure.

The general structure of a confidence interval is

Confidence interval = Sample mean or sample proportion
± Confidence coefficient
× Standard error of sample mean or sample proportion

Confidence coefficient is level of confidence desired.

$$\text{Standard error of mean} = \frac{\sigma}{\sqrt{n}}$$

$$\text{Standard error of proportion} = \sqrt{\frac{pq}{n}}$$

where p is proportion having a given characteristics;

$q = 1 - p$, proportion not having the characteristics.

Example: In a school survey covering 100 plus one children, the average IQ was found to be 120 with a standard deviation 25.What is value in the population.

$$\text{Standard error of mean} = \frac{25}{\sqrt{100}}$$
$$= \frac{25}{10}$$
$$= 2.5$$

95% confidence interval:

$$120 \pm 1.96 \times 2.5 = 115.1 - 124.9$$

The interpretation is that among the population of one students, the average IQ (parameter) will lie between these two values. In 5% of the cases, the interval may not contain the parameter.

Example: In a community survey of 900 antenatal mothers, 20% are anemic. Construct 99% confidence limits.

Here P = 80, q = 100 – 80 = 20

$$\text{Standard error of proportion} = \sqrt{\frac{pq}{n}}$$
$$= \sqrt{\frac{20 \times 80}{900}}$$
$$= \sqrt{1.98}$$
$$= 1.3$$

99% confidence interval:

$$20 \pm 2.58(1.3) = 20 \pm 3.35 = 16.7 - 23.3$$

The interpretation is that among antenatal mothers, the percentage of anemic (parameter) will lie between these two values. In 1% of the cases the interval may not contain the parameter. (If P is expressed as proportion, the confidence interval will be (0.17 – 0.23).

Testing of hypothesis

Types of hypothesis:

Null hypothesis: The hypothesis "no difference" in the population is called null hypothesis.

Alternative hypothesis: The alternative hypothesis (H_A) or research hypotheses states that a relationship or difference exists in the population. H_A can be directional or non-directional. Here the research question is presented as a declarative statement.

The word testing of hypothesis signifies testing the level of significance means at which it is significant; to estimate the chance of testing wrong decisions whether it is <5/100 (5%) or <1/100 (1%) or < 1/1000 (.01%).

1. The word testing hypothesis denotes the testing of one claim over other.
2. The testing of hypothesis is defined as the methodology that is used to see whether the difference between sample estimate and true value of population (parameter) or between two or more sample estimates themselves is due to sampling variation or otherwise.
3. It measures the strength of evidence to accept or reject the null hypothesis.

Types of test used for test of significance

1. Parametric test
   - t-test
   - z-test
   - ANOVA
2. Non-parametric test
   - Chi-square test
   - Mann-Whitney U test
   - Wilcoxon signed rank test

Parametric test: This test is used when data is having a normal probability distribution. It is also called normal distribution statistical test.

Table 16.8 Types of parametric and non-parametric tests

Application	Parametric test	Non-parametric test	Efficiency of non-parametric test with normal population
Matched pairs of sample data	Paired t-test	Sign test Wilcoxon signed rank test	0.63 0.95
Two independent samples	T-test/Z-test	Mann–Whitney U test	0.95
Several independent samples	ANOVA (F test)	Kruskall-Wallis test	0.95
Correlation	Linear correlation	Rank correlation test	0.91
Randomness	No parametric test	Run test	

Degrees of freedom

Degrees of freedom abbreviated as d.f. is a concept used in some statistical tests to refer to what extent the scores in a data set have the freedom to vary once certain restrictions are imposed. It may be recalled while computing variance; the sum of squared deviations is divided not by n but by n – 1. The quantity n – 1 is called degree of freedom. This happens because for computing variance, the researcher has to compute mean. For computation of mean, the scores have to be added and then divided by the sample size. Thus, after computing the mean number of independent scores, variance is reduced by 1.

Table 16.9 Some important statistical tests that need the calculation of d.f.

Name of the test	Information needed	d.f.
Two sample t-test	First sample size n_1; second sample size n_2	$(n_1 - 1) + (n_2 - 1)$
One sample t-test	Sample size n	n – 1
Paired t-test	Sample size n	n – 1
Chi-squared test	Number of rows (r); number of columns (c)	(r – 1)(c –1)
	Total d.f., if n is the total sample size	n – 1
One way ANOVA	Between group d.f., if number of independent groups is denoted by k	k – 1
	Within group d.f.	n – k

Theoretical Distributions

Normal distribution

Normal distribution is the most important distribution in statistics. It is a symmetrical distribution, which means the left half of the normal distribution is especially a photocopy of the right half. Most of the scores in a normal distribution tend to occur near the centre, while more extreme scores on either side of the centre become increasingly rare. If the distance from the centre increases, simultaneously the frequency of scores decreases. Under normal distribution, mean = median = mode. The normal distribution curve is a specific normal curve that has several characteristics.

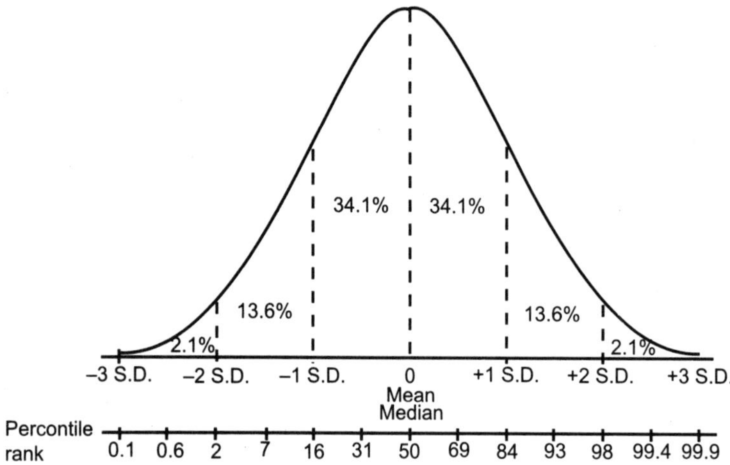

Figure 16.14 Normal distribution

Features of normal curve

1. The normal curve is unimodal, bell-shaped and symmetric.
2. Mean, median and mode are equal.
3. 68% of the observations lie in the interval $\mu = \pm 1SD$. 95% lie in the interval $\mu \pm 2SD$ and 99.7% of the observations lie in the interval $\mu \pm 3SD$.
4. It is a continuous-type probability curve.
5. The normal curve has two parameters, i.e. mean (μ) and standard deviation (σ).

Standard normal curve

There are an infinite number of normal curves depending upon mean and standard deviation. There is only one standardized normal curve.

The standardized normal distribution is extremely valuable because we can translate or transform any normal variable X into the standardized value Z. This has many practical implications for health researchers. The computation of standardized value Z of any measurement expressed in the original unit is simple. Subtract the mean from the value to be transformed and divide by the standard deviation.

$$Z = \frac{X - \mu}{\sigma}$$

where Z is standardized value, μ is the hypothesized or expected value of mean, X are values to be transformed, and σ is standard deviation.

Standard normal distribution

The standard normal curve is a normal distribution having mean zero and SD one. This curve is also called Z. When the mean of a normal distribution is not zero and standard deviation is not 1, a simple transformation called Z transformation must be made so that we can use the standard normal table. The Z transformation expresses deviation from the mean in SD units. That is, any normal distribution can be transformed into standard normal distribution by the following steps:

1. Move the distribution up or down the number line so that the mean is equal to zero. This can be accomplished by subtracting mean from the value for X.
2. Make the distribution either narrower or under so that standard deviation is equal to 1.This is accomplished by dividing by σ, i.e. $x - \mu$.

Importance of normal distribution

Normal distribution plays an important role in sampling theory. It has been found that:

1. Data obtained from biological measurements approximately follow normal distribution.
2. Binomial and Poisson distribution can be approximated to normal distribution.
3. For large samples, any statistics (i.e. sample mean, sample standard deviation) approximately follows normal distribution and it can be studied with the help of normal curve.
4. Normal curve is used to find confidence limits of population parameters.
5. Normal distribution also forms the basis for tests of significance.

t-distribution

It is similar to normal distribution. William Gosset found that when observations came from a normal population, the means are normally distributed only if the true SD in the population is known. When the true SD is known and the researcher has to use the sample SD in its place, the means are no longer normally distributed.

t-distribution is also symmetric like the normal or Z distribution. But it has a mean zero and SD > 1. When we use t-distribution to answer questions about one group, it has n – 1 difference.

As the t-distribution has SD > 1, it is wider and tails are higher than that for the Z distribution. As the sample size increases, the t-distribution almost tends to become the same as the standard normal distribution. Even if observations deviate from the normal distribution in a minor way, t-distribution can be used because it is robust for non-normal data. (Robustness means we can draw a proper conclusion even when all our assumptions are not met.)

Properties of 't' distribution

1. t-distribution is asymptotic to x-axis.
2. The shape of curve form of t-distribution varies with degrees of freedom.
3. t-distribution is a symmetrical distribution with mean zero.
4. t-distribution has greater spread than normal distribution.
5. t-distribution becomes closer to the Z distribution theorctically when d.f. increases and approaches the standard normal curve.

Types of t-tests

1. **Unpaired t-test:** It is applied when data is obtained from subjects of two independent groups of sample from two different populations.
2. **Paired t-test:** It is applied on paired data of independent observations made on the same sample before and after the intervention.

χ^2 distribution

χ^2 distributions have no negative value and the mean of distribution is equal to its degrees of freedom. As the degree of freedom increases, standard deviation increases and the shape of χ^2 curve becomes more like the normal curve.

Chi-squared test is a non-parametric test not based on any summary values of population. This test is most commonly used when the data are in frequencies, such as the number of responses in two or more categories. It can be used with any data which can be reduced proportions or percentages. Chi-squared test is denoted χ^2 and is pronounced by "kye square".

It is defined as

$$\chi^2 = \sum \frac{(O-E)^2}{E},$$

where O is the observed frequency and E is the expected frequency of the same event (or for the same cell).

Two-way classification or h × K table, in which observed frequencies occupy h rows and k columns, is called contingency table.

Expected frequency in a contingency table is calculated by the formula:

$$\text{Expected frequency} = \frac{\text{Row total} \times \text{Column total}}{\text{Grand total}}$$

Characteristics of χ^2 test

1. The total number of observations in each column (treatment and control) and the total observations in each row (positive and negative) are considered to be predetermined. These column and row totals are called marginal frequencies. The numbers in the cells are called observed frequencies.
2. If the rows and columns are assured as independent, then the number of expected frequencies can be calculated by multiplying the column total by the row total and dividing by the grand total.
3. The Chi-squared test compares the observed frequency in each cell with expected frequency. If no relationship exists between the row and column variable, then the value of χ^2 will be small. If there is relationship between the variables, then the value of χ^2 will be large. If $\chi^2 = 0$ there is perfect agreement between theory and observation.

$$\chi^2 = \sum_{i=1}^{n} \frac{(O_i - E_i)^2}{E_i}$$

where n is the number of classes, O_i observed frequency, E_i expected frequency and d.f. degrees of freedom.

4. The test is applied only for testing the hypothesis.

Properties of χ^2 distribution

1. Chi-square values increase with the increase in degrees of freedom.
2. The value of χ^2 lies between zero and infinity.
3. Chi-squared curve is always positively skewed.
4. The mean of χ^2 distribution is the number of degrees of freedom and the standard.

   Deviation = $\sqrt{2\theta}$, where θ is the degree of freedom

Application of χ^2 test

It is mainly applied

1. To test the goodness of fit.
2. To test the independence of attributes.
3. To test the homogeneity of attributes in respect of a particular characteristic or it may also be used to test population variance.

Significance tests

A significance test enables us to measure the strength of evidence which the data supply concerning some proposition of interest. To carry out the test of significance, we suppose that in the population, there is no difference between the two treatments.

Procedure for test of significance

1. Formulate a null hypotheses.
2. Formulate alternative hypotheses.
3. Decide appropriate and suitable test statistics.

4. Fix probability level (p less than 0.05, p less than 0.01, p less than 0.001).
5. Calculate the degree of freedom.
6. Compare the calculated value of test statistics with table values and interpret.

If the data do not support null hypotheses, we reject null hypotheses. If the data are consistent with null hypotheses we accept it.

Significance levels and types of error

Suppose we take a probability of 0.01 or less as constituting reasonable evidence against the null hypothesis, if the null hypothesis is true, we shall make a wrong decision one in a hundred times. Devising against true null hypothesis is called an error of the first kind (type-I error). We get an error of the second kind (type-II error) if we do not reject a null hypothesis which is in fact false. Now the smaller we demand the probability before we divide against the null hypothesis, the larger the observed difference must be, and so the more likely we are to miss real differences. By reducing the risk of an error of the first kind, we increase the risk of an error of the second kind.

One- and two-sided tests of significance

Whether a statistical test is one-sided or two-sided (also known as one-tailed or two-tailed) can be observed from research (or alternative) hypotheses. One-tailed test states that the parameters are different and also states the direction also. For example, average stress score is more for girls than for boys. The two-tailed test states only that the parameters are different. For example, the average stress scores for boys and girls are different. A researcher can opt for a one-tailed test when the previous studies establish a clear trend, or his/her clinical experience indicates a clear direction. When the previous studies establish contradicting results or when a study is conducted for the first time, a two-tailed test is appropriate. Whether to perform a one-tailed or two-tailed test must be fixed before the analysis of data.

Multiple significance tests

If we test a null hypothesis which is in fact true, using 0.05 as the critical significance level, we have a probability of 0.95 of getting a no significance conclusion (i.e. correct). If we test two independent true null hypotheses, the probability that neither test will be significant is $0.95 \times 0.95 = 0.903$.

If we test 20 such hypotheses, the probability that none will be significant is $0.95^{20} = 0.36$. This gives a probability of $1 - 0.36 = 0.644$ of getting at least one significant result; we are most likely to get one than not. The expected number of spurious significant result is $20 \times 0.05 = 1$.

Many medical research studies are published with a large number of significance tests. They are not usually independent, being carried out on the same set of subjects; so the above calculations do not apply exactly. However, it is clear that if we go on testing, we will find something which is significant.

Repeated significance tests and sequential analysis

A special case of multiple testing arises in clinical trials where patients are admitted at different times. Those can be a temptation to keep looking at the data and carrying out significant tests. This is liable to produce spurious significant differences, detecting treatment effects where none exists.

Large sample test

For a large sample ($n \geq 30$), sampling distributions of many statistics are approximately normal distributions. In such cases, Z-statistic is used in hypothesis testing. Some special tests are given below:

1. Test for a special mean or test significance of mean (large sample).
2. Test for quality of two means or test significance of difference between two means (large sample).
3. Test for specified proportions (large sample).
4. Test for equality of two proportions or test of significance of difference between two proportions (large samples).

Small sample test

For a sample of small size ($n < 30$), a new test of significance known as student's t-distribution is applied. This test is also known as t-test which involves an important expression of degree of freedom.

Testing of hypotheses

Case I: When population size is large and population standard deviation is known or when population size is small but population standard deviation is known

The researcher has to use tables of standard normal distribution and compute statistics. The common types of problems include:

1. Comparison of a sample mean with population mean or norm.
2. Comparison of two sample means.
3. Comparison of a sample proportion with a population proportion.
4. Comparison of two sample proportions.

These four situations are discussed hereunder. (All tests are two-tailed). While determining the statistical significance, the calculated value of Z must be compared with table value. An abstract of the same is shown below.

Z	1.65	1.96	2.3	2.58
P	0.10	0.05	0.02	0.01

For statistical significance in a two-tailed test, the calculated value of Z must be ≥1.96 ($p < 0.05$), and in a one-tailed test the calculated value of Z must be ≥1.65 ($p < .05$).

Sample mean vs. population mean (or norm)

Null hypothesis:

$$H_0 \quad = \quad \mu = x$$

$$H_A \quad = \quad \mu \neq x$$

Z statistics is obtained by:

$$Z = \frac{\bar{x} - \mu}{\frac{\sigma}{\sqrt{n}}}$$

where $\bar{x}$ is sample mean

μ is population mean (or norm)

σ is population standard deviation

n is sample size

If σ is not provided, then replace it with S, the sample standard deviation. The rational is that the sample standard deviation adequately represents population standard deviation when sample size is large.

Example: A random sample of 400 birth weights shows a mean value of 2.1 kg and standard deviation of 0.9 kg. Test whether this sample could have come from a normal population with mean 2.9 kg.

$H_0 \quad : \quad \mu = 2.9$ kg

$H_A \quad : \quad \mu \neq 2.9$ kg

$$Z = \frac{|2.1 - 2.9|}{\frac{0.9}{\sqrt{400}}}$$

$$= \frac{0.8}{\frac{0.9}{\sqrt{400}}}$$

$$= \frac{0.8}{\frac{0.9}{2.0}}$$

$$= \frac{0.8}{0.045}$$

$$= 17.7$$

From the table of Z distribution, the critical value at 5% level is 1.96 (or more) since the calculated value of Z is greater than the critical value. The observed difference is statistically significant and H_0 is rejected. The sample is from a different population (may be from a well-to-do community).

Comparison of two sample means

Let there be two different populations with means μ_1 and μ_2 and the standard deviations σ_1 and σ_2, respectively. Suppose the researcher draws two samples of sizes n_1 and n_2 from these populations and let $\bar{x}_1$ and $\bar{x}_2$ be the corresponding sample means, then

$H_0 \quad : \quad \mu_1 = \mu_2$

$H_A \quad : \quad \mu_1 \neq \mu_2$

The researcher wants to know whether the observed difference between $\bar{x}_1$ and $\bar{x}_2$ is statistically significant or not. If the difference is significant then the conclusion is that the difference is real and two samples are from different populations having means μ_1 and μ_2. Z statistics is obtained as

$$Z = \frac{|\bar{x}_1 - \bar{x}_2|}{SE(\bar{x}_1 - \bar{x}_2)}$$

where

$$SE(\bar{x}_1 - \bar{x}_2) = \sqrt{\frac{\sigma_1^2}{n_1} + \frac{\sigma_2^2}{n_2}}$$

$\bar{x}_1$ is first sample mean

$\bar{x}_2$ is second sample mean

σ_1 is standard deviation of first sample

σ_2 is standard deviation of second sample

$SE(\bar{x}_1 - \bar{x}_2)$ is standard error of difference of means

If σ_1 and σ_2 are not provided, use S_1 and S_2 (first and second sample standard deviations).

Example: To study the level of knowledge of mothers on nutrition, two groups were administered a questionnaire and the scores were obtained. The results are given below.

	Mothers from rural area	**Mothers from urban area**
Mean knowledge score	24.8	32.0
SD	6.0	5.0
Sample size	90	100

Can the researcher conclude that the maternal knowledge is different for mothers from rural and urban areas?

$H_0 \quad : \quad \mu_1 = \mu_2$

$H_A \quad : \quad \mu_1 \neq \mu_2$

$$Z = \frac{|24.8-32|}{\sqrt{\frac{6^2}{90}+\frac{5^2}{100}}} = \frac{7.2}{\sqrt{0.65}} = \frac{7.2}{0.806} = 8.93$$

Here the calculated value of Z is greater than the critical value for Z at 5% level, and for a two-tailed test (Z = 1.96); hence the observed difference is statistically significant and H_0 is rejected. The researcher can conclude that the average knowledge on nutrition is more for mothers hailing from urban areas.

Sample proportion vs. population proportion

When the level of measurement is nominal, the researcher can find either proportion or percentage. Let there be a population having a specific attribute or character and let the proportion having this attribute be denoted by P. Suppose the researcher draws a random sample of size n and let p denotes the proportion having a given characteristic in the sample. The researcher wants to know whether a given sample is drawn from a given population or not or whether the observed difference between sample proportion and population proportion is significant or not.

Null hypothesis:

H_0 : $P = p$

H_A : $P \neq p$

Z statistics is obtained as

where SE(p) is standard error of proportion

p, proportion having a given characteristic in the population $= \sqrt{\frac{pq}{n}}$

$$q = 1 - p$$

If p is expressed as percentage, then $q = 100 - p$

Example: After surveying 900 children, it was found that 12% have not completed their vaccination schedule. Can we conclude that this sample is taken from a population where 10% of children are unprotected?

$$p = 12$$

$$q = 100 - p = 88$$

$$P = 10$$

$$\text{SE of P} = \sqrt{\frac{12 \times 88}{900}} = \sqrt{1.17} = 1.08$$

$$Z = \frac{|10 - 12|}{1.08} = \frac{2}{1.08} = 1.85$$

Here the calculated value is less than the critical value of Z at 5% level and for a two-sided test. Here the researcher retains H_0 and concludes that the observed difference is due to chance. The sample was taken from the given population. The observed difference is not statistically significant.

Comparison of two sample proportions

Let there be two different populations and with P_1 and P_2 proportion having a given attribute P_1 and P_2. Suppose the researcher draws two samples from these populations with sample proportions P_1 and P_2, respectively. Let n_1 and n_2 be the sample sizes of first and second sample.

H_0 : $P_1 = P_2$

H_A : $P_1 \neq P_2$

The researcher wants to know whether the observed difference between P_1 and P_2 is statistically significant or not.

$$Z = \frac{P_1 - P_2}{SE(P_1 - P_2)}$$

Standard error of difference of proportions,

$$SE(p_1 - p_2) = \sqrt{\frac{p_1 q_1}{n_1} + \frac{p_2 q_2}{n_2}}$$

Example: To study the incidence of caesarian section, a community study was conducted. Two random samples were obtained from two villages. The results are given below. Test whether the CS rates are the same in the two villages.

	Village A	Village B
Number of women having multi gravida	600	450
Number of women undergone CS	18	30

$$\text{CS rate for village A} = \frac{18}{600} \times 100 = 3$$

$$\text{CS rate for village B} = \frac{30}{450} \times 100 = 6.7$$

$p_1 = 3$, $q_1 = 97$, $p_2 = 6.7$, $q_2 = 93.3$

H_0 : $p_1 = p_2$ (caesarian rates are the same)

H_A : $p_1 \neq p_2$ (caesarian rates are different)

$$\text{SE of difference} = \sqrt{\frac{3 \times 97}{600} + \frac{6.7 \times 93.3}{450}}$$

$$= \sqrt{1.874}$$

$$= 1.36$$

$$Z = \frac{|3 - 6.7|}{1.36} = \frac{3.7}{1.36} = 2.72$$

Since the calculated value of Z is greater than the critical value of Z at 5% level and for a two-tailed test, H_0 is rejected. The observed difference is statistically significant; hence caesarian rate is significantly more in village B.

Case II: When the sample size is small and population standard deviation is unknown

A sample is small if its size is less than 30. It may be noted that the tests of significance for small samples can be extended to large samples but the large sample tests cannot be applied for small samples. When the sample size is less than 30 and population standard deviation is unknown, the researcher has to compute t-statistic and use the table of t-distribution.

The common types of problem include:

1. Comparison of a sample mean with population mean (or norm)
2. Comparison of two sample means (independent 't' test)
3. One group pre-test–post-test ('t' test for paired data or related data)

These three situations are briefly discussed hereunder:

Sample mean vs. population mean (or norm)

H_0 : $\mu = \overline{x}$

H_A : $\mu \neq \overline{x}$

t is obtained as:

$$t = \frac{\overline{x} - \mu}{\frac{s}{\sqrt{n}}}$$

where

$\overline{x}$ is sample mean

σ is population mean or norm

s is standard deviation of sample

n is sample size

Degrees of freedom = n – 1

Here, first compute the value of t and compare with the table value of t at 5% level and for n – 1 degrees of freedom. If the calculated value is greater than the table value, the observed difference is statistically significant.

Example: A sample of 20 students in class 5 shows a mean 1Q of 120 with a standard deviation of 15. Can we consider it as a sample from a population with mean 110.

H_0 : $\mu = 110$

H_A : $\mu \neq 110$

Degree of freedom, $n - 1 = 20 - 1 = 19$

Critical value of t at 5% level and for 19 degrees of freedom (two-tailed) is 2.09 (from table of 't' distribution).

Calculated value of t:

$$t = \frac{120 - 110}{\frac{15}{\sqrt{20}}} = \frac{10}{3.35} = 2.98$$

Since the calculated value at t is greater than the critical value, H_0 is rejected. The sample may be taken from a population of higher IQ.

Comparison of two sample means

Let there be two different populations with means μ_1 and μ_2 and standard deviations S_1 and S_2. Suppose the researcher draws two samples of sizes n_1 and n_2 from these populations with means $\bar{x}_1$ and $\bar{x}_2$, then

H_0 : $\mu_1 = \mu_2$

H_A : $\mu_1 \neq \mu_2$

The researcher wants to know whether the observed difference between $\bar{x}_1$ and $\bar{x}_2$ is statistically significant or not. If the difference is significant, the researcher concludes that they are from different populations and the difference is real.

t is obtained as:

$$t = \frac{\bar{x}_1 - \bar{x}_2}{SE(\bar{x}_1 - \bar{x}_2)}$$

$$SE(\bar{x}_1 - \bar{x}_2) = s\sqrt{\frac{1}{n_1} + \frac{1}{n_2}}$$

Common population variance,

$$s^2 = \frac{(n_1 - 1)s_1^2 + (n_2 - 1)s_2^2}{n_1 + n_2 - 2}$$

Degrees of freedom $= n_1 + n_2 - 2$

Example: To study the effectiveness of different methods of teaching, 8 children were randomized to 2 groups. One group receives a class using OHP and the other group a class using LCD projection. The results are given below. Test which method is more useful?

	OHP	LCD
Mean score	3	5
SD	0.8	1.3
Sample size	4	4

Here,

$H_0 \quad : \quad \mu_1 = \mu_2$

$H_A \quad : \quad \mu_1 \neq \mu_2$

Degrees of freedom $= n_1 + n_2 - 2 = 4 + 4 - 2 = 6$

Critical value of t at 6 d.f. and at 5% level (two-tailed) is 2.45 (from table of 't' distribution).

Calculated value of t:

First calculate SE.

$$
\begin{aligned}
SE &= \sqrt{\frac{1}{4}+\frac{1}{4}} \times \sqrt{\frac{3 \times 0.8^2 + 3 \times 1.3^2}{4+4-2}} \\
&= \sqrt{0.50} \times \sqrt{1.17} \\
&= 0.707 \times 1.08 \\
&= 0.764
\end{aligned}
$$

Now,

$$
t = \frac{13-51}{0.764} = 2.62
$$

Since the calculated value of t is greater than the critical value, H_0 is rejected. Teaching programme using LCD projector is effective than OHP presentation.

Paired t-test (when observations are made on the same group for two times)

This test is appropriated for one group pre-test–post-test design. It can also be employed with matched samples like matched case-control study.

H_0 : $\mu_d = 0$ (no difference between initial and final scores)

H_A : $\mu_d \neq 0$ (there is difference between initial and final scores, d being the difference in the scores for each individual)

The researcher takes measurements at two different times, before and after administering an intervention (may be an educational programme or an exercise). If the intervention is effective, the scores obtained the second time will increase or (knowledge, for example) decrease (pain scores, for example).

t is obtained as

$$t = \frac{\bar{d}}{SE(\bar{d})}$$

where $\bar{d}$ is mean of differences.

Standard error of differences,

$$SE(\bar{d}) = \frac{s}{\sqrt{n}}$$

where s is standard deviation of differences and N is number of subjects.

Note: While finding the mean, negative differences and positive differences must be summed without ignoring the signs. Zero differences must also be taken into consideration in the calculation of $\bar{d}$.

Example: Five subjects were given exercises for reducing pain following a surgery. The scores are given below.

Subject	Pre-test score	Post-test score
A	6	4
B	7	6
C	7	7
D	5	4
E	8	6

First find the difference between scores. The differences are 2, 1, 0, 1, 2; mean of the differences is 1.2. Standard deviation of difference is 0.834.

Degrees of freedom $= n - 1 = 5 - 1 = 4$

H_0 : $\mu_D = 0$

(no difference between initial and final scores)

H_A : $\mu_D \neq 0$

Critical value of 't' at 5% level (two-tailed) and 4 degrees of freedom is 2.78.

Calculated value of 't':

$$t = \frac{\bar{d}}{\frac{s_d}{\sqrt{n}}} = \frac{1.2}{\frac{0.834}{\sqrt{5}}} = \frac{1.2}{\frac{0.834}{2.24}} = \frac{1.2}{0.372} = 3.22$$

Since the calculated value at t is greater than the critical value, H_0 is rejected. The observed difference is statistically significant; exercise programme reduces the pain significantly.

Analysis of variance (ANOVA)

ANOVA can be considered an extension of 't' test for independent samples which permit the researcher to compare more than two groups or experimental conditions. When there are more than two groups or experimental conditions, for each group sample, means and standard deviations can be obtained and any attempt to perform a series of t-tests to evaluate them will inflate type-I error.

ANOVA, on the other hand, permits multiple comparisons with the overall significance level at $\alpha = 0.05$. This method is also known as one-way ANOVA since the researcher is concerned with only one variable at a time.

In ANOVA, the researcher is concerned with the variability of data and uses the sum of squares: $\Sigma(x - \bar{x})^2$. In ANOVA, the first step is to find the total variability for the entire dataset, taking into account each and every single score irrespective of group membership or experimental condition.

The next step is to divide total variability into two components: (a) Between-treatments variance which refers to variation in the mean of each group from the total group and (b) within treatment variance which refers to the average variability of scores within each group. While t-test is based on t-distribution, ANOVA is based on F distribution. F is also called variance ratio and is defined as:

$$F = \frac{\text{between treatment variance}}{\text{within treatment variance}}$$

Before proceeding to learn the computational procedure, it is desirable to familiarize with the notional system.

k is the number of separate groups of experimental conditions;

n is the number of subjects or scores in each group or experimental conditions.

N is the total number of scores (sample size) in the study; this is obtained as nk.

T is the sum of scores in each group or experimental condition.

G is the sum of all scores in the study; this is obtained as ΣT.

Computation of ANOVA

Step I: Find the total sum of squares (SS_{total}):

$$SS_{total} = \sum \frac{X^2}{n} - \frac{G^2}{N}$$

Step II: Find within group sum of squares (SS_{within}) about mean:

$$SS_{within} = \sum \begin{matrix}\text{Sum of squares inside each group} \\ \text{or experimental condition}\end{matrix}$$

Step III: Between group sum of squares ($SS_{between}$):

$$SS_{between} = \sum \frac{T^2}{n} - \frac{G^2}{N}$$

Step IV: Total degrees of freedom:

$$df_{total} = N - 1$$

Step V: Within group degrees of freedom:

$$df_{within} = \sum N - K$$

Step VI: Between group degrees of freedom:

$$df_{between} = k - 1$$

Now the researcher can proceed to calculate mean square which is nothing but a terminology used in ANOVA to denote variance

$$\text{Mean square within groups} = \frac{SS_{within}}{df_{within}}$$

$$\text{Mean square between groups} = \frac{SS_{between}}{df_{between}}$$

and finally

$$F = \frac{MS_{between}}{MS_{within}}$$

The numerator of F-ratio indicates treatment effect, and the denominator indicates differences due to chance. In some textbooks, the denominator is indicated as MS error. This type of ANOVA is also called one-way ANOVA or single-factor ANOVA. In ANOVA, variables are called factors.

The ANOVA Summary Table

Source of variation	**Sum of squares**	**Degrees of freedom**	**Mean squares**	**F**	**Significance**
Between groups or conditions	$SS_{between}$	$df_{between}$	$MS_{between}$		
Within groups or conditions	SS_{within}	df_{within}	MS_{within}	$\frac{MS_{between}}{MS_{within}}$	
Total	SS_{total}	df_{total}			

To assess the effectiveness of different methods of teaching, twenty women were randomly allocated into four groups and each group received a class on first-aid using different methods of teaching. The scores are tabulated (fictitious data). To evaluate the observed differences, ANOVA can be used.

Subjects	Scores obtained			
	Lecture only	**Lecture + OHP**	**Lecture + LCD**	**Lecture + demonstration**
A	3	4	5	5
B	4	4	4	7
C	2	2	7	6
D	3	2	4	6
Mean	3	3	5	6
SS	2	4	6	2
T	12	12	20	24

$$\sum x^2 = 330; G = 68; N = 16; K = 4$$

Computation proceeds as follows:

1. Total sum of squares:

$$SS_{total} = \sum x^2 - \frac{G^2}{N}$$
$$= 330 - \frac{68^2}{16}$$
$$= 41$$

2. Within-treatments sum of squares:

$$SS_{within} = \sum \text{Sum of squares inside each treatment}$$
$$= 2 + 4 + 6 + 2 = 14$$

3. Between-treatments sum of squares:

$$SS_{between} = \sum \frac{T^2}{n} - \frac{G^2}{N}$$
$$= \frac{12^2}{4} + \frac{12^2}{4} + \frac{20^2}{4} + \frac{24^2}{4} - \frac{68^2}{16}$$
$$= 316 - 289$$
$$= 27$$

4. Total degrees of freedom:

$$df_{total} = N - 1 = 16 - 1 = 15$$

5. Within-treatments degrees of freedom:

$$df_{between} = N - K = 16 - 4 = 12$$

6. Between-treatments degrees of freedom:

$$df_{between} = k - 1 = 4 - 1 = 3$$

7. $MS_{between} = \dfrac{SS_{between}}{df_{between}} = \dfrac{27}{3} = 9$

8. $MS_{within} = \dfrac{SS_{within}}{df_{within}} = \dfrac{14}{12} = 1.2$

9. $F = \dfrac{MS_{between}}{MS_{within}} = \dfrac{9}{1.2} = 7.5$

Example ANOVA summary table

Source of variation	**SS**	**DF**	**MS**	**F**	**Significance**
Between treatment	27	3	9		
Within treatment	14	12	1.2	7.5	P <0.05 (also <0.01)
Total	41	15			

To find the critical value of F, the F table has to be consulted. To locate the critical value, d.f. values for between-treatments and within-treatments must be used. The d.f. between-treatments is printed across the top of table and d.f. within-treatments are printed as the first column of the table. Tables are usually separately available for 5% level and 1% level. Whether the researcher is using 5% level or 1% level, locate the value of d.f. at the intersection of two d.f.'s. In this problem, the critical value of F at 5% level is 3.49 and at 1% level is 5.95. Hence the observed differences are statistically significant. Null hypothesis is rejected. Now to determine which means are significant, post-hoc tests may be done. In the absence of a post-hoc test, the researcher can conclude that a combination of lecture class and demonstration is the most effective method of teaching.

Post-hoc tests

Once the F-ratio indicates statistical significance, additional hypothesis tests are done to determine which means are significant and which are not. These tests are called post-hoc tests. In psychological/educational research, the most commonly used post-hoc test is the Tukey's HSD test. Another test widely used is the Scheffe test. Students may refer standard statistical books to learn them.

Repeated measures of analysis of variance

Repeated measures ANOVA summary table

Source of variation	Sum of squares	Degrees of freedom	Mean squares	F	Significance
Between treatments	$SS_{between}$	$df_{between}$	$MS_{between}$		
Within treatments	SS_{within}	df_{within}			
(a) Between subjects	$SS_{between\ subjects}$	$df_{between\ subjects}$		$\frac{MS_{between}}{MS_{error}}$	
(b) Error	SS_{error}	df_{error}	MS_{error}		
Total	SS_{total}	df_{total}			

The repeated measures of ANOVA can be considered as an extension of paired t-test. While the paired t-test can evaluate a pre-test–post-test situation, the repeated measures of ANOVA can be used when two or more post-tests are performed. The computational procedure of repeated measures of ANOVA is slightly different from that of one-way ANOVA. Here also, the researcher calculates total sum of squares (SS_{total}), between-treatments sum of squares ($SS_{between}$), and within-treatments sum of squares (SS_{within}) but separates individual differences from within-treatments sum of squares. Once individual differences are removed, the remaining variance is called error variance. Now the d.f. between-subjects can be subtracted from d.f. within-subjects so that d.f. error is obtained. Now F is obtained as:

$$F = \frac{MS_{between\text{-}treatments}}{MS_{error}}$$

To study the effectiveness of an education programme, five women were given a class on breastfeeding practices. The results are given below. Test whether the intervention was effective.

Knowledge score

Subject	Pre-test	Post-test after 1 week	Post-test after 1 month	Post-test after year	Total
A	8	10	10	10	38
B	6	10	9	8	33
C	9	9	9	9	36
D	4	10	9	8	31
E	8	11	13	10	42
T	35	50	50	45	
SS	16	2	12	4	
Mean	7	10	10	9	

Computation of ANOVA for repeated measures is given below. First obtain the following values: N = 20; n= 5; K= 4; G = 180

Step 1: Total sum of squares:

$$\Sigma X^2 - \frac{G^2}{N} = 1684 - \frac{180^2}{20} = 64$$

Step 2: Within-treatments sum of squares:

$$SS_{within} = \sum \text{Sum of squares inside each treatment}$$
$$= 16 + 2 + 12 + 4 = 34$$

Step 3: Between-treatments sum of squares:

$$SS_{between\text{-}treatments} = \sum \frac{T^2}{n} - \frac{G^2}{N}$$
$$= \frac{35^2}{5} + \frac{50^2}{5} + \frac{50^2}{5} + \frac{45^2}{5} - \frac{180^2}{20}$$
$$= 1650 - 1620$$
$$= 30$$

Step 4: Between-subjects sum of squares:

$$SS_{between\text{-}subjects} = \sum \frac{P^2}{K} - \frac{G^2}{N}$$
$$= \frac{38^2}{4} + \frac{33^2}{4} + \frac{36^2}{4} + \frac{31^2}{4} + \frac{42^2}{4} - \frac{180^2}{20}$$
$$= 1638.5 - 1620$$
$$= 18.5$$

Step 5: $$SS_{error} = SS_{within\text{-}treatment} - SS_{betwen\text{-}subject}$$
$$= 34 - 18.5$$
$$= 15.5$$

Step 6: $df_{total} = N - 1 = 20 - 1 = 19$

Step 7: $df_{within\text{-}treatment} = K - 1 = 4 - 1 = 3$

Step 8: $df_{within\text{-}treatment} = N - K = 20 - 4 = 16$

Step 9: $df_{between\text{-}subject} = n - 1 = 4$

Step10: $$df_{error} = df_{within\text{-}treatment} - df_{betwen\text{-}subject}$$
$$= 16 - 4$$
$$= 12$$

Step 11: $$MS_{between\text{-}treatment} = \frac{SS_{between\text{-}treatment}}{df_{between\text{-}treatment}}$$
$$= \frac{30}{3}$$
$$= 10$$

Step 12: $$MS_{error} = \frac{SS_{error}}{df_{error}}$$
$$= \frac{15.5}{12}$$
$$= 1.29$$

Step 13: $$F = \frac{MS_{between}}{MS_{error}} = \frac{10}{1.29} = 7.75$$

For locating the table value of F (critical value), the d.f. for between-treatments and for error has to be used (usually called numerator d.f. and denominator d.f.). The d.f. between-treatments is given as the first row of the F table (usually termed numerator d.f.). The error d.f. is presented as first column of the F table, usually termed denominator d.f. The table value of F at 5% level for 3 and 12 degrees of freedom is 3.49 and at 1% level is 5.95. At 5% level and 1% level, the observed difference is significant (5% significance is sufficient). H_0 can be rejected and can conclude that the education programme was effective in enhancing the knowledge.

Non-parametric test: The statistical tests discussed so far are parametric tests. A parametric test requires interval ratio level data. Other important requirements include assumption of normality. When the level of measurement is nominal or parametric assumptions are not satisfied, the researcher can employ non-parametric tests of significance. Some important non-parametric tests are Chi-squared test, Mann-Whitney U and Wilcoxon Signed-Ranks test.

Conditions of validity of Chi-squared test

χ^2 test can be used only when:

1. Level measurement is nominal.
2. The total number of observations is large (N >50).
3. The observations are independent.
4. The expected frequency of any item of cell should not be less than 5. If it is less than 5, then frequency taken from the preceding or succeeding frequency be pooled together in order to make it 5 or more than 5.
5. Like t-distribution, χ^2 distribution has degrees of freedom.

   d.f. = (c −1) × (r − 1), where c is the number of columns and r is the number of rows.
6. Chi-square is obtained as

   $$\chi^2 = \sum_{i=1}^{n} \frac{(O_i - E_1)^2}{E_i}$$

   where n is the number of cells, O_i is observed frequency and E_i is expected frequency.

Expected frequency in a contingency table is calculated by the formula.

$$\text{Expected frequency} = \frac{\text{Row total} \times \text{Column total}}{\text{Grand total}}$$

Table 16.9 Hypothetical data for Chi-square showing the effectiveness of a new type of surgery

	Treatment	**Control**	**Total**
Positive	40 (25)^{E1}	10(25)^{E2}	50
Negative	60(75)^{E3}	90(75)^{E4}	150
Total	100	100	200

(Figure in brackets represents expected frequencies)

$$\chi^2 = \frac{(40-25)^2}{25} + \frac{(10-25)^2}{25} + \frac{(60-75)^2}{75} + \frac{(90-75)^2}{75}$$

$$= 9 + 9 + 3 + 3$$

$$= 24$$

$$\text{d.f.} = (2-1)(2-1) = 1$$

Table value of χ^2 at 5% level and for 1 d.f. is 3.84.

Since the calculated value is greater than the table value, the observed difference is statistically significant. Percentage having improvement in conditions is more in the treatment group (40%).

Alternatively, in a 2 × 2 table, the value of Chi-square can be obtained using the following equation.

	Treatment	**Control**	**Total**
Positive	40^{a}	10^{b}	50^{a+b}
Negative	60^{c}	90^{d}	150^{c+d}
Total	100^{a+c}	100^{b+d}	200

$$\chi^2 = \frac{N(ad-bc)^2}{(a+c)(b+d)(a+b)(c+d)}$$

If any of the cell value is less than 5, Yate's correction for discontinuity has to be applied. Now Chi-square becomes

$$\chi^2 = \frac{N\left[(ad-bc)-\frac{N}{2}\right]^2}{(a+c)(b+d)(a+b)(c+d)}$$

Mann–Whitney U test (Rank sum test)t

This test is an alternative to t test for independent samples. This test is ideal when the level of measurement is ordinal. It is also used with interval ratio level data when the assumption of normality is not true. The computational procedure starts with combining the scores in two groups and assigning ranks to them. Assign rank 1 to the lowest, rank 2 to the next lowest and so on. When two or more scores are the same, use the procedure for tied ranks. Now find the sum of ranks of each group separately. Now work out two U values as shown below.

$$U_1 = n_1 n_2 + \frac{n_1(n_1+1)}{2} - \Sigma R_1$$

$$U_2 = n_1 n_2 + \frac{n_2(n_2+1)}{2} - \Sigma R_2$$

where n_1 is first sample size, n_2 is second sample size, R_1 is sum of ranks of the first group, R_2 is sum of ranks of the second group

Now U is the minimum of (u_1, u_2). The table of U values is available for different levels of significance and for different values of n_1 and n_2. For statistical significance, the calculated value must be equal or lower than the table value.

Alternatively, Z statistic can be computed as follows:

$$Z = \frac{U - \frac{n_1 n_2}{2}}{\sqrt{\frac{n_1 n_2 (n_1 + n_2 + 1)}{12}}}$$

Now, the critical value of Z can be used to assess the statistical significance.

Example: A survey was conducted among mothers to ascertain their views on PNDT Act. One group consists of primi mothers and other multi gravid. The scores are as given below. Can the researcher conclude that the opinions are same for the two groups?

Opinion on PNDT Act

Subjects	Score of primi gravid	Rank	Score of multi gravid	Rank
	12	3.5	14	7
	14	7	25	18
	12	3.5	17	11
	13	5	18	12
	20	14	19	13
	16	10	21	15
	15	9	24	17
	14	7	22	16
	9	1		
	11	2		
	$n_1 = 10$	$\Sigma R_1 = 62$	$n_2 = 8$	$\Sigma R_2 = 109$

$$U_1 = n_1 n_2 + \frac{n_1(n_1+2)}{2} - \Sigma R_1$$

$$= 10 \times 8 + \frac{10(10+1)}{2} - 62$$

$$= 73$$

$$U_2 = n_1 n_2 + \frac{n_2(n_2+1)}{2} - \Sigma R_2$$

$$= 10 \times 8 + \frac{8 \times 9}{2} - 109$$

$$= 7$$

$$z = \frac{U - \frac{n_1 n_2}{2}}{\sqrt{\frac{n_1 n_2 (n_1 + n_2 + 1)}{12}}}$$

$$= \frac{7 - \frac{10 \times 8}{2}}{\sqrt{\frac{10 \times 8(10+8+1)}{12}}}$$

$$= \frac{7-40}{\sqrt{126.5}} = \frac{33}{11.25} = 2.93$$

The calculated value of Z is greater than the critical value at 5% level (1.96); the observed difference is significant. Multi gravid women favour the Act more than that of primi gravid women (find the mean and median for two sets for clarity).

Wilcoxon signed-rank test

This test is an alternative to paired 't' test. This test is ideal when the level of measurement is ordinal. It can also be used with interval ratio level data when an assumption of normality is failed. The computational procedure starts with finding the difference for each pair of observations. In the next step, the differences are ranked ignoring the positive or negative sign; zero differences are ignored and will not be ranked. Assign 1 to the lowest rank, 2 to the next lowest and so on. When two or more differences are the same, use the procedure for tied ranks. Now restore the signs to the ranks and find the sum of positive ranks and negative ranks separately. Let the letter T denote the smaller of these totals. For significance, the calculated value of T must be equal or lower than the table value.

Alternatively, Z statistics can be computed as:

$$Z = \frac{T - \frac{n(n+1)}{4}}{\sqrt{\frac{n(n+1)(2n+1)}{24}}}$$

Now the critical values of Z can be used to assess the statistical significance.

Example: Knowledge scores of 13 subjects before and after of an intervention programme are given. Test whether the education programme was effective.

Sub	Before	After	d	R
A	7	8	1	3
B	5	7	2	6.5
C	4	6	2	6.5
D	4	4	0	
E	3	7	4	9.5
F	4	3	−1	−3
G	5	8	3	8
H	9	8	−1	−3
I	3	7	4	9.5
J	2	7	5	11
K	3	4	1	3
L	3	3	0	0
M	6	7	1	3

$$z = \frac{T - \frac{n(n+1)}{4}}{\sqrt{\frac{n(n+1)(2n+1)}{24}}}$$

$$= \frac{6 - \frac{13 \times 14}{4}}{\sqrt{\frac{13 \times 14 \times 27}{24}}}$$

$$= 2.7$$

Since the calculated value is greater than table value (1.96), the observed difference is statistically significant.

Applications of Statistics in Health

Vital statistics

Vital statistics have great importance in public health. These are systematically collected information regarding events such as birth, marriages, deaths, etc. in a given population.

Vital statistics are statistics fundamental to events of life such as birth, death, marriage and sickness that occur in our community. These data are used to evaluate how effective the public health programmes are and for further planning and health administration.

Definitions

According to Benjamin, "Vital statistics are conventional numerical records of marriages, births, sickness and deaths by which the health and growth of a community may be studied."

Vital statistics have been defined as "the facts, systematically collected and compiled in numerical form, related to or derived from records of vital events".

Uses of vital statistics

1. For scheduling of health administration
2. For appraisal of the progress of health programmes
3. To assess the health status of a community
4. To compare the health status of one country with that of another
5. To find solutions to health problems
6. To settle on the health needs
7. To communicate the health issues

Measures of vital statistics

The common vital statistical rates and indices used in community health are:

1. Crude death rate
2. Fertility rate
3. Total fertility rate
4. Infant mortality rate
5. Neonatal mortality rate
6. Perinatal mortality rate
7. Under five mortality rate
8. Maternal mortality rate
9. Population growth rate

Crude death rate

It measures fertility in relation to the number of birth to the total population.

$$\text{Annual crude death rate} = \frac{\text{Number of deaths which occurred among the population in a given geographical area during one year}}{\text{Mid-year total population of the given year}} \times 1000$$

Fertility rate

The rate related to women in the reproductive period by relating the number of live births to the number of women in the child-bearing ages (15–49) years.

$$\text{General fertility rate (GFR)} = \frac{\text{No. of live births in one year}}{\text{No. of women of ages 15–49 years}}$$

Age-specific fertility rate (ASFR)

$$\text{ASFR} = \frac{\text{No. of live births to women in a given age during one year}}{\text{No. of women in that age group}} \times 1000$$

Total fertility rate (TFR)

It gives an estimate of the average number of children that would be born alive to a woman throughout her reproductive age span as per prevailing specific fertility rate.

$$\text{TFR} = 5\sum_{15}^{49} \text{ASFR, for 5 year age intervals}$$

$$\text{TFR} = \sum_{15}^{49} \text{ASFR, for single years of age}$$

Infant mortality rate (IMR)

It is the number of infant deaths under one year of age per 1000 live births in one year.

$$\text{IMR} = \frac{\text{No. of death under one year of age}}{\text{Total live birth in the year}} \times 1000$$

IMR is regarded as a most sensitive index of the health of the community.

Neonatal mortality rate (NMR)

Deaths occurring within 4 weeks or 28 days of birth are called neonatal deaths.

$$\text{NMR} = \frac{\text{No. of deaths under 28 days of age}}{\text{Total live birth}} \times 1000$$

Perinatal mortality rate (PMR)

It is the mortality of infants occurring during the period from 28th week of pregnancy to 7 days after birth per 1000 total births. In other words, it includes still births and deaths under one week.

$$\text{PMR} = \frac{\text{Late fetal deaths 28 weeks or more} + \text{Death under one week}}{\text{Total live} + \text{still birth}} \times 1000$$

Under five mortality rate

It is the annual number of deaths of children aged under 5 years, which is expressed on a rate per 1000 live births.

$$\text{Under five mortality} = \frac{\text{No. of deaths of children less than 5 years of age in a given year}}{\text{Total live births in the same year}} \times 1000$$

Maternal mortality rate (MMR)

It is the number of deaths from puerperal causes per 1000 live births.

$$MMR = \frac{\text{No. of death directly due to pregnancy of childbirth and occurs during pregnancy or within 42 days of delivery}}{\text{Total live birth in the year}} \times 1000$$

Population growth rate (PGR)

It is the rate at which the number of individuals in a population increases in a given time period as a fraction of the initial population. PGR ordinarily refers to the change in population over a unit time period.

$$PGR = \frac{\ln\left[P(t_2)\right] - \ln\left[P(t_1)\right]}{t_2 - t_1}$$

SUMMARY

Descriptive statistics are a means of describing and organizing data gathered in research. The four levels of measurement are nominal, ordinal, interval and ratio. Each has appropriate descriptive techniques associated with it. Measures of central tendency describe the average numbers of a sample. Mode is the most frequent score; median is the middle score; and mean is the arithmetic average of the scores. Inferential statistics are a tool to test hypotheses about populations from sample data. It allows researchers to estimate population parameters and to test hypothesis. If null hypothesis is accepted, this result indicates that the findings are likely to have occurred by chance.

Statistical hypothesis testing is subject to two types of errors, type-I and type-II. Type-I error occurs when the researcher rejects a null hypothesis that is actually true. Type-II error occurs when the researcher accepts a null hypothesis that is actually false. The researcher controls the risk of making a type-I error by setting the alpha level or level of significance. Unfortunately, reducing the risk of type-I error by reducing the level of significance increases the risk of making type-II error. The results of statistical tests are reported to be significant or non-significant statistically. Significant results are those whose probability of occurring is less than 0.05 or 0.01 depending on the level of significance set by the researcher. The commonly used parametric and non-parametric statistical tests include those that test for differences between means, such as the 't' tests and ANOVA, and those that test for differences in proportions such as chi-square test. Tests that examine data for the presence of relationships include Pearson correlation (r), sign test, Wilcoxon matched pairs, signed rank test and multiple regression.

Moreover, advanced statistical procedures include path analysis, LISPEL, and factor analysis.

MULTIPLE CHOICE QUESTIONS

1. The phenomenon in which sample values tends to be normally distributed around the population value is known as __________.
   (a) Hawthorne effect
   (b) central limit theorem
   (c) triangulation
   (d) time sampling
2. A theoretical frequency distribution based on an infinite number of samples is called __________.
   (a) analysis of variance
   (b) canonical correlation
   (c) critical value
   (d) sampling distribution
3. The ability of the test to reject a null hypothesis when it is false is known as __________.
   (a) power of a statistical test
   (b) canonical correlation
   (c) region of rejection
   (d) two-tailed test of significance
4. Which of the following is concerned with populations and using sample data to make an inference about a population?
   (a) descriptive statistics (b) inferential statistics
   (c) normative statistics (d) parametric statistics

5. Which of the following is also called skewed distributions?
   (a) non-symmetrical distribution
   (b) symmetrical distribution
   (c) formal distribution
   (d) frequency distribution
6. A graph that uses bars to represent the frequency distribution of variables measured at the ordinal interval or ratio levels is __________.
   (a) bar graphs
   (b) frequency polygons
   (c) frequency curves
   (d) histogram
7. Statistics that describe the average, typical or most common value for a group of data is __________.
   (a) percentage
   (b) parameters
   (c) frequency
   (d) measures of central tendency
8. Which of the following is a measure of standard deviation?
   (a) mean
   (b) percentile
   (c) variability
   (d) none of these
9. Square of standard deviation is __________.
   (a) mean (b) variance
   (c) mode (d) correlation
10. A non-parametric inferential technique appropriate for comparing sets of data that are in the form of frequencies or percentages is __________.
    (a) ANOVA
    (b) dependent t-test
    (c) chi-squared test
    (d) ANCOVA

11. Which of the following examines the difference between the mean scores of two or more groups on two or more dependent variables that are examined at the same time?
    (a) analysis of covariance (ANCOVA)
    (b) canonical correlation
    (c) multivariate analysis of variance (MANCOVA)
    (d) chi-squared test
12. The cut-off point that denotes the place in a theoretical distribution at which all obtained values from a sample that are equal to or beyond that point are said to be statistically significant is __________.
    (a) degrees of freedom
    (b) power of statistical test
    (c) mode
    (d) critical value

ANSWER KEY

1. (a) 2. (d) 3. (a) 4. (b) 5. (a) 6. (d)
7. (d) 8. (c) 9. (b) 10. (c) 11. (c) 12. (d)

REVIEW QUESTIONS

1. Define central tendency. Describe the various measures of central tendency and measures of variability.
2. Describe levels of measurements. Discuss the levels of measurement.
3. Explain type-I and type-II errors.
4. Write short notes on:
    (a) Point estimation
    (b) Sampling distribution
    (c) Critical ratio
    (d) Sources of vital statistics

(e) Attrition
(f) Bar diagram
(g) Statistical packages
(h) Scales of measurements

5. Explain confidence interval and normal probability curve.
6. Write short notes on:
   (a) Chi-square test
   (b) Normal probability curve
   (c) Type-II error
   (d) Latin squares
   (e) Uses of biostatistics
   (f) ANOVA
   (g) Measures of asymmetry
   (h) Parametric tests
   (i) Correlation study
   (j) Validity
   (k) Probability
   (l) Testing of hypothcsis
   (m) Population and samples
7. Explain frequency distribution and measures of central tendency.
8. Describe in brief the procedure for testing a hypothesis.
9. Describe "test of significance" or 't' test with examples.
10. Define chi-square test. Discuss its significance.
11. Describe the requisites for an ideal measure of central tendency.
12. Describe hypothesis formulation and testing in nursing research.
13. A hospital record indicates that out of 2020 births, 1050 were boys and the rest were girls. Do these figures confirm that the score ratio is 50:50? Test at 5% level of significance. (The two-tailed value at 5% level is 1.96.)

14 Differentiate between mean, median and mode for the following blood urea values: 15, 22, 40, 32, 30, 32, 30, 22, 32, 30.

15. Explain the application of statistical packages. Explain the various sources and methods of collection of vital and health statistics.

16. Explain briefly about the
    (a) Properties of normal distribution curve.
    (b) Weight (in kg) of 10 new borns is recorded as follows: 3.0, 2.5, 3.2, 1.8, 3.1, 2.0, 2.2, 2.8, 2.4, 3.0. Calculate the coefficient of variation.

17. The number of hours of volunteer services given by eight village health nurses (VHN) at an emergency station are as follows: 10, 8, 11, 9, 12, 10, 7 and 13. Compute mean and standard deviation.

18. A study of 150 pregnancies yielded the following data:

Pregnancy complication	**Mother hypertensive**	
	Yes	**No**
Present	20	40
Absent	10	80

    Is there any significant association between hypertensive states of mothers and complication of pregnancy? (Chi-square value for 1 d.f. at 5% level is 3.84.)

19. (a) Define standard deviation.
    (b) List out the relative merits over the various measures of dispersion.

20. Write short notes on:
    (a) Grounded theory
    (b) Cluster sampling
    (c) Threats to internal validity
    (d) Research proposal
    (e) Levels of measurement
    (f) Probability and non-probability sampling
    (g) Uses of biostatistics

21. Discuss the preparation of frequency distribution of a given set of raw scores.

22. List the various statistical measures used to summarize the data.
23. Define measures of variability. Write briefly about different measures of variability, its merits and demerits.
24. Explain Wilcoxon signed rank test. How it differs from Wilcoxon rank sum test.
25. Discuss the various methods of graphical representation of data and bring out the differences between histogram and bar diagram.
26. Discuss the importance of 't'-test in testing hypothesis drawing suitable illustrations from nursing practice.
27. The marks secured by a group of second year B.Sc. Nursing students are as follows: 10, 8, 11, 9, 12, 10, 7 and 13. Compute mean and standard deviation.

REFERENCES

Abplanalp, J. (1988). Psychosocial theories. In W.R. Keye (Ed.). The premenstrual syndrome (94–112). Philadelphia: WB Saunders.

Abraham, I.L., & Neundorfer, M.M. (1990). The design and analysis of time-series studies. In L.E. Mody (Ed.). *Advancing Nursing Science Research* (Vol. 2, 145–175). Newbury Park, CA: Sage.

Allison, P.D. (1984). Event history analysis: Regression for longitudinal event data. Beverly Hills, CA: Sage.

Barnett, V., & Lewis, T. (1978). Outliers in statistical data. New York: Wiley.

Bland, J.M., & Altman, D.G. (1986). Statistical methods for assessing agreement between two methods of clinical measurement. Lancet, 1(8476), 307–310.

Box, G.E.P., & Jenkins, G.M. (1976). Time-series analysis: Forecasting and control (Rev. ed). San Francisco: Holden–Day.

Crawford, G. (1982). The concept of pattern in nursing conceptual development and measurement. *Advances in Nursing Science*, 5(1), 1–6.

Ferketich, S., & Verran, J. (1986). Technical notes: Exploratory data analysis-Introduction. Part 1: *Western Journal of Nursing Research*, 8(4), 464–466.

Fox, H., & Long, J.S. (1990). Modern methods of data analysis. Newbury Park, CA: Sage.

Glass, G.V., Willson, W.L., & Gottman, J.M. (1975). Design and analysis of time-series experiments. Boulder, CO: Colorado University Associated Press.

Gouman, J.M. (1981). Time-series analysis: A comprehensive introduction for social scientists. Cambridge, MA: Cambridge University Press.

Gross, A.J., & Clark, V. (1975). Survival distributions: Reliability applications in the biomedical sciences. New York: Wiley.

Hintz, J.L. (1990). Survival analysis. Number cruncher statistical system version 5.5. Kaysville, UT: Hintze.

Jirovec, M.M. (1986). Time-series analysis in nursing research: ARIMA modeling. *Nursing Research*, 35(5), 315–319.

Kazdin, A. (1982), Single-case research designs. New York: Oxford University Press.

Lee, E.T. (1984). Statistical methods for survival data analysis. Belmont, CA: Wadsworth.

Lentz, M.J. (1990). Time-series issues in sampling. *Western Journal of Nursing Research*, 12(1), 123–127.

__________. (1990). Time-series analysis-Cosinor analysis: A special case. *Western Journal of Nursing Research*, 12(3), 408–412.

McCain, L.J., & McCleary, R. (1979). The statistical analysis of the simple interrupted time-series quasi-experiment. In T.D. Cook & D.T. Campbell (Eds.). Quasi-experimentation: Design and analysis issues for field setting (233–293), Chicago: Rand McNally.

McCleary, R., & Hay, R.A., Jr. (1980). Applied time-series analysis for the social sciences. Beverly Hills, CA: Sage.

McDowall, D., McCleary, R., Meidinger, E.E., & Hay, R.A., Jr. (1980). Interrupted time-series analysis. Beverly Hills, CA: Sage.

Metzger, B.L., & Schultz, S., II (1982). Time-series analysis: An alternative for nursing. *Nursing Research*, 31(6), 375–378.

Mitchell, E., Woods, N., & Lentz, M. (1985). Methodologic issues in the definition of perimenstrual symptoms. Proceedings of the Society for Menstrual Cycle Research. Chicago: Chicago University Press.

__________. (1991). Distinguishing among menstrual cycle symptom severity patterns. In D. Taylor & N. Woods (Eds.). Menstruation, health and illness (89–101). Washington, D.C.: Hemisphere.

APPENDIX I

USEFUL REFERENCES FOR WRITING AND PRESENTING RESEARCH

- American Psychological Association (2010). Publication manual of the American Psychological Association (7th ed.). Washington D.C.: American Psychological Association.
- Bernstein, T. (1997). Do's, don'ts & maybes of English usage. New York: Times Books.
- Carpinello, S., & Caley, L. (1993). Preparing research results for journal submissions. *Journal of New York State Nurses Association*, 24(1), 5–7.
- Day, R.A. (1983). How to write and publish a scientific paper (2nd ed.). Philadelphia: ISI.
- Fitzpatrick, J. (1995). The making of a manuscript [editorial]. *Applied Nursing Research*, 8, 1–2.
- __________. (1998). Encyclopedia of nursing research. New York: Springer Publishing Co.
- Jackie, M. (1989). Presenting research to nurses in clinical practice. *Applied Nursing Research*, 2, 191–193.
- Lester, J.D., & Lester, J.D. Jr. (2002). Writing research papers: A complete guide. (10th ed.). New York: Longman.
- Klausmeier, H.J. (2001). Research writing in education and psychology-from planning to publication: A practical handbook. Springfield, IL: Charles C. Thomas.
- Locke, L. (1987). Proposals that work: A guide for planning dissertations and grant proposals. Newbury Park, CA: Sage.
- Maggio, R.E. (1987). Nonsexist word finder: A dictionary of gender free usage. Phoenix, AZ: Oryx Press.
- Martin, P. (1994). Poster session tips for the novice viewer. *Applied Nursing Research*, 7, 208–210.

- Meloy, J.M. (2001). Writing the qualitative dissertation. (2nd ed.). Mahwah, NJ Lawrence Erlbaum.
- Miracle, V., & King, K. (1994). Presenting research: Effective paper presentations and impressive poster presentations. *Applied Nursing Research*, 7, 147–151.
- Rempusheski, V. (1990). Resources necessary to prepare a poster for presentation. *Applied Nursing Research*, 3, 134–137.
- Robinson, A., & Notter, L. (1982). Clinical writing for health professionals. Bowie, MD: Robert J. Brady.
- Ryan, N.M. (1989). Developing and presenting a research poster. *Applied Nursing Research*, 2, 52–55.
- Selby, M.L., Tornquist, E.M., & Finerty, E.J. (1988). How to present your research. *Nursing Outlook*, 37, 172–175.
- Sherbinski, L., & Stroup, D. (1992). Developing a poster for disseminating research findings. *Journal of the American Association of Nurse Anesthetists*, 60, 567–572.
- Sheridan, D., & Dowdney, D. (1997). How to write and publish articles in nursing (2nd ed.). New York: Springer Publishing Co.
- Sigma Theta Tau International. (1984). Why write? Why publish? A collection of papers from the Sigma Theta Tau writers' seminars. Indianapolis, IN: Author.
- Skillin, M., & Gay, R. (1986). Words into type (3rd ed.). Englewood Cliffs, NJ: Prentice-Hall.
- Torquist, E.M. (1986). From proposal to publication: An informal guide to writing about nursing research. Menlo Park, CA: Addison Wesley.
- Ventura, M. (1992). Guidelines for writing for publication. *Journal of the New York State Nurses Association*, 23(2).

APPENDIX II

LIST OF FUNDING SOURCES FOR NURSING RESEARCH

Professional Organizations/Foundations

- American Academy of Nurse Practitioners (AANP)
- American Association of Critical-Care Nurses (AACN)
- American Association for the History of Nursing, Inc. (AAHN)
- American Association of Neuroscience Nurses (AANN)
- Neuroscience Nursing Foundation (NNF)
- American Association of Occupational Health Nursing Foundation (AAOHN)
- American Nurses Foundation (ANF)
- American Psychiatric Nurses Association (APNA)
- American Society of Diabetes Educators (AADE)
- American Psychiatric Nurses Association (APNA)
- American Society of Diabetes Educators (AADE)
- American Society of Peri-anesthesia Nursing (ASPAN)
- Indian Council for Medical Research (ICMR)
- National Institute for Nursing Research
- National Institute for Occupational Safety and Health
- Sigma Theta Tau International
- State Board of Medical Research

Foundations

- California Healthcare Foundation
- California Wellness Foundation
- Lance Armstrong Foundation

- Bill & Melinda Gates Foundation
- Robert Wood Johnson Foundation
- The Hearst Foundation
- The Lalor Foundation
- The Lupus Research Institute
- Michael and Susan Dell Foundation
- Doris Duke Charitable Foundation
- Jay and Rose Phillips Family Foundation
- The Charles A. and Anne Morrow Lindbergh Foundation

APPENDIX III

IMPORTANT WEBSITES FOR SCIENTIFIC NURSING RESEARCH

- Alan Guttmacher Institute: http://www.agi-usa.org
- American Academy of Nurse Practitioners: http://www.aanp.org
- American Association of Colleges of Nursing: http://www.aacn.nche.edu
- American Association of Critical-Care Nurses: http://www.aacn.org
- American College of Nurse Practitioners: http://www.Nurse.orgacnp
- American Holistic Nurses Association: http://www.ahna.org
- American Journal of Nursing Company Online: http://www.ajn.org
- American Nurses Association: http://www.nursing.world.org
- American Psychiatric Nurses Association: http://www.apna.org
- Association of Reproductive Health Professions: http://www.arhp.org
- Cancer Net-International Cancer Information Centre: http://cancernet.nci.nih.gov
- Cumulative Index for Nursing and Allied Health Literature: http://www.cinahl.com
- National Centre for Health Statistics: http://www.cdc.gov/nchs
- National Institute for Nursing Research (NINR): http://www.hih.gov/ninr/index.html
- National Institutes of Health: http://www.nih.gov
- Nursing World: http://www.nursingworld.org
- Sigma Theta Tau International: http://www.stti.iupui.edu

APPENDIX IV

EXPERIENCES OF POST-GRADUATE STUDENTS IN THEIR NURSING PROJECTS

Presently, nursing research is included in the syllabus of Diploma in Nursing Course, GNM Course, Post-Basic B.Sc. Nursing, B.Sc. Nursing and M.Sc. Nursing Course. Often the experiences of senior researchers are valuable. Here an account of real-life experiences of post-graduate students is given. These tips will help you plan your project effectively.

Planning

It is important to plan each and every aspect of the research project from the introduction right down to the reference section. Proper planning gives you the overall idea about the research project.

Even if your results do not work out as you first anticipated, this in itself adds to the learning experience. Planning is a key part of the research project and discussion. Planning is of extreme importance to an experiment, yet not everything of an experiment.

Thorough enquiry or review

A detailed investigation of books, journal-articles, consulting friends and supervisors should be done before starting a research project. Starting the literature review early is important as it is a time-consuming process.

Choosing an appropriate method for research project is a difficult task for researchers. In such cases, opinions from colleagues or friends can be resorted. This might help to provide many alternatives and options. This brainstorming method is of extreme importance in research studies and it helps in weighing the pros and cons of each possible option.

Be prepared for unexpected

During research, be prepared for the unexpected which may be that the research methods did not work properly, or sometimes the participants did not cooperate with the research study. Sometimes, even the research results may be just opposite than expected. Conducting a few pilot studies and test runs will greatly help in these situations. This will allow to recognize the potential problems that come during the research process.

Discussion of results

The discussion of results is an important step. It summarizes the whole research study and evaluates the outcome. It also identifies the drawbacks and points out the actual situation in the research area. This helps in suggesting further researches in the same area. The discussion of results suggests valuable advise for future research.

Discrepancy between theory and practice

One should always keep in mind that there may be a vast discrepancy between theory and practice. It is not always possible to put the theory into practice. As research process is largely about testing theory in practice, it should be done in a comprehensive and well-planned manner.

Theoretically, anything is possible and feasible since human creativity and imagination is unlimited. In reality there is limitation in terms of time and resources. The research methods should be adaptive to the unexpected.

Research is a daunting task

The researcher may think there is a whole world of topics to choose from and will have no idea which topic to choose. The researcher is always in a dilemma. Even when the researcher eventually picks a topic, hearing what others have opted can often create confusion and doubt. The researcher may wonder if he has gotten it wrong because everyone else is doing something different.

Be creative

To make your project stand out and get noticed, choose a topic carefully. Try to be imaginative and creative as it will help to impress the examiner.

Selection of topic

The topic you select should be in an area of your interest. Before choosing the topic, think about the possible problem areas in it. Make sure you are well equipped with the ways to encounter and tackle issues or problem areas. The possible issues include availability of samples, resources, etc. The topic should contribute to the body of knowledge.

Timeline

As the research study includes a series of steps, setting a realistic timeline is of extreme importance. Every section of the project is of importance; so try to allocate time evenly. If time limit is not followed strictly, it ruins the whole research process. It is useful to construct a timetable. A timetable ensures that you spend time productively on one object.

Relationship with supervisors

Listen to the supervisors' advice and take advantage of their experience. Maintain a good relationship with your supervisors so that you can approach them whenever you encounter a problem in the research process. They are there to help students. Meetings with supervisors are invaluable for keeping your research project on right track. Acknowledging the research supervisor is important while presenting or publishing the research work.

Theory into practice

Research study is an opportunity to put into practice the theoretical and practical knowledge that you have gained over the past. So make sure that you make full advantage of it.

Start early

Putting things on the long finger is one of the worst things expected from a researcher. At the start of research process, the researcher may feel he has plenty of time ahead and keep aside all things till end. Every single day counts when carrying out a research project. Thus, it is useful to start thinking about the potential research topics in advance so that you can begin the literature review in advance.

Use internet

Most literature searches are carried out in internet these days. However, not all articles from the internet are authoritative. The use of internet should be as that of an additional guide.

Backup

Proper backing up is important. Make sure you have a practice of backing up your work at the end of day and keep the backups in a safe place. A safe way of backing up your work is to email it every week. If your laptop or PC breaks down, your work can still be accessed through your email account.

APPENDIX V

EVALUATION CRITERIA FOR DISSERTATION AND VIVA FOR M.Sc. NURSING

SECTION A: Dissertation (Book)

Criteria	Marks	Register number			
1. Research problem Background Objectives Operational definition Hypothesis/Assumption	5				
2. Review of literature inclusion of recent references Citation of primary source Style of writing	5				
3. Research methodology Research approach and design Population and sample Ethical consideration Data collection	15				
4. Interpretation of data and results	10				
5. Discussion	5				
6. Summary and conclusion Bibliography Abstract	10				
Total marks	50				

Signature of Examiner:

Name:

Designation:

Address:

SECTION B: Viva Voce

Criteria	Marks	Register number			
1. Presentation of the study - Language - Clarity - Systematic and organized	5				
2. Research problem and objective	5				
3. Methodology Research approach Research design Population, sample ethical consideration Data collection	15				
4. Interpretation of data and results	10				
5. Ability to defend the study - Ability to clear the doubts	5				
6. Ability to critique the study - Ability to present - Strength and weakness of the study	5				
7. Knowledge about research methodology	5				
Total marks	50				

Signature of Examiner:

Name:

Designation:

Address:

APPENDIX VI

't' TABLE VALUE

d.f.	Probability level (P value)					
	.20	.10	.05	.02	.01	.001
1.	3.078	6.314	12.706	31.821	63.567	636.62
2.	1.886	2.920	4.303	6.965	9.925	31.60
3.	1.638	2.353	3.182	4.541	5.841	12.92
4.	1.533	2.132.	2.776	3.747	4.604	8.61
5.	1.476	2.015	2.571	3.365	4.032	6.87
6.	1.440	1.943	2.447	3.143	3.707	5.96
7.	1.415	1.895	2.365	2.998	3.499	5.41
8.	1.397	1.860	2.306	2.896	3.355	5.04
9.	1.383	1.833	2.262	2.821	3.250	4.78
10.	1.372	1.812	2.228	2.764	3.169	4.59
11.	1.363	1.796	2.201	2.718	3.106	4.44
12.	1.356	1.782	2.179	2.681	3.055	4.32
13.	1.350	1.771	2.160	2.650	3.012	4.22
14.	1.345	1.761	2.745	2.624	2.977	4.14
15.	1.341	1.753	2.131	2.602	2.947	4.07
16.	1.337	1.746	2.120	2.583	2.921	4.02
17.	1.333	1.740	2.110	2.567	2.898	3.97
18.	1.330	1.734	2.101	2.552	2.878	3.92
19.	1328	1.729	2.093	2.539	2.861	3.88
20.	1.325	1.725	2.086	2.528	2.845	3.85
21.	1.323	1.721	2.080	2.518	2.831	3.82
22.	1.321	1.717	2.074	2.508	2.819	3.79
23.	1.319	1.714	2.069	2.500	2.807	3.77
24.	1.318	1.711	2.064	2.492	2.797	3.76
25.	1.316	1.708	2.060	2.485	2.787	3.73
26.	1.315	1.706	2.056	2.479	2.779	3.71
27.	1.314	1.703	2.052	2.473	2.771	3.69
28.	1.313	1.701	2.048	2.467	2.763	3.67
29.	1.311	1.699	2.045	2.462	2.756	3.66
30.	1.310	1.697	2.042	2.457	2.750	3.65
40.	1.303	1.684	2.021	2.423	2.704	3.55
60.	1.296	1.671	2.000	2.390	2.660	3.46
120.	1.289	1.658	1.980	2.358	2.617	3.37
∞	1.282	1.645	1.960	2326	2.576	3.29

APPENDIX VII

SIGNIFICANT VALUES OF χ^2

d.f.	Probability level (P value)								
	0.990	0.950	0.900	0.500	0.1000	.050	0.025	0.010	0.001
1.	0.00016	0.00393	0.0158	0.455	2.71	3.84	5.02	6.63	10.83
2.	0.0201	0.103	0.211	1386	4.61	5.99	7.38	9.21	13.82
3.	0.115	0.352	0.584	2.366	6.25	7.82	9.35	11.34	16.27
4.	0.297	0.711	1.064	3.357	7.78	9.49	11.14	13.28	18.47
5.	0554	1.145	1.61	4.251	9.24	11.07	12.83	15.09	20.52
6.	0.872	1.64	2.20	5.35	10.64	12.59	14.45	16.81	22.46
7.	1.24	2.17	2.83	6.35	12.02	14.07	16.01	18.48	24.32
8.	1.65	2.73	3.49	7.34	13.36	15.51	17.53	20.09	26.13
9.	2.09	3.33	4.17	8.34	14.68	16.92	19.02	21.67	27.88
10.	2.56	3.94	4.87	9.34	15.99	18.31	20.48	23.21	29.59
11.	3.05	4.57	5.58	10.34	17.28	19.68	21.92	24.73	31.26
12.	3.57	5.23	6.30	17.14	18.55	21.03	23.34	26.22	32.91
13.	4.11	5.89	7.04	12.34	19.81	22.36	24.74	27.69	34.53
14.	4.66	6.57	7.79	13.31	21.06	23.68	26.12	29.14	36.12
15.	5.23	7.26	8.55	14.34	22.31	25.00	27.40	30.58	37.70
16.	5.81	7.96	9.31	15.34	23.54	26.30	28.85	32.00	39.25
17.	6.41	8.67	10.09	16.34	24.77	27.59	30.19	33.41	40.79
18.	7.01	9.39	10.86	17.34	25.99	28.87	31.53	34.81	42.31
19.	7..63	10.12	11.65	78.34	27.20	30.14	32.85	36.19	43.82
20.	8.26	10.85	12.44	19.34	28.41	31.41	34.17	37.57	45.32
21.	8.90	11.59	13.24	20.34	29.62	32.67	35.49	33.93	46.80
22.	9.54	12.34	14.04	21.34	30.81	33.92	36.78	40.29	48.27
23.	10.20	13.09	14.85	22.34	32.0	35.17	38.03	41.64	49.73
24.	10.86	13.85	15.66	23.34	33.20	36.42	39.36	42.98	57.18
25.	11.52	14.61	16.47	24.34	34.38	37.65	40.65	44.31	52.62
26.	12,20	15.38	17.29	25.34	35.56	38.89	41.92	45.64	54.05
27.	12.83	16.15	18.11	26.34	36.74	40.11	43.19	46.96	55.48
28.	13.56	16.93	18.94	27.34	37.92	41.34	44.46	48.28	56.89
29.	14.26	17.71	19.77	28.34	39.09	42.56	45.72	49.59	58.30
30.	14.95	18.49	20.60	29.34	40.26	43.77	46.98	50.89	59.70
40.	22.16	26.51	29.05	39.31	51.81	55.76	59.34	63.69	73.40
50.	29-71	34.76	37.69	49.33	63.17	67.50	71.42	76.15	86.66
60.	37.43	43.19	46.46	59.33	74.40	79.09	83.30	88.33	99.61
70.	45.44	51.74	55.33	69.33	85.53	90.53	95.02	100.4	112.3

GLOSSARY

Abstract (research abstract) A brief summary of a completed research or a proposal. It contains purpose, method and major findings of the study, located at the beginning of a report or proposal.

Accidental sampling (convenience sampling) Selection of most readily available people as study participants.

Adjusted mean The mean group value for the dependent variable, after statistically removing the effect of covariates.

After only design An experimental design in which data are collected only after introducing experimental intervention.

Alpha (α) In tests of statistical significance, the level designating the probability of committing a type-I error. Alpha is commonly set at 0.05, 0.01 or 0.001.

Alternative hypothesis A statement indicating the opposite of the null hypothesis.

Analysis of covariance (ANCOVA) A statistical procedure used by the researcher to control source variables that may have an effect on the dependent variable.

Analysis The process of synthesizing data in order to answer research questions and test hypothesis.

Analysis of variance (ANOVA) A statistical procedure used to collate (compare) the difference between the means of two or more groups or tests of values.

Analysis triangulation The use of two or more analytic techniques to analyze the same set of data.

Anonymity Protecting the identity of research subjects such that even the researcher cannot touch individual's information provided.

Applied research Research which is conducted to find a solution to an immediate practical problem.

Assent The affirmative agreement of a subject (e.g. child >7 years who is not able to give an informed consent) to participate in a research study.

Associate relationship An association between two variables that cannot be described as casual.

Assumption A basic principle/belief that is held true in basis of logic or reason but without any scientific proof or verification.

Asymmetric distribution A distribution of skewed data values that is having two halves that are not mirror images of each other.

Attitude scale A data collection instrument where the respondents (subjects) are asked to report their attitudes or feelings on a continuum.

Attrition The loss of study participants over the course of study which can cause a bias.

Audio CASI (computer-assisted self interview) An approach of collecting self-reporting information in which the subjects listen to questions over a headphone and respond by entering the data directly into a computer.

Basic research (pure research) Research conducted to widen the base of knowledge in a discipline rather than to solve an immediate problem.

Bar graph A pictorial representation of frequency distribution of nominal or ordinal data.

Baseline measure A measure of the dependent variable before introducing an experimental intervention.

Basic social process The central social process emerging out of an analysis of grounded theory data.

Before-after design An experimental design in which the data are collected before and after introduction of an intervention.

Behavioural objective An expected outcome of a programme, stated in terms of the behaviour of those at whom the programme is aimed.

Beneficence An ethical principle that prevents harm and exploitation of the study subjects.

Bias Any error that creeps into the data. Bias can be introduced by the researcher, the respondent, the questionnaire, the sample and so on.

Bibliography A listing of books, articles and other relevant materials, alphabetically arranged according to the last name of authors, referring the title of their works, and indicating where they can be located.

Bivariate statistics The research study in which the statistics is derived by comparing two variables simultaneously to assess the empirical relationship between them.

Blind review The review of the proposal such that the author and reviewer is not identified to each other.

Borrowed theory A theory borrowed from another disciplines to guide nursing practice of research.

Calendar question A question used to obtain information about the chronology of events or activities in peoples lives.

Call for abstract A request for a brief summary of study that the researcher wishes to present at the research conference.

Canonical analysis A statistics procedure for examining the relationship between two or more independent variables and two or more dependent variables.

Case control design A non-experimental research design involving the comparison of a case and a matched control.

Case study A research method involving a thorough, in depth analysis of an individual, group institution or other social unit.

Causal relationship A relationship between two variables such that presence or absence of one variable (the cause) determines the presence or absence or value of the other (the effect).

Census A survey covering entire population.

Central tendency Indication of the centre of data in a distribution (mean, median and mode).

Chi-square test (χ^2) A non-parametrical test of statistical significance used to assess whether a relationship exists between two nominal level variables.

Clinical relevance The extent to which a study addresses a problem of significance to nursing practice.

Clinical research Research designed to generate knowledge in nursing practice.

Clinical trial Research studies conducted to evaluate new treatments, new drugs or improved medical equipment.

Closed-ended question A question that offers respondents a set of mutually exclusive and jointly exhaustive alternative replies, from which 'right' answer must be chosen.

Cluster analysis A multivariate statistical procedure used to cluster people or things based on patterns of association.

Cluster sampling A type of sampling where large groups of samples are selected first with successive sub sampling of smaller units.

Code of ethics The fundamental ethical principle established by a discipline or institution to guide researcher's in conducting research on human/animals.

Coding The process of transforming raw data into standardized form for data processing and analysis in quantitative research, the process of attaching numbers to categories in quantitative research.

Coercion In a research context, the explicit or implicit use of threat or excessive rewards to gain compliance from the subjects to participate in the study.

Cognitive test An instrument designed to assess cognitive skills or cognitive functioning.

Cohort comparison design A design that compares two or more age cohorts.

Cohort study A kind of trend study that focuses on specific population at different periods of time.

Comparison group A group of subjects in an experimental study who does not receive any experimental treatment, who are used to compare the outcome of the group of primary interest.

Component design A study design for a mixed method study with qualitative and quantitative aspects are implemented as judicious components of the overall inquiry.

Computer-assisted personal interviewing (CAPI) In personal interviewing in which the interviewer reads the questions from a computer investigator and enter responses onto, a laptop computer.

Computer-assisted telephone interviewing (CATI) Interviewing done over the telephone in which the interviewer read questions from the computer enter response onto a computer.

Concealment A technique involving collection of research data without knowledge or consent of participants, for obtaining an accurate view of naturalistic behaviour.

Concept An abstraction or mental idea of a phenomenon.

Conceptual definition The theoretical meaning of the concept being studied.

Conceptual model Symbolic presentation of concepts and the relationship between these concepts.

Concurrent validity A type of criterion validity in which a determination is made of the instruments ability to obtain a measurement of subjects behaviour that is comparable to some other criticism used to indicate that behaviour.

Confidence interval The array of values within which a population parameter is predicted to lie, at specific probability.

Confidence levels The estimated probability that a population parameter lies within a confidence interval.

Confidentiality The protection of the identity of study subjects, such that identity is known only to the researcher.

Confirmability A criterion for evaluating data quality with qualitative data, referring to the objectivity or neutrality of the data.

Consent form A written agreement signed by the subject and the researcher concerning the terms and conditions of participation in a study.

Consistency check A procedure in which a set of data is checked to ensure that the data are internally consistent.

Constant comparison In grounded theory analysis, newly collected data are compared in ongoing fashion with data obtained earlier.

Construct validity The degree to which an instrument measures the construct under investigation.

Construct A concept that is deliberately invented by researcher for a scientific purpose.

Contamination The undesirable influence of one experimental intervention on another intervention.

Content analysis The process of organizing and integrating the communication messages that are usually in written forms.

Content validity The degree to which the items in an instrument represents the concept being measured.

Contingency table A two dimensional table that displays a relationship between sets of nominal data.

Continuous variable A variable that can assume an infinite range of values along a continuum.

Control group A group of subjects in an experimental study that does not receive an experimental intervention.

Convenience sampling (accidental sampling) Selection of most readily/easily available persons as study participants.

Core category In a grounded theory study, the central phenomenon i.e. used to integrate all categories of data.

Correlational studies Research studies that examine the strength of relationships between variables.

Correlation coefficient An index summarizing the degree of relationship between variables, typically ranging from +1.00 (for a +ve relationship) through 0.0 (for no relationship) to −1.00 (for a perfect negative relationship).

Correlation The extent to which the values of one variable are related to values of the other variable. It may be either positive or negative.

Correlational matrix A two dimensional display showing the correlation coefficient between all combinations of study variables.

Correlational research Research that explores the interrelationship among variables of interest without any active intervention by the researcher.

Covariate A variable that is statistically controlled in analysis of covariance.

Credibility The process of evaluating the data quality in qualitative studies.

Data The pieces of information obtained in the courses of study.

Data analysis The systematic organization and synthesis of research data and testing of hypothesis using the data.

Data collection The collection of information to address a research problem.

Data entry The process of entering data.

Data set The total collection of data on all variables for all subjects.

Data transformation A process of arranging the data in a form that can be meaningfully analyzed.

Data triangulation Using multiple data sources for the purpose of validating conclusions.

Debriefing Communication with the study participants after completion of study.

Deductive reasoning A reasoning process that proceeds from the general to specific.

Degrees of freedom (d.f.) A term used in statistical testing, referring to the number of sample values face to very; degrees of freedom is often N – 1, but different formulas are relevant for different tests.

Delphi technique A method of obtaining written judgements from a panel of experts about an issue of concern; experts are questioned individually in several rounds, with a summary of the panels views, in order to achieve some consensus.

Dependability A criteria for evaluating data quality in qualitative data, referring to the stability of data over time or over conditions.

Dependent variable The "effect" A response or behaviour that is influenced by the independent variable.

Descriptive statistics Statistics used to describe or summarize information about a population or sample.

Descriptive studies Research studies in which phenomena are described or the relationship between variables are examined.

Discrete variable A non-continuous variable containing discrete categories with clear boundaries between categories.(e.g. male and female).

Discriminate validity An approach to construct validation that involves assessing the degree to which a single method of measuring two constructs yields different results.

Disproportionate sample A sample in which the different proportion of study participants are selected from different population static to ensure adequate representation.

Double blind experiment An experimental study in which neither the subject nor the researcher know who is in the experimental or control group.

Effect size A statistics statement of the magnitude of the relationship between two variables, or the magnitude of difference between groups with regard to some attribute of interest.

Electronic database Bibliographic files that can be assessed through computer for conducting a literature review.

Element Single member or basic unit of a population.

Eligibility criteria Criteria used to designate the specific attributes of the target population on the basis of which people are selected for participation in the study.

Emergent design A design that unfolds in the course of a qualitative study as the researcher makes ongoing design decisions reflecting what was already been learned.

Empirical evidence Evidence gathered by using one's senses as the basis of generating knowledge.

Endogeneous variable A variable whose variation is by other variables within the governed/controlled model.

Equivalence The degree of similarity between alternate forms of a measuring instrument.

Error The mathematic expression that represents all unknown or immeasurable attributes that can affect the dependent variable.

Ethics A system of moral values that pertains with the degree to which research procedures adhere to proof essential, legal and social obligations to the study participants.

Ethnic perspective A term used by ethnographers to refer to the outsiders, view of the experiences of a cultural group.

Evidence-based practice Nursing practice that is based on best available evidence, with an emphasis on evidence from disciplined research.

Exclusion criteria The criteria that specify characteristics that a population does not have.

Exogenous variable In path analysis, a variable whose determinants lie outside the model.

Experimental group The subjects who receive the treatment or intervention in a research study.

Exploratory factor analysis A factor analysis undertaken to determine the underlying dimensionality of a set of variables.

Exploratory research A study that explore the dimensions of a phenomenon when little is known about the phenomenon.

External criticism A criticism used in historical approach to validate the genuineness or authenticity of the data.

External validity The degree to which study results can be generalized to other people.

Extraneous variable A variable that is not the variable of interest to the researcher but may influence the results of the study.

Extreme case sampling A sampling approach used in qualitative research that involves purposeful selection of the most extreme cases.

Extreme response set A bias in self report instruments, especially in psychosocial scales, created when participants select extreme response alternatives (e.g. strongly agree), independent of the item's content.

Factor analysis Type of validity used to identify cluster of related terms on an instrument or scale.

Factor loading In factor analysis, the weight associated with a variable on a given factor.

Factorial design An experimental design in which two or more independent variables are simultaneously manipulated permitting a separate analysis of the main effects of the independent variables, plus the interaction effects of those variables.

Face validity A subjective determination that an instrument is adequate for obtaining the desired information, on the surface or the face of instrument it appears to be an adequate means of obtaining the desired data.

Feasibility study A small scale study to determine the feasibility of a large study.

Field study Research studies conducted in real life situations.

Findings Result of the analysis of research data.

Fisher's exact test A statistical procedure, used to test the significance of the difference in proportions used when the sample size is small or cells in contingency table have no observations.

Focus group A small group of individuals who meet together and are asked questions by a moderator about certain topics.

Framework The conceptual underpinnings of a study, often called a theoretical framework in studies based on a theory; or conceptual framework in studies rooted in specific conceptual model.

Functional relationship A relationship between two variables in which it cannot be assumed that one variable caused the other, but it can be said that one variable changes values in relation to changes in the other variable.

Galley proofs Sheets of paper that show how an article/book will appear in type set form.

Generalizability The degree to which research methods justify the interface that the findings are true for a broader group than study participants, from a sample to a population.

Grand theories A broad theory aimed at describing large segments of the physical, social or behavioural world, also called a macro theory.

Grant A financial award made to a researcher or team of researcher to conduct a proposed project.

Grantsmanship The combination of set of skills and knowledge needed to secure financial support for a research idea.

Graphic rating scale A scale which the responses are rated along are ordered continuum and subjects are asked to select one.

Grounded theory A study in which data are collected and analyzed and a new theory is developed which is having the real life value.

Hawthorne effect The effect on the dependent variable resulting from subject's awareness that they are participants under study.

Heterogeneity Degree to which the dissimilarity of objects with respect to some attribute.

Histogram Graphic representation of frequency distribution data.

Historical research Systematic research studies designed to discover facts and relationship about past events.

Homogeneity The degree to which objects are similar.

Homogenous sampling A sampling approach used by qualitative researchers involving the deliberate solution of cases with limited variation.

Hypothesis A statement of predicted relationship behaviour between two or more variables.

Identical replication An exact duplication of the original methods used in a prior study to determine if similar results are obtained.

Impact analysis An evaluation of the effects of an intervention and outcomes of interest net of other factors influencing those outcomes.

Implied consent Consent to participate in a study that a researcher assumes has been given based on certain actions of the participant.

IMRAD format The organization of a research report into four sections; the introduction, method, the result and discussion sections.

Incidence rate The rate of new cases with a specified condition, determined by dividing the number of new cases over a given period of time by the number at risk of becoming a new case.

Independent variable The variable thought to influence the dependent variable in experimental research.

Inductive reasoning The process of reasoning from specific observations to more general rule.

Inferential statistics Statistics concerned to the use of sample data to make an inference about a population.

Informed consent An ethical principle that requires researcher to obtain voluntary participation of subjects, after informing them about possible risks.

Institutional review board Every agency or institution that have a committee that review each research proposals and ensure the research is conducted ethically.

Instrument Tool for collecting data.

Integrative review An integrative or systematic review is a scientific approach that combines results from a group of original research studies and looks at the studies as a whole.

Internal consistency The degree to which the components of instruments are measuring the same characteristics or dimension, as a measure of the instrument's reliability.

Internal validity The degree to which it can be inferred that the experimental treatment, rather than uncontrolled, extraneous factors, is responsible for observed effects.

Intervention protocol The specification of exactly how the treatment and alternative condition will be carried out, used in experimental research.

Interview schedule An instrument containing a set of questions, directions for asking these questions, and space to record the respondent's answers.

Interview A method of data collection in which the interviewer obtains responses from a subject in a face to face encounter or through phone.

Joint interview An interview where two or more people are interviewed simultaneously, typically using either semi-structured or unstructured interview.

Judgemental sampling A type of non-probability sampling method in which the researcher selects study participants based on personal judgement about who will be most representative. This is also called purposive sampling.

Kendall's tau A correlation coefficient used to indicate the magnitude of a relationship between ordinary level variables.

Key informant A person who is knowledgeable of the culture studied, in ethnographic research.

Known group technique A technique for estimating the construct validity of an instrument through an analysis of the degree to which the instrument separate groups produced to differ based on known theory or characteristics.

Level of significance The probability of rejecting a null hypothesis when it is true, symbolized by α and p.

Likert scale A measure of attitudes designed to allow respondents to indicate how strongly they agree or disagree with carefully constructed statements that range from very positive or very negative towards an attitudinal object.

Limitation Limitations are those which can limit the study from generalizability. Eg. Uncontrolled variables.

Linear regression An analysis for predicting the value of dependent variable by determining a straight line fit to the data that minimizes deviation from the line.

Literature review A critical summary of research on a topic of interest, often prepared to put a research problem in constant.

Longitudinal study A study conducted over time in contrast to cross sectional study conducted at our point in time to answer research question.

Manipulation How the researcher exposes the subjects to the independent variable to determine cause-effect relationships in experimental designs.

Maturation effect An effect on the results of a research experiment caused by changes in the experimental subjects over time.

Maturation A threat to the internal validity of a study that results when changes to the outcome measure result from passage of time.

Mean A description statistic that is a measure of central tendency, computed by summing all scores and dividing by number of subjects.

Measurement A process in scientific research that uses rules to assign number to objects.

Median A descriptive statistic that is a measure of central tendency, representing the exact middle value in a score distribution, the value above and below which 50% of the scores lie.

Meta-analysis A technique of analyzing and integrating result of several similar studies on a topic and determine what is known and what is unknown about a particular area of interest.

Meta synthesis The theories or interpretive translations produced from the integration or compassion of findings from qualitative studies.

Methodological research Research studies concerned with development, testing and evaluation of research instruments and methods.

Modality threat A threat to the internal validity of a study, referring to the differential loss of participants from different groups.

Mode A descriptive statistics that is a measure of central tendency, the score or value that occurs most frequently in a distribution of a score.

Model A symbolic representation of some phenomenon.

Multiple regression A statistical procedure used to determine the influence of more than one independent variable on the dependent variable.

Multivariate study A research study in which more than two variables are examined.

Negative relationship A relationship between two variables in which there is a tendency for the values of one variable to increase as the values of the other variable decrease.

Negatively skewed A frequency distribution in which the tail of distribution points to the left.

Non-probability sampling A sampling process in which a sample is selected from elements or member of a population through non-random methods; includes purposive sampling, quota sampling etc.

Nominal level of measurement The lowest level of measurement, data are named or categorized such as race, marital status, etc.

Non-directional research hypothesis A type of research hypothesis in which prediction is made that a relationship exist between variables, but the type of relationship is not specified.

Non-equivalent control group design A type of quasi experimental design, similar to the pre-test–post-test-control group experimental design, except that there is no random assignment of subjects to groups.

Non-experimental research Research in which researcher does not manipulate or control the dependent variable.

Non-parametric tests Types of inferential statistics that are not concerned with population parameters, can be used with nominal and ordinal data and small sample size.

Non-participant observer (covert) Researcher does not identify herself or himself to the subjects who are being observed.

Non-participant observer (overt) Researcher identifies himself to the subjects who are being observed and provides information about the type of data that will be collected.

Non-significant results Study results do not allow rejection of the null hypothesis.

Normal curve A bell-shaped curve that graphically depicts a normal distributed frequency distribution.

Normal distribution A symmetrical bell-shaped theoretical distribution, has one central peak or set of values in the middle of distribution.

Null hypothesis A statistical hypothesis that predicts there is no relationship between variables; the hypothesis that is subjected to statistical analysis.

Nursing research A systematic, objective process of analyzing phenomena of importance to nursing.

Objectivity The extent to which two independent researcher would arrive at similar judgements or conclusions.

Observation research A data collection method in which data are collected through visual observation.

Odds ratio The ratio of two probabilities namely the probability of an event occurring to the probability that will not occur.

Operational definition The definition of a variable that identifies how the variable will be observed or measured.

Operationalization The method of translating research concepts into measurable phenomena.

Ordinal measure A level of measurement that rank order phenomena along some dimension.

Outcome research Research designed to document the effectiveness of health care services and the end results of patient care.

Outliers Values that lie outside the normal values for other cases in a data set.

Parametric statistical test Types of inferential statistics that are concerned with population parameters. When parametric tests are used assumptions are made that (a) The level of measurement of the data is interval or late (b) Data are taken from population that are normally distributed on the variable being measured and (c) Data are taken from population that have equal variances on the variable being measured.

Parametric A numerical characteristic of a population.

Participant observation The participants directly observes and records information in a study and it requires that researcher become a part of the setting in which person, group or culture is being observed.

Participant observer (covert) Research observer interacts with the subjects and observes their behaviour without their knowledge.

Participant observer (overt) Research observer interacts with subjects openly and with the full awareness of those people who will be observed.

Peer review The review of a research manuscript by professional colleagues who have content or mythological expertise concerning the material presented in the manuscript.

Phenomenological studies Research studies that examine human experiences through the description of the meaning of these experiences provided by the people involved.

Pilot study Small-scale version of the research study used as a trial to make decisions about the best way to conduct the major study.

Population A complete set of persons or objects that possess some common characteristics of interest to the researcher.

Positive relationship A relationship between two variables in which the variable tend to vary together, as the values of one variable increase or decrease, the values of the other variable increase or decrease.

Positively skewed A frequency distribution in which the tail of the distribution points to the right.

Post-test only control group design True experimental design in which subjects in the experimental groups are given a post-test after the experimental group receives the study treatment.

Post-test Data collected after the administration of the intervention.

Power analysis A procedure that is used to determine the sample size needed to prevent a type-II error.

Power of a statistical test The ability of a statistical test to reject a null hypothesis when it is false.

Predictive validity A type of criteria validity of an instrument in which a determination is made of the instrument's ability to predict behaviour of subjects in the future.

Pre-test Data collected before the administration of the intervention in an experimental research.

Primary source It is the first hand information or direct evidence of an event.

Principal investigator The lead researcher, the person who has the prime responsibility for the study.

Probability sampling The use of a random sampling procedure to select a population; includes simple, stratified, cluster and systematic random sampling techniques.

Projective techniques Self report measure in which a subject is asked to respond to stimuli that are designed to be ambiguous or to have no definite meaning. The responses reflect the external feelings of the subject that are projected on the external stimuli.

Proposition A statement or assertion of the relationship between concepts.

Prospective studies Studies in which the independent variable is identified at the present time of then subjects are followed for some time in the future to observe the dependent variable or effect.

Purposive sampling A non-probability sampling procedure in which researcher uses personal judgement to select subjects considered to be representative of the population.

Q-sort (Q methodology) A data collection method in which subjects are asked to sort statements into categories according to their attitude towards, or rating of the statements.

Qualitative research Research that is concerned with the subjective meaning of an experience to an individual.

Quantitative research Research that is concerned with objectivity, light controls over the research situation, and the ability to generalize findings.

Quasi-experimental design A type of experimental design in which there is either no comparison group or no random assignment of subjects to groups, includes the non-equivalent control group design of time series design.

Questionnaire A paper and pencil self report instrument used to gather data from subject.

Quota sampling A non-probability sampling procedure in which the researcher selects the sample to reflect certain characteristics of the population.

Random assignment A procedure used in an experimental study to ensure that each study subject has an equal chance of being placed into the study groups.

Random sampling Refer probability sampling.

Range The distance between highest and lowest value in a group of values or scores.

Reactive effects of pre-test A threat to the external validity of a research study that occurs when subjects are sensitized to the experimental treatment by the pre-test.

Reliability The consistency and dependability of a search instrument to measure a variable, type of reliability and stability equivalence and internal consistency.

Research design The overall plan for gathering data in a research study.

Research hypothesis (H_1) An alternative hypothesis to the statistical null hypothesis predicts the researcher actual expectations about the outcome of a study; also called scientific, substantive and theoretical.

Research question Statement of the relationship between variables stated as a question.

Research report A written or oral summary of a research study.

Research utilization The implementation of research findings into practice.

Respondent A person in a study who provides answers or responses to the researcher.

Retrospective studies Studies in which the dependent variable is identified in the present and an attempt is made to determine the independent variable.

Sample A subset of the population that is selected to represent the population.

Sampling bias (i) The difference between sample data and population data that can be attributed to a facility selection process (ii) a threat to the external validity of a research study that occur when subjects are not randomly selected from the population.

Sampling distribution A theoretical frequency distribution that is based on an infinite number of samples. Sampling distribution are based on mathematical formulas and logic.

Sampling error • Random fluctuations in data that occur when a sample is selected to represent a population.

Sampling frame A listing of all elements of the population from which a sample is to be chosen.

Saturation The researcher has repetition of ideas from several participants in a qualitative study.

Scatter plot (Scatter diagram, scattergram) A graphic presentation of the relationship between two variables. The graph contains variables plotted on an X axis and Y axis. Pairs of scores are plotted by the placement of dots to indicate where each pair of X's and Y's interact.

Secondary source In the research relative, an account of a research study that has been written by someone other than the study investigates in historical studies, secondary sources are second hand information or data provided by some one who did not observe the event.

Selection bias A threat to the internal validity of an experimental research study that occurs when study results are attributed to the experimental treatment when, infact, the results may be related to pretreatment differences between the subjects in the experimental and comparison group.

Semantic differential Attitude scale that asks subjects to indicate their position or attitude about some concept along a continuum between two adjectives or phrases that are presented in relation to the concept being measured.

Semi-quartile range Determined by dividing the inter quartile range in half.

Semi-structured interviews Interviewers ask a specified number of questions but additional or probes are used at the discretion of the interviewer.

Simple hypothesis A hypothesis that predicts the relationship between one independent and one dependent variable.

Simple random sampling A method of random sampling in which each element of the population has an equal and independent chance of being chosen for the sample.

Simulation studies Laboratory studies in which subjects are presented with a description of a case study or situation intended to represent a real-life situation.

Skewed A frequency distribution that is nonsymmetrical.

Snowball sampling A sampling method that involves the assistance of study subjects to help obtain other potential subjects.

Solomon 4-group designs True experimental design that combines both the pre-test–post-test with control groups and post-test only with control group design, thereby providing a means for controlling the interactive testing effect and other sources of extraneous variables.

Stability reliability The consistency of a research instrument one time, test re-test procedures and repeated observations are methods to test the stability of an instrument.

Standard deviation (SD) A measure of variability, the static that indicate the average derivation or variation of all values in asset of data from the mean values of that data.

Standard error of the mean (S_n) The standard deviation of the sampling distribution of the mean.

Stratified random sampling A random sampling process in which a sample is selected after the population has been divided into subgroups or strata according to some variable of importance to the research study.

Study limitations Weakness in a study that is not controlled by the researcher.

Survey studies Research studies in which self report data are collected from a sample to determine the characteristic of a population.

Symmetrical distribution Frequency distribution in which both halves of the distributions are the same.

t-test A parametric statistical test that examines the differences between the means of two groups of values. Types of t-test are the independent t-test and dependent t-test.

Target population The entire group of people or objects to which the researcher wishes to generalize the findings of a study.

Telephone interviews Data are collected from subjects through the use of phone calls rather than in face to face encounter.

Testing A threat to the internal validity of a research study that occurs when a pre-test is administered to subjects; the effects of taking a pre-test on responses on the post-test.

Theoretical framework A study framework based on propositional statements from a theory.

Theory A set of inter-related statements that explains phenomena systematically.

Time sampling Observations of events or behaviour that are made during certain specified time periods.

Time series design Quasi-experimental design in which the researcher periodically observes subjects and administers an experimental treatment between two of the observations.

Triangulation Combining both qualitative and quantitative methods in one study.

Two-tailed test of significance A test of statistical significance in which critical values are sought in each of the sampling distribution, used when the cescaseling has not predicted the discretion of the relationship between the variable.

Type-I error Rejection of a true null hypothesis.

Type-II error Acceptance of a false null hypothesis.

Unimodal A frequency distribution that contains one value that occur more frequently than any other.

Univariate study A research study in which only one variable is examined.

Unstructured interview The interviewer is given a great deal of freedom to direct the course of the interview. The interviewers main goal is to encourage the responder to talk freely about the topic being explored.

Unstructured observation The researcher describes behaviour as they are viewed, with no preconceived ideas of what will be seen.

Validity The ability of an instrument to measure the variable that it is intended to measure.

Variable An attribute of a person or object that differs among the persons or objects being studied.

Variance A measure of variability the standard deviation squared (SD^2, S^2).

Visual analogue scale Subjects are presented with a straight line anchored on each end with words or phrases that represent the extremes of some phenomena, such as pain. Subjects are asked to match on the scale on the basis of their experience.

Wilcoxon signed ranks test A non-parametric test of significance which is used to test whether two independent groups have been drawn from the same population, with ordinal level variables.

Z score A standard score that indicates how many standard deviation that a particular value is from the mean of set of values.

INDEX